Fundamentals of
Chest Radiology

FUNDAMENTALS OF CHEST RADIOLOGY

Second Edition

Loren H. Ketai, MD
Associate Professor, Department of Radiology
University of New Mexico
Chief of Thoracic Radiology, Department of Radiology
University of New Mexico Health Science Center
Albuquerque, New Mexico

Richard Lofgren, MD, M.P.H.
Chief Medical Officer, Professor of Medicine
Department of Medicine, University of Kentucky
Lexington, Kentucky

Andrew J. Meholic, MD
Associate Professor, Department of Radiology
University of New Mexico Hospitals and Clinics
Albuquerque, New Mexico

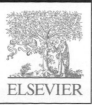

SAUNDERS

ELSEVIER

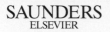

1600 John F. Kennedy Blvd.,
Ste 1800
Philadelphia, PA 19103-2899

FUNDAMENTALS OF CHEST RADIOLOGY (A Volume in the
Fundamentals of Radiology Series edited by Fred A. Metter, Jr., MD)
Copyright © 1996, 2006, Elsevier Inc.

ISBN-13: 978-0-7216-1016-0
ISBN-10: 0-7216-1016-1

Library of Congress Cataloging-in-Publication Data

Ketai, Loren.
    Fundamentals of chest radiology / Loren H. Ketai, Richard Lofgren, Andrew J.
Meholic.-- 2nd ed.
        p. ; cm.
    Meholic's name appears first on the earlier edition.
    Includes bibliographical references and index.
    ISBN 0-7216-1016-1
        1. Chest--Radiography.   I. Lofgren, Richard.   II. Meholic, Andrew.   III. Title.
        [DNLM: 1. Radiography, Thoracic. WF 975 K428f 2006]
    RC941.M36 2006
    617.5'40752--dc22

2005047249

Acquisitions Editor: Allan Ross
Publishing Services Manager: Tina Rebane
Project Manager: Norm Stellander
Interior Design Direction: Steve Stave
Cover Design: Steve Stave

Printed in the United States of America

Last digit is the print number: 9 8 7 6 5 4 3 2 1

"To Yuko, Matt and David, may they write their own books someday and to my Dad, may he live to read them all"
(*LHK*)

"To my essential support system – my wife Lynn and patient children Martha, Andrea and Emma"
(*RL*)

To my loving, patient wife, Judy, to our children, and to the memory of my parents.
(*AJM*)

Preface

Like the previous edition, this book is written for novice radiology residents and for residents in internal medicine, general surgery, family practice, and emergency medicine. Our primary goal remains that of helping these clinicians use thoracic imaging to solve clinical problems.

Since the first edition was published striking advances have occurred in thoracic imaging using multidetector CT and MRI, particularly in the realm of cardiovascular disease. These modalities have permanently changed the work-up for diagnosing and evaluating pulmonary emboli, thoracic aortic disease, and chest trauma, and we have included information about these techniques in the current edition. Nevertheless, chest radiographs remain the starting point for most evaluations of cardiopulmonary disease, and chest radiography remains the emphasis of this book. In addition to displaying CT and MR images that are keys to diagnosis, we have also tried to use CT and MR images to better explain findings seen on chest radiography.

Although the current edition contains more illustrations and text than did the first edition, this book remains a very much abridged version of chest radiology. There are excellent in-depth thoracic radiology texts available, several including material on cardiac imaging. We hope readers view the materials in our text as Churchill viewed quotations from Bartlett's—as words that "give you good thoughts . . . and also make you anxious to read . . . and look for more."

Loren H. Ketai, MD
Richard Lofgren, MD, M.P.H
Andrew J. Meholic, MD

Acknowledgments

We are grateful to RuthAnne Bump for her cheerful willingness to print the "just one more last final last image" that every chapter seemed to need so desperately. Once again, Loren Ketai would like to thank Yuko Komesu, MD, who, after editing this second edition, undoubtedly knows more thoracic radiology than any other urogynecologist in the world. Last, the authors would like to thank non-government relief organizations for their efforts in 2005. We will be donating all author royalties from the sale of the second edition of this book to assist victims of natural disasters here in the US and abroad.

Contents

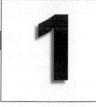

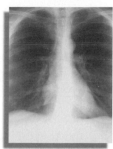

The Basics

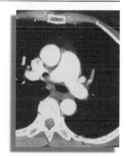

This chapter introduces the clinically important methods of chest imaging: plain radiography, computed tomography (CT), and magnetic resonance imaging (MRI). Discussion of invasive angiography is notably absent. Over the past decade, angiography performed by CT (termed computed tomography angiography, CTA) and MRI (termed magnetic resonance angiography, MRA) has supplanted catheter-directed angiography for most diagnostic studies of the chest other than coronary angiography. For example, diagnostic pulmonary angiography is now reserved for the evaluation of pulmonary emboli in the rare cases in which the CTA has been nondiagnostic.

☐ PLAIN RADIOGRAPHY

Plain radiography remains the most common method used to evaluate patients with complaints or problems related to the chest. It is important to know when routine plain images will suffice and how radiographic techniques can be modified to increase their yield. Traditional chest radiography uses a film-screen method for making the radiograph. With this method, x-ray photons that pass through the patient are converted to light as they strike the material in the screen.

The light generated when photons strike the screen exposes the adjacent film, creating an image. Digital chest radiography is a newer alternative to the film-screen method. Although several different types of digital systems are in use, all share the ability to use the energy of the x-ray photons to generate an electrical signal that is in turn used to create a radiographic image. Each of the digital systems uses a different intermediate step during which the x-ray photons are converted into light or electrical charge before their energy can be used to generate the electrical signal.

Digital images can be viewed on a monitor or printed on film and offer several advantages over images created with the film-screen technique. These systems can generate a readable image despite large variations in the quantity of x-ray photons penetrating the patient, making underexposed or overexposed radiographs much less common. Images can also be transmitted or stored electronically and can be manipulated after they are taken to improve image interpretation (e.g., magnified, made darker or lighter).

Regardless of imaging technology, the upright posterior-anterior (PA) chest radiograph remains the preferred initial study whenever it is clinically feasible. With this view, the artifacts that are associated with the anterior-posterior (AP) view are avoided (to be discussed further). The addition of a lateral view is crucial in identifying abnormalities in the posterior costophrenic angles, within the mediastinum, and in areas related to the spine. These relatively "blind" areas on frontal views make up 40% of the lung area and 25% of the lung volume. Masses as large as 2 cm can easily be missed in these locations (Fig. 1-1).

About one half of all plain chest radiographs are taken at the bedside. Typically, these studies are done to evaluate line and tube placement, and the portable chest radiograph meets such needs well. In some cases, bedside radiography can also detect acute disease; however, changes

in heart size and mediastinal width can be misleading (Table 1-1).

On the AP view, the heart and mediastinum appear about 15% wider than on the PA view. Most of the magnification occurs because portable radiography is performed with the x-ray tube closer to the patient than radiography done in the radiology department. This is a necessary evil when a portable machine is used. Placing the radiographic plate in back of the patient magnifies anterior chest structures, primarily the heart and great vessels, more than posterior structures. Because of these factors, comparison of an AP projection with a prior PA projection can falsely suggest an enlarging cardiac silhouette or a widened mediastinum (Fig. 1-2). The latter can,

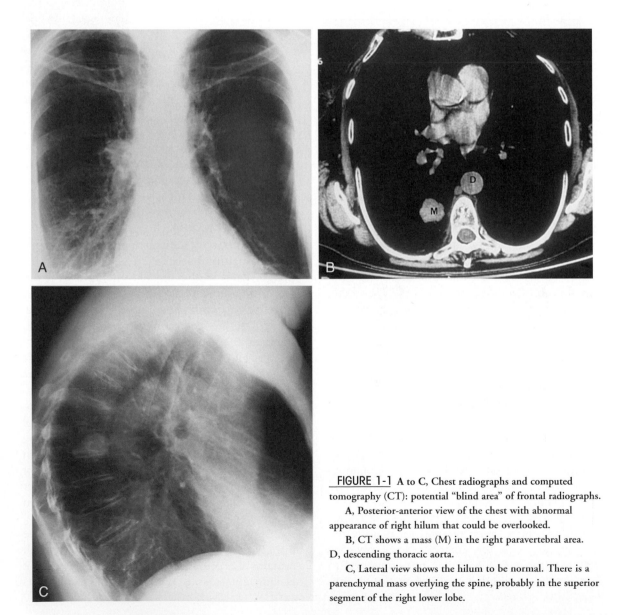

FIGURE 1-1 A to C, Chest radiographs and computed tomography (CT): potential "blind area" of frontal radiographs.

A, Posterior-anterior view of the chest with abnormal appearance of right hilum that could be overlooked.

B, CT shows a mass (M) in the right paravertebral area. D, descending thoracic aorta.

C, Lateral view shows the hilum to be normal. There is a parenchymal mass overlying the spine, probably in the superior segment of the right lower lobe.

TABLE 1-1
Portable Chest Radiographs

Uses

Routine assessment of ICU patients, tube and line placement, pneumothoraces, etc.

Non-ICU patients immediately following an invasive procedure (e.g., central venous access or thoracentesis)

Unstable patients, to exclude large pneumothorax, large effusion, perforated viscus,* acute pulmonary edema, etc.

Limitations

Poor visualization of mediastinal structures

Magnification of cardiac silhouette

Incomplete visualization of lung parenchyma (e.g., the lung bases)

Supine position further impairs assessment of vasculature, effusions, etc.

---

*Need upright or decubitus views.
ICU, intensive care unit.

for instance, raise the specter of aortic rupture in trauma patients.

There are other, less widely known, technical problems with AP portable radiography. Because these radiographs are usually made with lower energy x-rays, they often do not show good anatomic detail in the thickest parts of the chest. This makes it hard to examine the thoracic spine on portable radiographs. One may not see catheters or tubes well if they overlie the thickest

portions of the mediastinum. In addition, the decreased number and energy of the photons produced by portable equipment must be compensated for by longer exposure times. This leads to more blurring of the radiograph because of motion and is a particular problem in large patients, who require the longest exposure times.

Some of the difficulties associated with bedside radiography can be ascribed to the fact that many images are taken when the patient is in the supine position. These difficulties can be prevented by the physician's insisting that the patient be upright when the radiograph is taken. Unless the patient is hypotensive and in the Trendelenburg position, it is worth making this effort. Pleural effusions can easily be missed on supine AP radiographs because they layer posteriorly. The meniscus seen on upright radiographs is absent, and all one may see is a diffuse haziness through which blood vessels are visible (Fig. 1-3). Equally important, with the patient in a supine position blood flow does not favor the lower lobes. Instead, blood flow may appear equally distributed to the upper and lower lobes. This pattern mimics that seen in volume overload and can be mistaken for that seen in heart failure (Fig. 1-4; see Chapter 12).

There are other subtle differences between PA and AP views that are less clinically important.

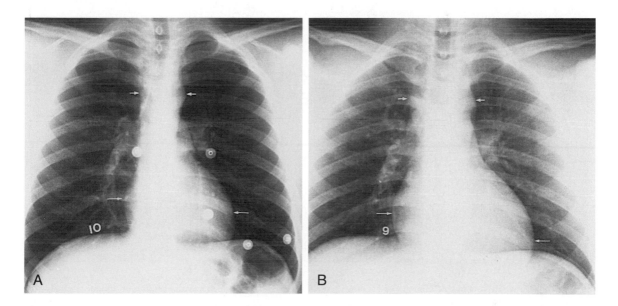

FIGURE 1-2 Posterior-anterior (PA) and anterior-posterior (AP) views of the chest, upright: positional effect on the appearance of cardiomediastinal structures.

A, The PA projection demonstrates a normal appearance of the cardiomediastinal silhouette. Note the width of the upper mediastinum *(small arrows)* and of the heart *(long arrows)*.

B, AP view of the same patient taken at the same time as the study shown in part A. There is increased width of the mediastinal *(small arrows)* and cardiac *(long arrows)* silhouettes, and the hilar structures appear larger.

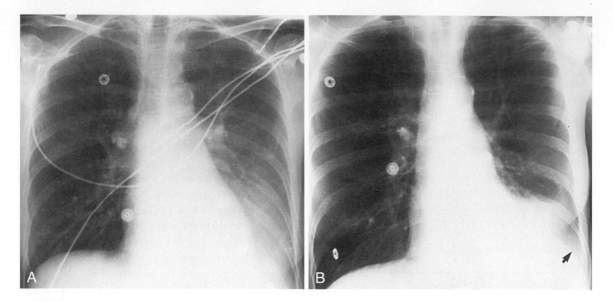

FIGURE 1-3 Anterior-posterior supine chest view: pleural effusion.

A, Increased opacity is seen at the left base that gradually diminishes as it reaches the level of the hilum, which is indicative of free pleural effusion in the major fissure or dependent pleural effusion along the pleural space posteriorly. The inferior pulmonary vessels are clearly defined through the fluid density, indicating the extraparenchymal location of the fluid.

B, An upright frontal view of the same patient at the same time shows a change in appearance, as the effusion now accumulates at the left base *(arrow)*.

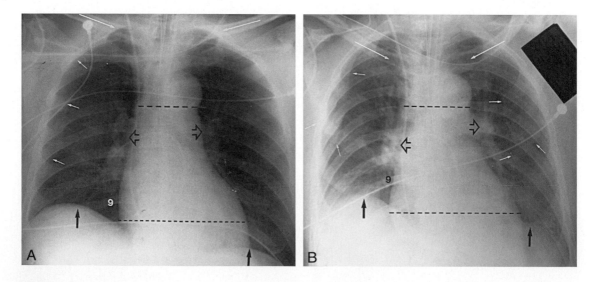

FIGURE 1-4 Anterior-posterior (AP) upright and supine chest radiographs: variation in vascular redistribution and mediastinal width caused by change in patient's position.

A, The AP upright chest radiograph shows the normal appearance of the cardiomediastinal *(dashed lines)* and hilar *(arrowheads)* structures. The AP position is evident, as the scapulae overlie the upper lung fields *(short white arrows)*. The *long white arrows* point to the clavicles and the *black arrows* to the diaphragm. Nine ribs are visible above the right diaphragm.

B, The AP supine chest radiograph shows increased prominence in the hilar vasculature *(open arrows)*, increased suprahilar mediastinal width, and increased cardiac silhouette size. Note: There is no change in excursion (nine ribs visible on right) between the views shown in parts A and B.

For instance, a PA projection shows the anterior ribs more clearly than an AP projection because better resolution is achieved in areas closer to the radiographic plate. Also, because the patient's arms are usually raised on a PA projection, less scapula overlies the lung parenchyma. These observations may help in determining whether an unlabeled radiograph is an AP or PA projection.

Lateral decubitus studies are the most commonly ordered additional views of the chest. They are usually performed when pleural effusions are suspected and are discussed further in Chapter 11. If decubitus views are needed, even if it is suspected that the pleural fluid is only unilateral, both right and left side down images should be requested. Bilateral decubitus films give a better look at the lung parenchyma underlying the effusion than a single view provides. Views with the affected hemithorax "up" (nondependent) can also determine whether the fluid is loculated. Furthermore, signs of pleural effusion can be subtle on routine radiographs, especially if the fluid is subpulmonic (below the lung). Assessment of both decubitus views sometimes shows an apparently unilateral effusion to be truly bilateral, a finding that can change the differential diagnosis (Fig. 1-5).

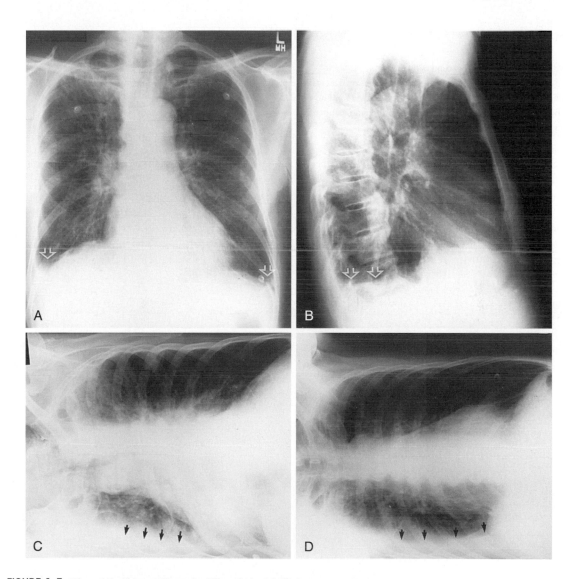

FIGURE 1-5 Bilateral decubitus radiographs: bilateral pleural effusions.

Posterior-anterior upright (**A**) and lateral (**B**) chest views show minimal blunting of costophrenic angles and sulci as evidence of effusions *(open arrows)* because they are mostly subpulmonic. As much as 300 mL of fluid can be hidden in the subpulmonic space.

Left (**C**) and right (**D**) lateral decubitus films (named for the side of the patient that faces down) demonstrate sizable free effusions layering along dependent thoracic gutters *(arrows)*. Nondependent costophrenic angles are sharp, indicating the fluid is not loculated.

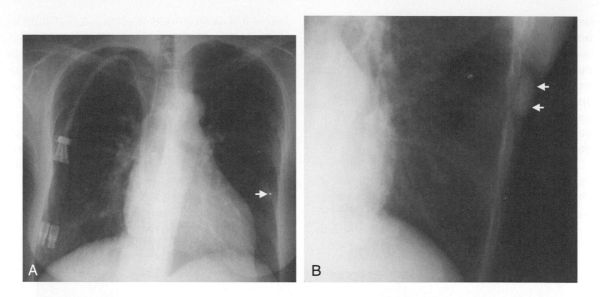

FIGURE 1-6 Skin mole and metallic marker.

A, An apparent nodule was seen on a posterior-anterior radiograph (not shown). Because the nodule was not seen on lateral view, a radiopaque marker *(arrow)* was placed over a mole found on the skin.

B, An oblique view better illustrates the exophytic nature of the skin mole *(arrows)*. (The radiopaque marker is present but difficult to see on this view.)

Lateral decubitus radiographs can also help demonstrate a pneumothorax in patients who cannot sit upright.

Nipples and large moles occasionally mimic lung nodules. The simplest way to confirm that an apparent nodule is caused by one of these extrapulmonary structures is to localize the skin lesion with a metallic marker and repeat the radiograph. These views are still commonly performed (Fig. 1-6). Other nonstandard views are occasionally used in chest radiology but are not commonly performed because of the widespread use of CT scanning. The apical lordotic view is designed to evaluate the upper convexities of the

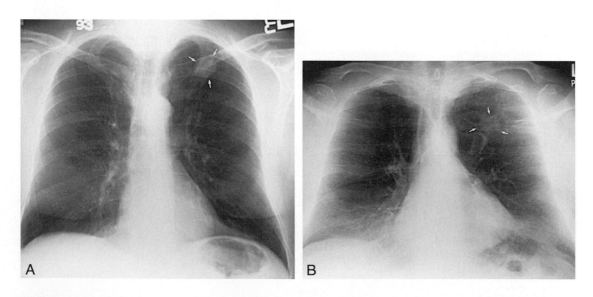

FIGURE 1-7 Posterior-anterior (PA) and apical lordotic chest radiographs: left apical mass, a bronchogenic carcinoma.

A, A routine PA chest view shows asymmetry in apparent "calcifications" of the first anterior costochondral junction *(arrows)*.

B, The apical lordotic view shifts the ribs and clavicles upward, exposing the apical area of lung parenchyma and revealing the presence of an irregular spiculated mass *(arrows)* within the lung parenchyma.

lung parenchyma by projecting the clavicles and first rib above the lung apices. This view is still occasionally used, most often to confirm the suspicion that an opacity seen in the apex is really part of the anterior aspect of this first rib. If the apical lordotic view shows that the opacity is definitely part of the first rib, no further evaluation is needed. If there is any doubt, it is best to proceed to chest CT (Fig. 1-7).

Oblique views or fluoroscopy can also be helpful in the evaluation of a pulmonary nodule (see Chapter 9) but are now rarely performed. For instance, if the area of opacity consistently projects within the same part of a rib during fluoroscopy or on oblique views, it proves that the nodule is within the rib rather than within the lung parenchyma. Note that the radiographic technique used to obtain these oblique views is different from the technique routinely used to examine the ribs. The latter uses an x-ray beam of lower energy than that used for routine chest radiography, enhancing bone detail at the expense of diminished contrast in the lung parenchyma (Fig. 1-8; see Chapter 14).

Lastly, expiratory views are useful in detecting pneumothoraces and endobronchial obstruction. Cross-table lateral projections are occasionally used to confirm a pneumothorax in an intensive care unit (ICU) patient but are difficult to interpret in adults. A decubitus film (pneumothorax side up) is another alternative, but at times it may be necessary to resort to

CT to find a pneumothorax in ICU patients with diffuse parenchymal disease and stiff lungs.

☐ ANATOMY

In general, readers with in-depth knowledge of chest anatomy can gather more information from plain radiographs. Sometimes this knowledge can obviate the need for additional studies, such as chest CT or MRI. Normal PA and lateral chest radiographs are shown in Figures 1-9 and 1-10, with important anatomic landmarks labeled. Throughout the book, we refer to these illustrations. More detailed explanations accompany important clinical points presented in later chapters.

The use of chest anatomy varies from physician to physician. In general, clinicians and radiologists approach chest radiographs differently. Radiologists are trained to look at each radiograph systematically and to evaluate the entire image (Table 1-2). This is analogous to an internist's history and physical, a mixture of a routine checklist and a more thorough search for associated findings when an abnormality is discovered. For most clinicians this global approach is not practical. Although it is painful for chest radiologists to admit, some details of chest anatomy are not clinically important. Moreover, the chest x-ray is often obtained to answer a specific clinical question, for instance, "Is the patient

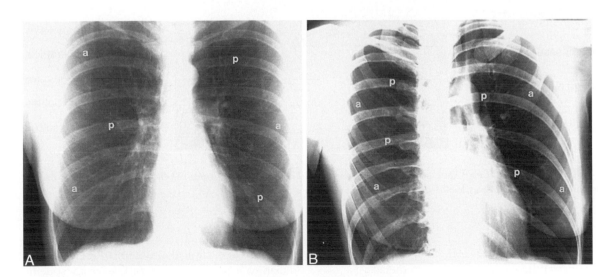

FIGURE 1-8 Comparative appearance of ribs: routine chest view versus rib detail technique.

A, Routine posterior-anterior chest radiograph demonstrates diminished bone detail of the anterior (a) and posterior (p) ribs when compared with a rib study (B).

B, Changes in exposure factors and positioning account for good anterior as well as posterior rib detail.

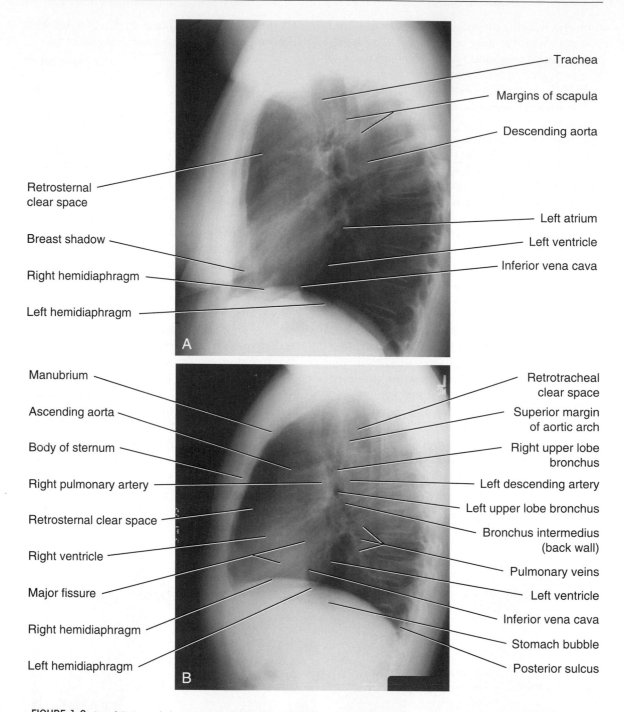

FIGURE 1-9 A and B, Lateral chest view: normal radiographic anatomy. Important structures usually seen are labeled. Note the specific position of the cardiac chambers, clear spaces, and pulmonary arteries.

in congestive failure?" or "Is a bronchogenic carcinoma the source of the brain metastasis?"

Occasionally, however, this focused approach can cause the observer to miss clinically important findings on a chest radiograph. A hybrid system of chest radiograph analysis, wherein each clinical problem triggers the clinician to look for a series of five or six specific findings, may be the best compromise. A short list of plain chest radiographic findings to look for with each of four clinical problems is given in Table 1-3. These key observations are defined

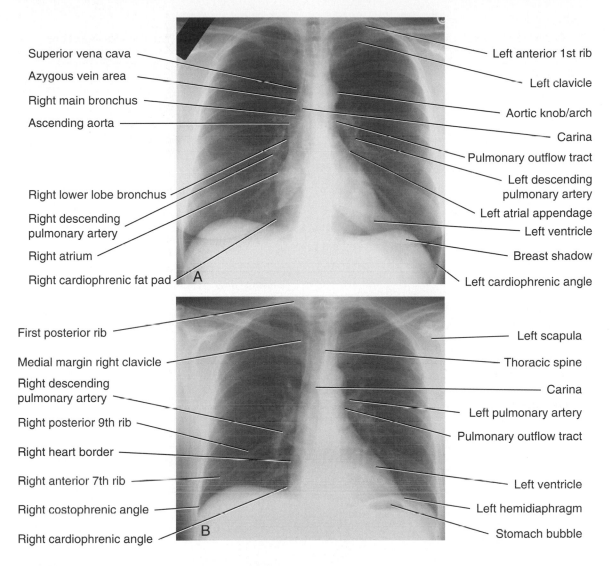

Superior vena cava
Azygous vein area
Right main bronchus
Ascending aorta

Right lower lobe bronchus
Right descending pulmonary artery
Right atrium
Right cardiophrenic fat pad

A

Left anterior 1st rib
Left clavicle
Aortic knob/arch
Carina
Pulmonary outflow tract
Left descending pulmonary artery
Left atrial appendage
Left ventricle
Breast shadow
Left cardiophrenic angle

First posterior rib
Medial margin right clavicle
Right descending pulmonary artery
Right posterior 9th rib
Right heart border
Right anterior 7th rib
Right costophrenic angle
Right cardiophrenic angle

B

Left scapula
Thoracic spine
Carina
Left pulmonary artery
Pulmonary outflow tract
Left ventricle
Left hemidiaphragm
Stomach bubble

FIGURE 1-10 A and B, Frontal chest views: normal radiographic anatomy. Important structures usually seen are labeled. Note important landmarks of the mediastinum and cardiac borders.

and their relevance discussed later in the appropriate chapters. Please remember that these lists are not meant to be exhaustive. For example, in a patient with a primary lung neoplasm, it is critical to detect the lytic rib lesion (not listed in the table) that may prevent a fruitless thoracotomy.

☐ SPECIFIC SIGNS

Abnormal Opacities

In reviewing a chest radiograph, it is important to identify areas of the chest that are too opaque

(too white). The increased opacity indicates increased absorption of x-ray photons and can be caused by abnormalities in the mediastinum, pleura, or parenchyma. In order to narrow the differential diagnosis, it is helpful to decide which of these components of the chest is the site of the abnormality. This can be difficult to do using the chest radiograph, but there are some helpful clues such as the appearance of air bronchograms (Table 1-4). The presence of air bronchograms in an abnormal opacity localizes disease to the lung parenchyma. Bronchograms occur when air-filled bronchi are outlined by fluid-filled alveoli (Fig. 1-11). The course of the

TABLE 1-2
Sites Examined in a Radiologist's Evaluation of the Chest Radiograph

Frontal view
Bones
  Ribs: posterior ribs, anterior ribs, axillary margin
  Spine
  Clavicles/scapula
Mediastinum
  Aortic arch
  Aortopulmonary window
  Pulmonary outflow tract
  Tracheal air column and right paratracheal
    soft tissues
  Area of azygous vein
  Paraspinous lines
Hilum
  Relative height and size of right and left hilum
  Hilar angle
  Bronchial wall thickness and vascular distribution
Heart
  Silhouette size
  Apex configuration
  Left atrium (e.g., carinal angle, double density)
  Calcifications
Diaphragms/pleura
  Contour, including costophrenic angles
  Upper abdomen
  Apices (e.g., thickening, pleural line)
Parenchyma
  Entire lung field, including a repeated examination
    of the portions already seen at the sites listed
    above

Lateral view
Bones
  Spine
  Sternum
Mediastinum
  Retrosternal space
  Tracheal air column
  Retrotracheal space
Hilum
  Interlobar arteries size and shape
  Posterior wall of bronchus intermedius
Heart
  Posterior margin (including inferior vena cava
    junction)
  Retrosternal space
Diaphragm/pleura
  Pleural fissures
  Contour, including costophrenic angles
  Upper abdomen (free gas and surgical clips)
Parenchyma
  Examine entire lung field, as on frontal view

TABLE 1-3
Key Observations in Four Clinical Questions

Is the patient in early congestive heart failure?
Cardiac silhouette size and shape
Left atrial size
Hilar contour (e.g., indistinctness)
Vascular redistribution
Azygous vein (vascular pedicle)
Linear opacities (e.g., Kerley's lines)
Effusions

What is the etiology of the patient's chest pain?
Aortic contour
Cardiac silhouette size and shape
Check for abrupt enlargement, sandwich sign
Signs of congestive failure (above)
Air bronchograms (pleural based)
Effusions
Pneumothoraces

Does the patient have pneumonia?
Reticular (net-like) opacities
Air bronchograms
Silhouette signs
Effusions
Hilar contour (adenopathy or mass)
Volume loss

Does the patient have a lung tumor (primary)?
Parenchymal mass (include apices)
Tracheal margin (frontal) and retrotracheal space
  (lateral)
Mediastinal nodes (azygous and aorticopulmonary
  window)
Hilar contour (check for increased opacity as well as
  change in contour)
Volume loss
Effusions

distal bronchial tree, not normally seen, is then easily traced and appears as dark bronchi superimposed on a light background. When air space disease is not as uniform, normal air-containing alveoli appear as very small radiolucencies within the opacified lung. These normal areas, interspersed between opacified alveoli, are known as air alveolograms. Unfortunately, it is sometimes hard to decide whether tiny radiolucencies are air alveolograms or represent small spaces in the net-like (reticular) opacity that is often caused by fibrosis. In contrast, air bronchograms are "bulletproof" evidence of disease causing alveolar filling. Both findings are discussed at length in Chapter 5.

TABLE 1-4
Focal Opacities Seen on Chest Radiographs—Location in the Thorax

Origin of the Opacity	Chest Radiograph Observations
Mediastinum	Smooth, well-defined contours
	Contiguous with mediastinum on posterior-anterior and lateral
	No air bronchograms
Pleura	No definable edge, or a smooth sharp contour on one side only
	Contiguous with the chest wall on at least one view
	No air bronchograms
Parenchyma	Any kind of contour (i.e., smooth, irregular, sharp, or indistinct)
	Located anywhere in the chest
	Can have air bronchograms

Abnormal Lucencies

Although less common than abnormal opacities, sometimes areas of the chest appear too radiolucent, "too black." These radiolucencies indicate areas where abnormally large amounts of x-ray photons penetrate the thorax. These too black areas may have definable borders and in these cases can be described as ring shadows, cysts, or cavities. These type of radiolucencies are discussed in several portions of this book, including Chapters 4, 5, and 7. Alternatively, increased radiolucency can be more generalized, involving one hemithorax or both lungs. Although large areas of radiolucency are frequently caused by abnormalities of the chest wall (e.g., mastectomy), they may also reflect obstructive or vascular lung disease. This is discussed further in Chapters 4 and 10 (see Table 4-3). Last, pneumothoraces may cause large areas of radiolucency. Usually, large pneumothoraces are easy to detect, but it may be difficult to determine that a large radiolucency is caused by air in the pleural space when the pneumothorax is loculated or imaged with the patient supine (see Chapter 11).

Localizing the Abnormality

Silhouette Sign

The silhouette sign can be used when reading a radiograph to help localize an opacity in relation to structures in the chest. The silhouette sign is present if the border of a structure normally seen on the chest radiograph (such as the diaphragm, heart, or aorta) is obscured by fluid or abnormal tissue. We normally see the mediastinal, hilar, and diaphragmatic contours well on chest radiographs because they are bordered by air-containing lung that stops only a few photons and therefore appears black. If aerated lung no longer forms the border of the diaphragm, mediastinum, or hilum, their margins are obscured.

For example, when the lung is filled with water or pus it stops more photons and appears more opaque (whiter) on the chest radiograph. Wherever it touches the diaphragm, the opacities of the abnormal lung and diaphragm blend together and the border of the diaphragm is no longer visualized. When the border of a normal structure such as the diaphragm is obscured, a silhouette sign is present. (Some physicians

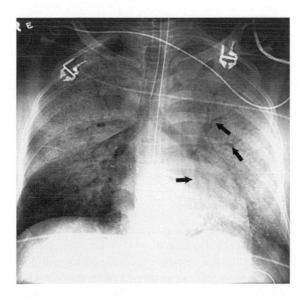

FIGURE 1-11 Posterior-anterior chest view: air bronchograms in adult respiratory distress syndrome. Air bronchograms *(arrows)* indicate the presence of airless alveoli with patent bronchi. The tubular branching pattern formed indicates that the abnormality is definitely in the lung parenchyma.

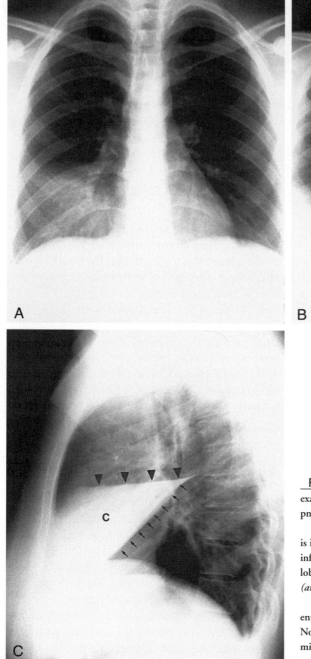

A

B

C

FIGURE 1-12 **A,** Posterior-anterior and lateral chest examination: silhouette sign seen in right middle lobe pneumonia.

In the frontal projection (**A**), the right lateral cardiac margin is indistinct. The silhouette is obscured by a right middle lobe infiltrate. This is not the case if the pneumonia is in the lower lobe (**B**), where the right cardiac margin is easily visible *(arrows).*

C, The lateral film of the same patient as in A shows the entirety of the middle lobe occupied by the air space disease. Note the position of the minor fissure *(arrowheads)* separating middle from upper lobe and the major (oblique) fissure *(arrows)* separating middle lobe from lower lobe. C, consolidation.

say "the diaphragm is silhouetted out." Not only is this confusing but also it misuses the noun, silhouette, as a verb.)

The silhouette sign is present only if the fluid or abnormal tissue is in direct contact with normal structure. For example, if a mass appears to overlie the hilum on the frontal projection but does not obscure its borders, the mass must not directly touch the hilum. The silhouette sign is absent, and a lateral view will show that the mass is actually located in front of or behind the hilum.

The silhouette sign can be used to evaluate the location of pulmonary collapse (atelectasis), encapsulated pleural fluid, tumors, and pneumonias. On frontal radiographs, loss of the right or left cardiac border can indicate middle lobe or lingular disease, respectively (Fig. 1-12). A lower lobe pneumonia causes increased opacity over the same area on the

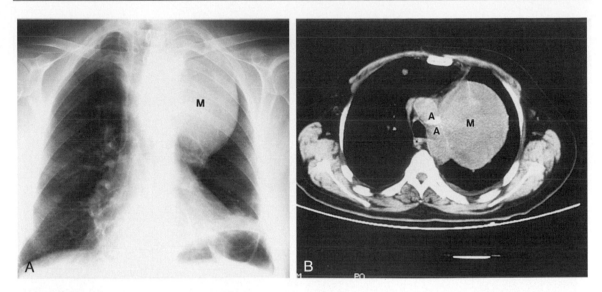

FIGURE 1-13 Posterior-anterior (PA) chest and computed tomography (CT) scan: middle mediastinal mass obscures aortic arch silhouette.

A, PA chest view shows a large mass projecting adjacent to the left upper lobe and obscuring the silhouette of the aortic knob/arch.

B, A CT scan at the level of the arch shows the large mass (M) abutting the lateral margin of the entire aortic arch (AA).

frontal view but does not obscure the heart border. (A lower lobe pneumonia that involves the anterior aspect of the lower lobe may obscure the diaphragm silhouette instead.)

The silhouette sign can also be applied to mediastinal structures other than the heart or aorta. For instance, opacities that obscure the lateral border of the aortic arch usually lie within the apical posterior segment of the left upper lobe or in the middle mediastinum (Fig. 1-13). If the opacity overlies the aortic arch but does not obscure its lateral border, it must lie anterior or far posterior in the chest (e.g., in the posterior portions of the mediastinum). In this case, the opacity of the abnormal tissue is added to that of the aorta and the aorta appears more radiopaque than usual. Some radiologists call this type of finding a "summation sign" (Fig. 1-14). This is the same effect that makes the heart look more opaque on frontal projection when left lower lobe pneumonia or atelectasis is behind it. Table 1-5 lists further applications of the silhouette sign.

In addition to localizing disease in the chest, the loss of a silhouette can help confirm the presence of disease when other radiographic findings are equivocal. For instance, the loss of the silhouette of the descending aorta on frontal projection makes it much more

likely that a subtle increased opacity behind the heart is significant and likely to represent pneumonia or atelectasis. Unfortunately, only about 10% of the lung touches the heart or diaphragm, limiting the sensitivity of these silhouettes in detecting disease.

There are also other limitations to the utility of the silhouette sign. The cardiac border can be obscured by nonpathologic structures, such as pectus excavatum deformities (which obscure the right cardiac border). Abundant pericardial fat may obscure the right or the left cardiac border, and vessels running parallel to the heart may also obscure its border (Fig. 1-15). Radiographic technique affects the accuracy of the silhouette sign. If the x-rays are too few or the photons are too low in energy to penetrate the heart and mediastinum, these midline structures appear uniformly white. This can artifactually obliterate the silhouette of the diaphragm and other structures. In a similar manner, if the spine projects over the right heart border, it can obscure the cardiac silhouette by preventing adequate penetration of x-rays.

Lobar Fissures

If it can be determined that an abnormal opacity lies within the lung parenchyma, it may be useful to localize it to a specific lobe of the lung.

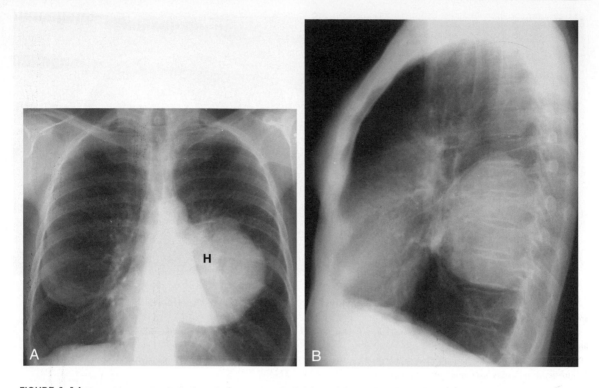

FIGURE 1-14 Posterior-anterior (PA) chest: Large mass in the left lower lobe overlies the cardiac border and left hilum but does not obscure their margins.

A, PA radiograph of a patient with non–small cell lung carcinoma. A large mass is present in the left lung. The mass overlies the cardiac border and hilum but does not obscure either silhouette. Therefore, the mass must be in back of the heart and hilum. Note that the left hilum and a portion of the heart appear more opaque than usual. This is an example of a summation sign. H, hilum.

B, Lateral radiograph shows the mass to be in the left lower lobe, posterior to the hilum and heart.

For instance, in a patient with chronic cough and sputum production, bilateral lower lobe parenchymal disease raises the question of aspiration. On the other hand, disease limited to the posterior segments of the upper lobes or to the superior segment of the lower lobe suggests reactivation tuberculosis. Identifying the pleural fissures helps to localize the abnormal opacity.

Also, observing that one of the fissures is abnormally positioned is key to recognizing that a lobe has lost volume (lobar atelectasis), potentially a sign that a cancer has obstructed a central bronchus.

The minor (horizontal) fissure separates the right upper lobe from the right middle lobe and is often seen on both lateral and PA projections.

TABLE 1-5
Applications of the Silhouette Sign

Finding on Frontal Radiography	Location of Abnormality
Loss of right heart border	Right middle lobe, anterior pleura or anterior mediastinum
Loss of left heart border	Lingula, anterior pleura or anterior mediastinum
Overlies heart border (border not lost)	Lower lobes, posterior pleura or mediastinum
Loss of aortic arch (lateral border)	Left upper lobe or middle/posterior mediastinum
Overlies aortic arch (border not lost)	Anterior or far posterior pleura or mediastinum
Loss of descending aorta lateral border	Left lower lobe or posterior mediastinum or pleura
Loss of diaphragm	Lower lobes (anterior segments)* or pleura

*Contrary to conventional wisdom, disease in the middle lobe and lingua can also obscure the diaphragm silhouette, probably dependent on where the adjacent major fissure intersects the diaphragm.

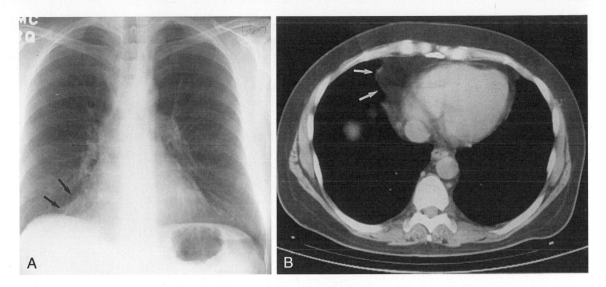

FIGURE 1-15 Posterior-anterior chest radiograph and non–contrast-enhanced conventional computed tomography (CT): pericardial fat pad.

A, On the radiograph, the cardiophrenic fat pad *(arrows)* is well defined and may be present at both right and left cardiophrenic angles. In this case it obscures part of the cardiac silhouette.

B, Non–contrast-enhanced chest CT is diagnostic *(arrows)*, showing the characteristic appearance of fatty tissues. Attenuation (Hounsfield) numbers are tissue specific for diagnosis of fat (−40 to −100).

The major (oblique) fissures separate the lower lobes from the upper lobes bilaterally and are seen best on lateral radiographs (see Fig. 1-10). The right major fissure can be differentiated from the left by its intersection with the minor fissure. The left major fissure is identified by its junction with the left hemidiaphragm, the latter often losing its silhouette as it comes into contact with the left ventricle anteriorly. On upright films, the gastric bubble can also be used to confirm the identity of the left hemidiaphragm.

☐ COMPUTED TOMOGRAPHY AND MAGNETIC RESONANCE IMAGING

Despite optimal views and optimal interpretation, plain radiography sometimes cannot answer the clinical question. Further evaluation of the chest usually falls to CT. Most imaging is now performed with spiral CT (explained later). MRI has traditionally been preferred for imaging structures where views in multiple planes are helpful. Images can be obtained that show cross sections perpendicular to the spine (axial), parallel to the spine running from right to left (coronal), or parallel to the spine

running from front to back (sagittal) (Fig. 1-16). The development of multidetector CT scanning has improved the ability of CT to image multiple planes, such that it now rivals MRI. MRI still maintains the important advantage of being free from ionizing radiation. General indications for these techniques are listed in Table 1-6.

Computed Tomography

Although CT scanning may be done by acquiring individual "slices," most CT scanning is now performed using spiral technique. In spiral CT, the x-ray tube makes continuous 360-degree revolutions without interruption while the patient is slowly moved through the circling x-ray beam. Imaging information is obtained as a virtual cylinder instead of one slice at a time (Fig. 1-17). This "cylinder" of data is usually divided into individual slices that are the same thickness as the x-ray beam. These axial cross-sectional images are displayed for viewing with the patient's right to the viewer's left (as if looking at the anatomy from the foot of the patient's bed) (see Fig. 1-16). The number and location of the axial CT slices can be selected so that the slices are contiguous ("stacked side by side") or overlap. Overlapping sections are useful in

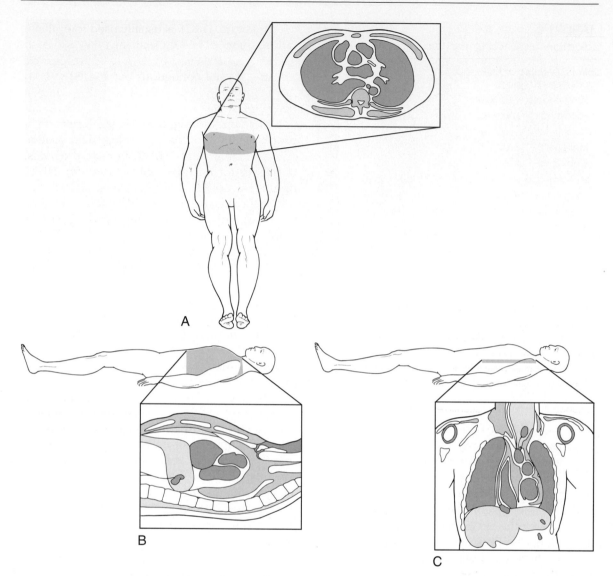

FIGURE 1-16 Drawings of a routine cross-sectional imaging planes for computed tomography (CT) and magnetic resonance (MR).

A, Inset shows an axial (transverse) section through the thorax. Axial CT or MR sections are displayed as if viewing the patient from the foot of the bed. Routine CT scanning is usually displayed only in this plane.

B, Inset shows a sagittal MR or CT section through the thorax. MR images can be obtained in this plane by manipulating the magnetic field in the MR scanner. In order to create a sagittal CT image, however, scanning is first performed in the axial plane and the data are then reformatted to produce a sagittal image. Thinner axial sections make for better spatial resolution in the reformatted images. Accordingly, reformatted images are of higher quality when created with a multidetector scanner than with a single-detector CT scanner.

C, Coronal MR or CT section through the thorax. As with the section in B, this imaging plane can be obtained directly with an MR scanner. Creation of coronal images with a CT scanner requires reformatting of imaging information initially obtained in the axial plane.

detecting lesions that are smaller than the slice thickness (see volume averaging, Chapter 2).

In general, the thinner the slices the better. Thinner slices generate more detailed images, particularly if the imaging data are used to construct images in sagittal and coronal planes. In order to obtain images of the chest that are free of motion artifact, however, the best images are obtained during a single breath-hold. For many patients the scan time then needs to be limited to 20 to 30 seconds. Because of this time limit, there has often been a trade-off between slice thickness and the amount of the chest that is imaged during a single spiral CT acquisition. For instance, if the x-ray tube can make only one revolution per second, the radiologist can

TABLE 1-6
Indications for Chest Computed Tomography

Spiral CT—single or multidetector
Evaluation of masses
    Lung nodule or nodules
    Hilar/mediastinal mass*
Evaluation of pleural disease
    Malignant
    Empyema*
Staging/treatment/follow-up for neoplastic disease
Large airway disease
    Hemoptysis (with negative chest radiograph)
    Persistent atelectasis
Thoracic vascular disease
    Aortic dissection/aneurysm[†]
    Pulmonary emboli[†]
Cardiac imaging
    Detection of pericardial calcification or effusion
    Coronary artery or valvular calcifications—
        multidetector spiral CT only

High-resolution CT
Evaluation of patients with signs and symptoms of lung
    disease but normal chest x-rays (dyspnea of
    unknown origin)
Immunocompromised patients (e.g., acquired
    immunodeficiency syndrome) with suspected
    pneumonia
Characterization of diffuse infiltrative pulmonary disease

*Intravenous contrast agent helpful.
[†]Intravenous contrast agent required.

choose to make 30 revolutions using 1-mm-thick collimation and image only 3 cm of the chest or choose to make 30 revolution using 10-mm-thick collimation and image 30 cm of the chest.

Most recently, multidetector spiral CT (MDCT) scanners have become widely available. Instead of using a single row of x-ray detectors to receive x-ray photons from an x-ray beam, these scanners use multiple rows of x-ray detectors to receive photons from a fan-shaped x-ray source. This has nearly the same effect as rotating multiple thin x-ray beams around the patient at the same time. It allows the CT image to be acquired much faster and allows the cylinder of data to cover more area yet still be divided into thin slices. Because MDCT scanners can create very thin slices over long sections of the body, they are particularly useful in accurately imaging blood vessels and large airways of the chest (see Chapter 12).

High-resolution CT (HRCT) of the chest is an exception to the widespread use of spiral CT technique. HRCT is usually used to evaluate diffuse lung disease. Because it is meant to survey lung involved by a diffuse process, CT sections are not contiguous but spaced at 1- to 2-cm intervals. To capture small anatomic detail, very thin sections (1 to 1.5 mm) are obtained and the digitized x-ray information is processed in a different manner than routine images of the lung. The computer programs, or reconstruction algorithms, used for HRCT produce a noisier (grainier) image in order to obtain better spatial resolution (the ability to see smaller objects). With this trade-off, we can gain a more detailed look at the lung parenchyma architecture. Often HRCT findings can limit the differential diagnosis for the diffuse lung disease to two or three possibilities (e.g., miliary tuberculosis, miliary fungal disease, or metastases). HRCT can also suggest whether the most likely diseases are those that can be diagnosed with closed lung biopsy (e.g., sarcoid) or are likely to require a surgical biopsy for diagnosis.

HRCT can also be useful in detecting early or occult parenchymal disease seen in patients with acquired immunodeficiency syndrome and in the early stages of fibrotic lung disease such as asbestosis and usual interstitial pneumonitis (see Table 1-6). When viewing an HRCT image, however, it is important to remember that the lung is only surveyed, and large sections between the slices are not examined. Usually a conventional spiral CT study is needed to make sure that nodules or other important findings do not "fall between the slices." Using MDCT, it is possible to obtain both conventional CT and HRCT thin slices simultaneously.

After the imaging data are collected, the CT images are compiled by the assignment of numeric values to different tissues based on the amount of x-rays they absorb. All tissues have CT numbers that are referenced to the electron density of water, which is arbitrarily assigned 0 Hounsfield units (HU). CT numbers of other tissues range from −1000 HU (air) to +1000 HU (dense bone). All other tissue densities— muscle, fat, blood, cerebrospinal fluid, and so forth—fall somewhere in between. A "window level" is centered at the appropriate CT number to highlight the tissue of interest. For instance, lung windows (air) are set at a level between −350 and −700 HU, whereas mediastinal windows (soft tissue and water) are set at a level of approximately 0 to 50 HU.

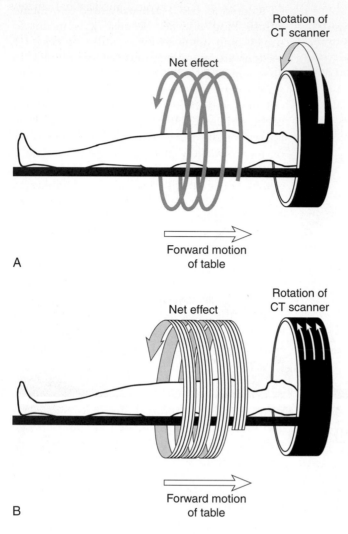

FIGURE 1-17 Line drawings of spiral computed tomography (CT) with single-detector and multidetector scanners.

A, The CT x-ray tube is activated continuously as the table and patient move through the scanner. During this process, the x-ray detector follows a spiral course with respect to the patient, acquiring a cylinder of data.

B, Spiral CT scanning with a multidetector scanner. The use of multiple detectors allows the CT image to be acquired with very thin slices without slowing down the scanning process.

Window width determines the range of tissue densities that are displayed on the image. All tissues with densities that are too great appear white and cannot be distinguished from one other. All tissues with densities that are too low appear black. For instance, the width on lung windows is often approximately 1500 HU (750 HU to either side of the level selected). If the level chosen is −500 HU, all tissues with CT numbers above 250 HU (−500 + 750) appear white. The tissues below −1250 HU (−500 − 750) appear black.

The range of absorption of x-rays is wider in the thorax than in any other area of the body. This is because tissue densities in the thorax range from very near air in the lungs to bone in the vertebrae. This range in densities cannot be well displayed in a single image. Therefore, chest CT images are viewed in at least two different levels and windows (one optimized for lung and the other for the mediastinum). In special cases, we add a third image optimized for bone. These images are all created from the same x-ray exposure. The different appearances are produced by changing the manner in which the computer displays the original data. If the CT images are read on an electronic monitor rather than on film, the data can actually be viewed at an infinite number of window and level configurations.

Normal lung windows that show the segmental bronchi, arteries, fissures, and peripheral pulmonary parenchyma at key anatomic levels are shown in Figure 1-18. The lung window setting is used primarily to evaluate parenchymal lung disease and tracheobronchial anatomy—the mediastinal structures and the thoracic envelope appear nearly white with these particular settings. Mediastinal windows better define the superior vena cava, the great vessels, the hila, the pleura, and the surrounding soft tissue structures. The esophagus is often seen immediately anterior and to the left of the anterior thoracic spine, and the cardiac chambers are sometimes well defined. Abnormal lymph nodes resulting from metastatic disease, such as the paratracheal area, are also seen well

(see Chapter 12). Typical mediastinal images are shown in Figure 1-19.

Routine CT evaluation of the chest can be done with or without intravenous administration of contrast media. Intravenous contrast is essential for the detection of pulmonary emboli and the assessment of aortic disease, such as dissection. CT scans with intravenous contrast are often useful for evaluating possible mediastinal

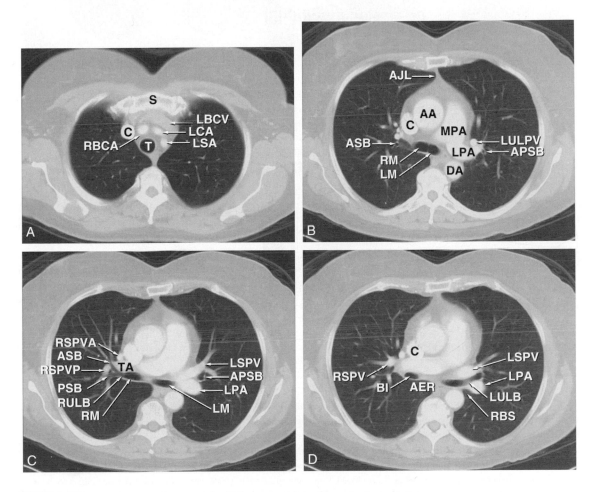

FIGURE 1-18 Normal computed tomography (CT) anatomy of the chest using lung windows.

A, Section above the level of the carina. C, superior vena cava; LBCV, left brachiocephalic vein; LCA, left carotid artery; LSA, left subclavian artery; RBCA, right brachiocephalic artery; S, sternum; T, trachea. Note that vessels lie against the left tracheal wall but not against the right tracheal wall. This causes the outer margin of the right tracheal wall to be clearly seen on chest radiographs.

B, Section at the level of carina. AA, ascending aorta; AJL, anterior junction line; APSB, left upper lobe apical posterior segmental bronchus; ASB, right upper lobe apical segment bronchus; C, superior vena cava; LPA, left pulmonary artery; LULPV, left upper lobe pulmonary vein; MPA, main pulmonary artery; RM, LM, right and left main bronchi.

C, Section 1-2 cm below carina. Note the well-defined upper lobe segmental anatomy, particularly on the right at this level. ASB, anterior segment bronchus; LM, left main bronchus; LSPV, left superior pulmonary vein and anterior segmental artery; PSB, posterior segment bronchus; RM, right main bronchus; RSPVA, right superior pulmonary vein anterior; RSPVP, right superior pulmonary vein posterior; RULB, right upper lobe bronchus; TA, truncus anterior.

D, Axial image at the level of the bronchus intermedius and left upper lobe bronchi. AJL, anterior junction line; BI, bronchus intermedius; LDPA, left descending pulmonary artery; LSPV, left superior pulmonary vein. Note the horizontal course of the left main bronchus as it proceeds laterally and bifurcates at the left upper lobe bronchus (LULB) level. Aerated lung is normally present in the azygoesophageal recess (AER) and adjacent to the retrobronchial stripe (RBS).

Illustration continued on following page.

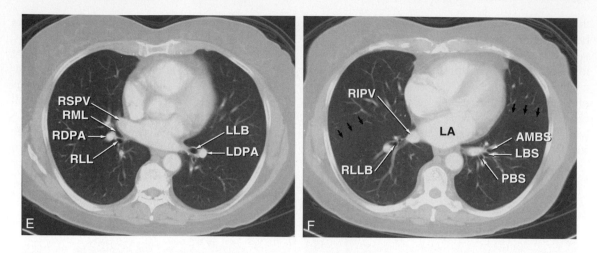

FIGURE 1-18, Cont'd E, Axial CT scan at the level of the middle lobe and lower lobe bronchi. LDPA, left descending pulmonary artery; RDPA, right descending pulmonary artery; RSPV, right superior pulmonary vein. Note the bifurcation of the bronchus intermedius into the lower lobe bronchus (RLLB) and middle lobe bronchus (RML) on the right. The lingual (not shown) arises from the left main bronchus slightly above the level of this section.

F, Axial CT section through the lower lobes. AMBS, anterior-medial basal segment bronchus; LA, left atrium; LBS, lateral basal segment bronchus; PBS, posterior basal segment bronchus; RIPV, right inferior pulmonary vein; RLLB, right lower lobe basal segment bronchi.

or hilar masses as well as possible empyemas. Intravenous contrast is usually *not* necessary for the evaluation of a lung nodule, detection of metastatic pulmonary disease, or the evaluation of diffuse lung disease.

Magnetic Resonance Imaging

The role of MRI in the evaluation of chest disease continues to change as the technology improves. MR images are derived by computer from the interactions of strong magnetic gradients and multiple radiofrequency energy pulses. In the past, the utility of MRI was limited by the length of time needed to perform the study, often several minutes to acquire each set of images This is particularly problematic in the chest, where there is a great deal of cardiac and respiratory motion over the time needed to collect the image data.

FIGURE 1-19 Normal computed tomography (CT) anatomy of the chest using mediastinal windows. Mediastinal and cardiovascular anatomy is well defined with this window. Key anatomic levels are selected from thoracic inlet to diaphragm.

A, Contrast-enhanced CT just above the lung apex demonstrates right and left jugular veins (RJV, LJV) and carotid arteries (CA). The right subclavian artery (RSA) is seen threading between the anterior and middle scalene muscles. The left subclavian vein (LSV) is seen before it joins with the left internal jugular vein. The esophagus (E) is directly behind the trachea.

B, Contrast-enhanced CT demonstrates well-opacified left brachiocephalic vein (LBV) and unopacified right brachiocephalic vein (RBV); the contrast agent was injected through the left arm. The brachiocephalic artery (BA), left subclavian artery (LSA), and left common carotid artery (LCA) are visible at this level. There are a few, normal-appearing lymph nodes in the axillae.

C, Contrast-enhanced CT from a different patient than in B, section just above the arch. Left brachiocephalic vein (LBV) crosses the mediastinum to join right brachiocephalic vein (RBV) and form the superior vena cava. Also visualized are the brachiocephalic artery (BA), left subclavian artery (LSA), left common carotid artery (LCA), trachea (T), and esophagus (E). Anterior chest wall soft tissues are asymmetric because of prior mastectomy.

D, Arch. Contrast-enhanced CT through the aortic arch (AA). Other structures identified at this level are the superior vena cava (SVC), trachea (T), and esophagus (E).

E, Intravenous contrast-enhanced CT at the level of the aorticopulmonary window. Structures seen include the ascending (A) and descending (D) aorta, the superior vena cava (BV), and the azygous vein (AV). The area above the pulmonary artery (not seen on this section) and beneath the arch is the aorticopulmonary window *(arrows)*. This area is normally filled with fat and may contain small (<1 cm diameter) lymph nodes.

F, Contrast-enhanced CT just below the tracheal bifurcation. Major structures seen at this level are the main pulmonary artery (MPA), left pulmonary artery (LPA), ascending aorta (A), descending aorta (D), and left superior pulmonary vein (LSPV). There is streak artifact caused by the SVC because of the high concentration of iodinated contrast material within it.

Long-established MRI techniques compensated respiratory motion by monitoring the patient's breathing and matching the image acquisition to the respiratory cycle in various ways. Newer MRI techniques allow imaging of the chest that is fast enough to be completed during a breath-hold. These techniques have markedly improved MRI's ability to image the heart and great vessels, particularly the thoracic aorta (Figs. 1-20 and 1-21). Faster image acquisitions and better methods to match the image acquisition to the patient's electrocardiogram (cardiac gating) can be used to record serial images of the heart through the cardiac cycle (Fig. 1-22). Because of these advances, state-of-the-art MRI equipment can perform a comprehensive cardiac examination that assesses cardiac wall motion, wall ischemia, coronary artery blood flow, and valvular function.

There are still limitations to the applications of MRI in the chest. The spatial resolution of MRI in the chest remains inferior to that of CT, and the high magnetic field strength needed for MRI can also pose a problem when patients

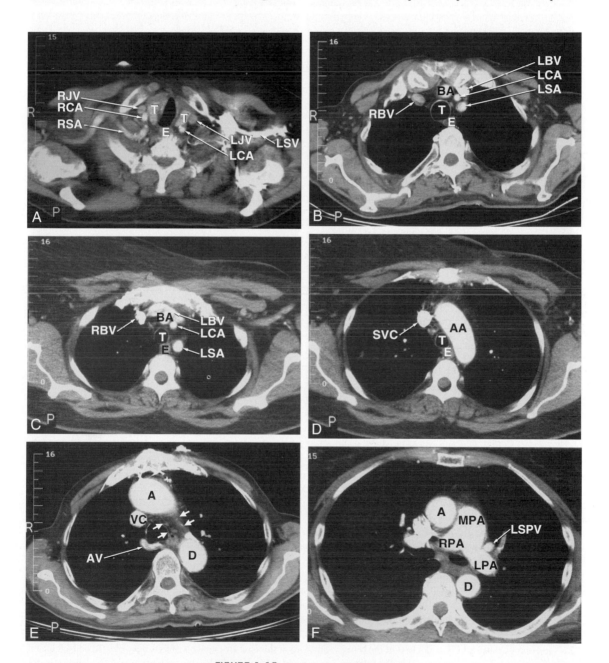

FIGURE 1-19 *See legend on previous page.*

Illustration continued on following page.

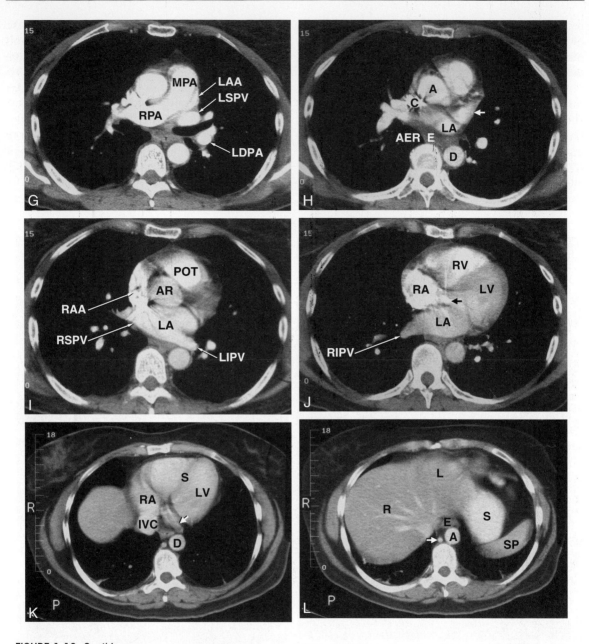

FIGURE 1-19, Cont'd G, Contrast-enhanced CT slightly more inferior than F shows the main pulmonary artery (MPA) and the right pulmonary artery (RPA). The descending left pulmonary artery (LDPA) is seen behind the left upper lobe bronchus. The left superior pulmonary vein (LSPV) is seen again and the left atrial appendage (LAA) is seen just in front of it.

H, Contrast-enhanced CT slightly inferior to image G. Ascending aorta (A), superior vena cava (C), descending aorta (D), and esophagus (E) are all well seen. The left atrium (LA) and left atrial appendage *(arrow)* are visible. Adjacent to the esophagus, the azygoesophageal recess (AER) is concave, which is normal.

I, The left atrium (LA) is the highest and most posterior cardiac chamber, seen here accepting left inferior (LIPV) and right superior pulmonary venous (RSPV) inflow. Also seen are the body of the left atrium and the right atrial appendage (RAA), aortic root (AR), and the main pulmonary outflow tract (POT).

J, Contrast-enhanced CT showing portions of all four cardiac chambers: left atrium (LA), right atrium (RA), left ventricle (LV), and right ventricle (RV). A very small portion of the aortic root is seen *(arrow)*. The right inferior pulmonary vein (RIPV) is also seen.

K, Contrast-enhanced CT at the level of the coronary sinus *(arrows)*. The coronary sinus *(arrow)* is seen posterior to the left ventricle (LV) and medial to the right atrium (RA) and inferior vena cava (IVC). The descending aorta (D), left ventricle (D), and interventricular septum (S) are also well seen.

L, Non–contrast-enhanced CT at the level of the hepatic veins. Seen at this level are segments of liver right lobe (R) and left lobe (L), stomach (S), spleen (SP), and esophagus (E). The inferior vena cava and portions of the hepatic veins are seen at the superior margin of the liver. The descending aorta (A) and azygous vein *(arrow)* are also seen.

require life support or complex physiologic monitoring. MR examinations also still take much more time than spiral CT of the chest, particularly if multidetector CT scanners are used.

It is generally agreed that patients who need further evaluation after plain chest radiography should usually be studied with chest CT. At this time, MRI should be used as a secondary imaging modality in patients who have confusing CT findings or in whom specific information is desired, for example, evaluation of thoracic cage invasion by tumors (Table 1-7). MRI and multidetector spiral CT are both very effective in imaging the heart and vascular system. The ability of MRI to evaluate the cardiovascular system without nephrotoxic contrast media or ionizing radiation is weighed against the greater speed and ease of spiral multidetector CT. The choice of modality varies between institutions and is often tailored to the patient.

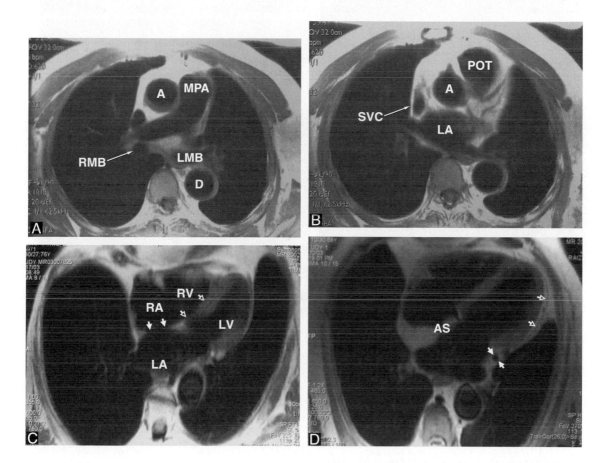

FIGURE 1-20 Magnetic resonance imaging of the chest and heart. These are "black blood" images in which flowing blood appears black. These can be obtained with a T1 spin echo technique or with a single shot fast spin echo technique with a double inversion pulse. Using either technique, fat is white (increased signal), blood/air/calcium is black (without signal), and muscle/fascia is gray (intermediate signal). Images are obtained with cardiac gating that "freezes" the motion of the heart and allows more accurate measurement of chamber size and wall thickness than with conventional CT (performed without cardiac gating).

A, Axial image just below the level of the aortic arch. A, ascending aorta; D, descending aorta; LMB, left main bronchus; MPA, main pulmonary artery; RMB, right main bronchus. Note that both blood vessels and bronchi appear black (signal voids).

B, Axial image at the level of the aortic root showing the aortic root (A), pulmonary outflow tract (POT), left atrium (LA), and superior vena cava (SVC).

C, At the level of the ventricles: the right and left ventricles (RV and LV), right and left atria (RA and LA), and the ventricular septum *(open arrows)*. Note that the atrial septum is so thin that it is imperceptible *(solid arrows)*.

D, At the level of the ventricles in a different patient than in C. The atrial septum in infiltrated by fat (called fatty hypertrophy, a finding without clinical importance). The portion of the septum without fat is the fossae ovalis. The great cardiac vein *(solid arrows)* and the pericardium *(open arrows)* appear as signal voids and low signal (dark), respectively. E through G, Coronal images obtained from posterior to anterior.

Illustration continued on following page.

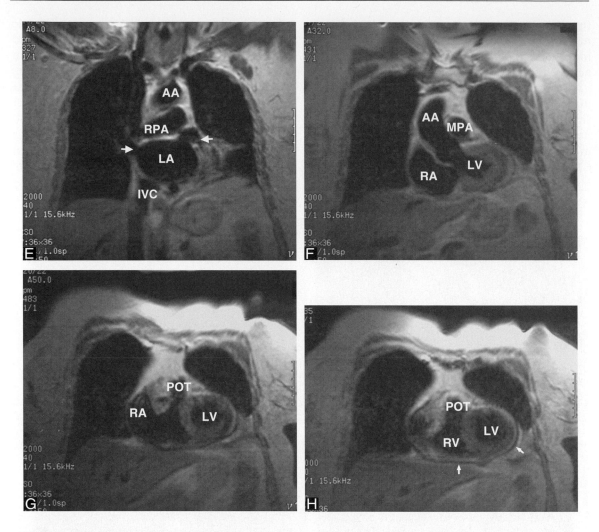

FIGURE 1-20, Cont'd **E,** Coronal image in the plane of the left atrium (LA), aortic arch (AA), right pulmonary artery (RPA), and a small portion of the inferior vena cava (IVC). Note the superior pulmonary veins entering the atrium *(arrows)*.

F, Coronal image slightly anterior to section E. This shows the right atrium (RA), ascending aorta (AA), left ventricle (LV), and main pulmonary artery (MPA).

G, Coronal image anterior to F shows the right atrium (RA), a portion of the pulmonary outflow tract (POT), and the left ventricle (LV).

H, Coronal image just behind the sternum shows the body of the right ventricle (RV), the infundibulum of the right ventricle or pulmonary outflow tract (POT), and the left ventricle (LV). The low-signal pericardium *(arrows)* is well seen. Note that the right ventricle does not make up any portion of the right or left cardiac border.

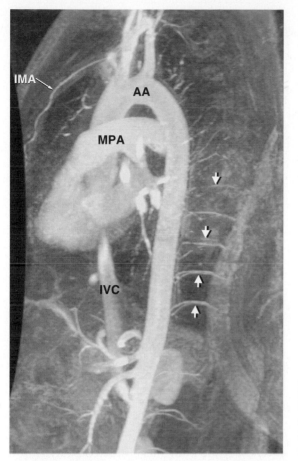

FIGURE 1-21 Magnetic resonance angiogram, created using fast gradient echo images following the administration of gadolinium intravenously. The entire thoracic aorta and the upper portion of the abdominal aorta are shown as well as the inferior vena cava (IVC), main pulmonary artery (MPA), aortic arch (AA), internal mammary artery (IMA), and intercostals *(arrows)*.

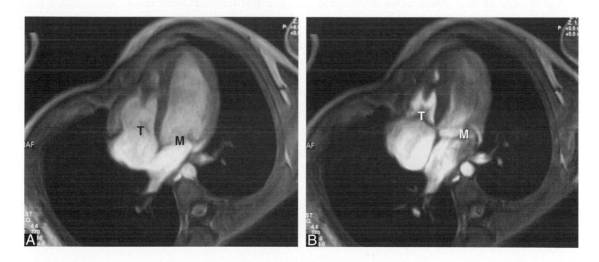

FIGURE 1-22 Gradient echo images of the heart on which blood is high in signal (white). These images are usually obtained at one anatomic site during multiples phases of the cardiac cycle.

A, Oblique axial image of the heart. The image is angled off the horizontal plane to better show all four cardiac chambers. This image is obtained in diastole and the tricuspid (T) and mitral (M) valves are open.

B, Oblique axial image of the heart at the same site as image B. This image was obtained during systole. Both the tricuspid (T) and mitral valves (M) are closed.

TABLE 1-7
Chest Pathology for Which Magnetic Resonance Imaging Is Preferable to Computed Tomography

Evaluation of mediastinum for vascular abnormality in patient who cannot receive intravenous contrast agent

Evaluation of aortic coarctation, chronic dissections*

Evaluation of Pancoast's tumors and tumors with suspected chest wall invasion

Cardiac imaging (except where detection of calcifications is important)*

*Multidetector CT may be comparable to CT for many cardiovascular indications, except in cases where radiation exposure is a major concern (children and young adults).

Pearls for Clinicians—The Basics

1. One view of the chest is like a physical examination without the history. Two views should be obtained whenever possible (e.g., PA and lateral). This goes for decubitus views as well, even if only unilateral disease is suspected.

2. If you are interested in the volume status of your patient, the portable radiograph must be taken with the patient upright.

3. Hilar shadows are difficult to assess but harbor important information. Give yourself a chance to get it right by not relying on the frontal projection alone. Learn the hilar anatomy on the lateral projection.

4. Both the summation and silhouette signs can help confirm the presence of an abnormal opacity in the chest. Loss of the left hemidiaphragm silhouette (caused by left lower lobe atelectasis) is the most common example and is seen in the ICU daily.

5. In order to see fine detail of isolated small structures, such as small lung nodules, CT scanning must be done using thin contiguous slices. This is *not* termed high-resolution CT (HRCT). The latter technique is usually used to sample a *diffuse process* in the lung and consists of thin slices that are widely spaced through the lung parenchyma

6. Multislice CT and MRI can both produce excellent images of the vasculature in the chest. Aside from imaging the coronary arteries, diagnostic angiography of the chest is (almost) an anachronism.

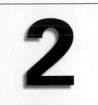

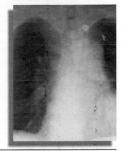

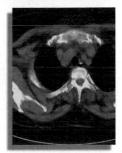

Normal Variants and Artifacts

Normal variants and artifacts are common on chest radiographs and can simulate disease. Early recognition of an abnormality as a normal variant or artifact can eliminate additional testing and treatment. Rib companion shadows, for instance, mimic pneumothoraces but do not warrant treatment with chest tubes. In this chapter, we present a few examples that are important because they occur frequently.

☐ ANATOMIC VARIANTS

Variations in chest wall morphology often mimic disease. Costochondral calcifications of the first rib can simulate an apical mass but can usually be differentiated from real pathology on an apical lordotic view. (On a lordotic view the first rib projects over the soft tissues but apical masses remain visible within the lung.) Vertebral osteophytes can mimic an intraparenchymal nodule on lateral projection or mimic mediastinal masses when seen on frontal chest radiographs (Fig. 2-1). Often this confusion is dispelled by connecting the abnormal opacity to the spine on both frontal and lateral views, but occasionally computed tomography (CT) is required.

Intraparenchymal anatomic variants can also mimic disease. One variant, the azygous lobe, occurs in approximately 1% of the population. It is caused by invagination of the pleura by the descent of the azygous vein in the right apex (Fig. 2-2). The portion of the lung that lies between this pleural fissure and the mediastinum forms the azygous lobe. Occasionally, this lobe appears more opaque than the adjacent lung parenchyma, simulating a paratracheal mass. Paratracheal opacities can also be caused by ectatic arterial vasculature (Fig. 2-3).

☐ ARTIFACTS ON CHEST RADIOGRAPHS

Nipple shadows are a common artifact. Fortunately, they are often readily identified by their location. Nipple shadows are usually seen near the fifth intercostal space at approximately the midclavicular line. Characteristically, their lateral margin appears sharper than the medial margin because the lateral margin is better defined by the surrounding air (Fig. 2-4).

Sometimes the appearance of nipple shadows is atypical. For instance, although

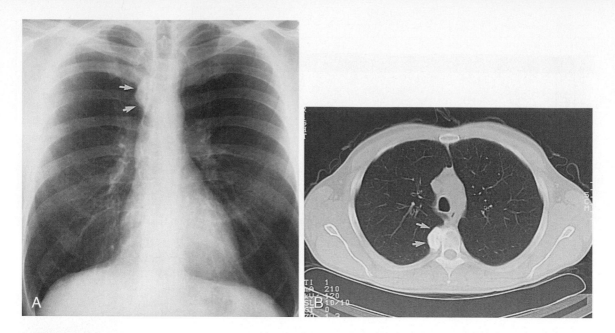

FIGURE 2-1 Posterior-anterior (PA) chest radiograph and computed tomography (CT) scan: paravertebral osteophyte mimicking mediastinal mass.

A, The frontal chest view shows an asymmetric density medially *(arrows)* that was imperceptible on a lateral film.

B, The CT scan (lung windows) through the level of the abnormality demonstrates a large paravertebral osteophyte *(arrows)*.

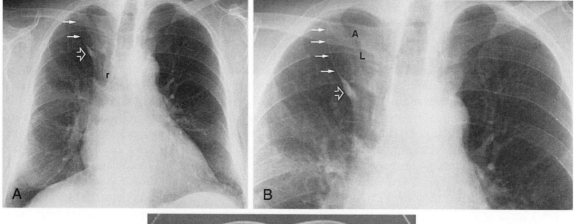

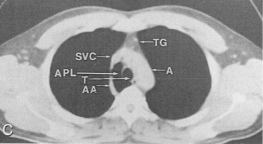

FIGURE 2-2 Posterior-anterior chest radiograph, detail of radiograph, and contrast-enhanced computed tomography (CT) scan: azygous pseudolobe.

A and B (detail), A curvilinear line *(arrows)* extends from the right apex inferomedially. A coalescence of two visceral and two parietal layers formed as the azygous vein *(arrowhead)* migrated (cephalad to caudal) toward the right tracheal–main stem bronchus angle *(r)*. The lung medial to the pleural line is the azygous pseudolobe. A, azygous; L, lobe.

C, Contrast-enhanced CT section (mediastinal windows) demonstrates relative positions of the trachea (T), azygous pseudolobe (APL), and azygous arch (AA) as the vein proceeds anteriorly to drain into the superior vena cava (SVC), the thymus gland (TG), and the aortic arch (A).

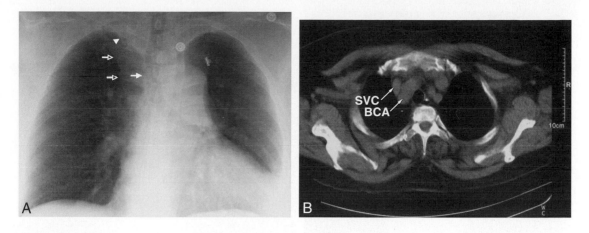

FIGURE 2-3 Posterior-anterior (PA) chest radiograph: superior vena cava (SVC) and tortuous right brachiocephalic artery.

A, PA chest radiograph shows an opacity that obscures the outer border of the trachea. The superior border of the opacity is smooth, suggesting that it is caused by vasculature *(arrowhead)*. Below this opacity the outer border of the trachea is sharply defined *(solid arrow)*. The outer border of the SVC is seen laterally *(open arrows)*. The vena cava does not obscure the margin of the trachea because it lies anterior rather than adjacent to it. (See silhouette sign in Chapter 1.)

B, CT section through the upper chest in the same patient shows that the brachiocephalic artery (BCA) is tortuous, extending along a portion of the right tracheal border. The SVC is anterior and lateral to both the artery and trachea.

anatomically symmetric, both nipple opacities may not be identifiable on the same radiograph. If there is any doubt about the identity of a nodular opacity in the expected area of the nipple, the simplest solution is to place metallic markers on the nipples and retake the radiograph. If the

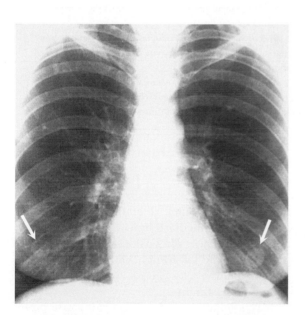

FIGURE 2-4 Posterior-anterior chest radiographs: nipple shadows. The nipples *(arrows)* are often seen at the fifth intercostal space midclavicular line but occasionally can vary in position. Typical nipple shadows have lateral edges that are well defined by air.

nodular opacity seen is actually the nipple, the metal marker should be superimposed on the soft tissue density. Remember, however, a single radiograph can be misleading and "bulletproof" confirmation requires two views (Fig. 2-5).

Other skin lesions (for example, moles) have an appearance similar to that of nipple shadows and can also be identified with skin markers. Opacities that overlie the thorax (for example, dressings, ribbons) can cause confusing soft tissue shadows. Most of these opacities can be traced past the pleura and external to the thorax. Hair braids are a common cause of such an artifact (Fig. 2-6).

Rib companion shadows are frequently troublesome. These shadows are caused by extrapleural fat and muscle that lie adjacent to the ribs. They form a faint linear opacity that parallels the inferior margin of a segment of a rib. This is most commonly seen at the level of the first or second ribs and is often bilateral (Fig. 2-7). The linear opacities can be misread as either pleural thickening or small pneumothoraces.

Positional changes in cardiac, vascular, and mediastinal contours are the artifacts most commonly associated with portable chest radiography (see Chapter 1). Although it is optimal to radiograph patients in the upright position, even the best efforts to position very ill patients properly may be unsuccessful. The patient often leans backward, resulting in an apical lordotic

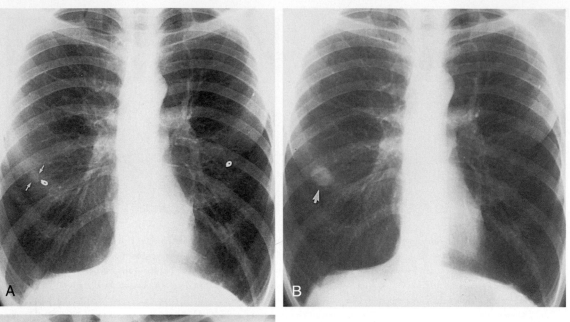

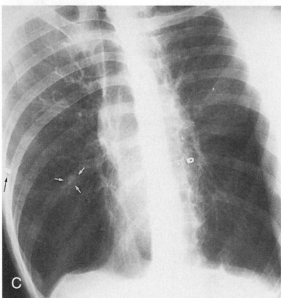

FIGURE 2-5 Serial chest radiographs: misleading nipple markers.

A, Chest radiograph with nipple markers shows superimposition and apparently confirms nipple identity.

B, A preoperative chest radiograph taken 6 months later suggests a slight increase in the size of the right "nipple" over this time interval *(arrow)*.

C, Oblique radiographs with nipple markers are obtained and show the nodule *(white arrows)* as separate from the right nipple marker *(black arrow)*. Primary bronchogenic carcinoma was diagnosed.

film that enlarges and distorts the cardiac silhouette. One can identify this artifact by noting that the clavicles project above the lung apices.

The position of the clavicles is a useful sign of a patient's rotation. Even subtle rotation causes the clavicular heads to project unequal distances from the pedicles of the thoracic spine. More marked rotation causes one clavicle to appear shorter than the other. This degree of rotation also causes the anterior segment of the ribs to appear shorter on the side of the apparently shortened clavicle. Recognizing rotation is important because the patient's rotation may artifactually cause one hemithorax to appear more opaque ("whiter") than the other (Fig. 2-8). Because the mediastinum is wider in the anterior-posterior dimensions (sagittal plane) than it is in the left-to-right dimension (coronal plane), rotation also causes apparent widening of the mediastinum.

Hypoinflation of the lungs can cause other problems. Normal inspiratory radiographs in adults should show at least 9, and preferably 10, posterior ribs above the diaphragm. On supine portable radiographs, the diaphragm is usually elevated, which causes compressive changes of

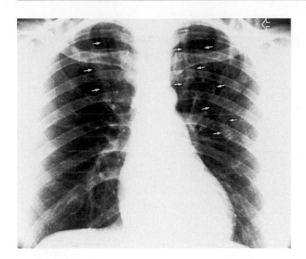

FIGURE 2-6 Posterior-anterior (PA) chest radiograph: hair braids. Routine PA chest radiograph of a 32-year-old woman shows vertically oriented linear opacities projecting over the upper lung fields asymmetrically *(arrows)*. They can be traced beyond the confines of the thorax *(arrowhead)*, above the left lung. (Similarly, skin folds and stretcher board artifacts can be traced beyond the confines of the thorax.)

the lower lung fields. Inadequate depth of inspiration on upright views can cause similar changes, crowding together vascular shadows and obscuring up to one third of the lower lobes. As a result of these changes, an expiratory radiograph of a physiologically normal chest can closely mimic the radiographic appearance of congestive heart failure or basilar pneumonia (Fig. 2-9).

☐ ARTIFACTS ON COMPUTED TOMOGRAPHY AND MAGNETIC RESONANCE IMAGING

CT and magnetic resonance imaging (MRI) are accompanied by their own unique artifacts. A complete discussion of many of the artifacts specific to these modalities is beyond the scope of this book. However, there are artifacts common to these two modalities: (1) motion artifacts (usually respiratory or cardiovascular), (2) artifacts associated with metallic objects, and (3) partial volume artifacts.

Motion Artifacts

Motion artifacts are the most frequently encountered artifacts seen in CT and MRI images and can cause enough distortion to obscure much

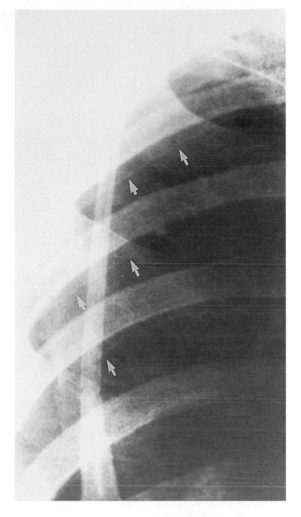

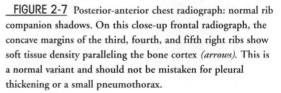

FIGURE 2-7 Posterior-anterior chest radiograph: normal rib companion shadows. On this close-up frontal radiograph, the concave margins of the third, fourth, and fifth right ribs show soft tissue density paralleling the bone cortex *(arrows)*. This is a normal variant and should not be mistaken for pleural thickening or a small pneumothorax.

of the diagnostic information. Gross movements of the body can cause severe motion artifacts (i.e., the patient actually moves a body part during scanning). Sedation can help to diminish these movements. Chloral hydrate is commonly used in pediatric patients, and a variety of benzodiazepines are used in adults. Motion artifact can also be caused by physiologic processes, such as bowel peristalsis, vascular or cardiac pulsation, and respiratory motion (Fig. 2-10). The amount of distortion has traditionally been greater for MRI than CT because of the longer MRI scan times. Respiratory motion artifact can be reduced if the MR or CT study can be completed in a single breath-hold.

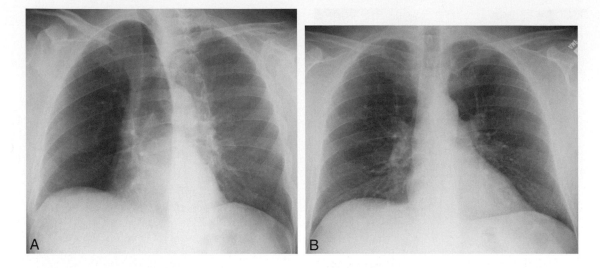

FIGURE 2-8 Anterior-posterior (AP) radiographs showing the effect of rotation.

A, Patient is rotated to the right, as can be seen from the position of the trachea and clavicles relative to the spine. The left hemithorax appears uniformly more opaque than the right. The apparent width of the mediastinum is slightly increased. In many patients, this degree of rotation causes greater apparent widening.

B, The same patient, AP radiograph taken within 24 hours of A. The patient is not rotated and both hemithoraces are approximately the same opacity.

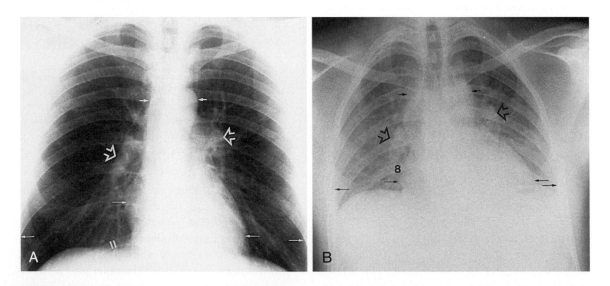

FIGURE 2-9 Serial posterior-anterior (PA) radiographs: effects of hypo-aeration.

A, Routine inspiratory PA chest view shows 11 ribs above the right hemidiaphragm posteriorly, normal peripheral and basilar vascular markings, and a normal cardiomediastinal silhouette. Note the hilar vessels *(open arrows)*, the mediastinal width at the level of the aortic arch *(small arrows)*, and the normal cardiothoracic ratio *(long arrows)*.

B, Frontal radiograph on expiration demonstrates obvious diaphragmatic elevation with only eight ribs visualized above the right hemidiaphragm posteriorly. A significant increase in bronchovascular markings (middle and lower lung fields) and prominence in the hilar vasculature *(open arrows)* are associated with compressive changes of hypo-aeration. There is increased width of the mediastinum at the level of the aortic arch *(short arrows)* and an increase in the cardiothoracic ratio *(long arrows)*. The increased opacity at the lung bases can be mistaken for congestive heart failure or basilar pneumonia.

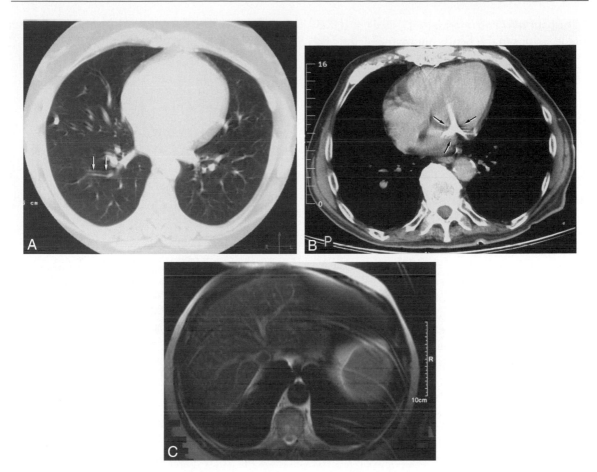

FIGURE 2-10 Motion artifacts with computed tomography (CT) and magnetic resonance imaging (MRI).

A, Axial image from a chest CT study with lung parenchymal windows performed at the level of the ventricles. Motion artifact is evident with blurring of the cardiomediastinal borders. A "double vessel" artifact is seen in the right lower lobe *(arrows)*. This finding and similar observations such as a "double major fissure" are diagnostic of motion artifact on CT.

B, Axial image of chest CT with mediastinal windows from a different patient. On mediastinal windows, motion artifact may be more difficult to detect by looking at the margins of the heart and great vessels. On this image there is a streak artifact caused by calcifications of the mitral annulus *(arrows)*. This artifact is due in part to the high density of the calcification but is exaggerated by the motion of the annulus caused by cardiac pulsation.

C, MRI motion artifact from respiratory motion. This is a T2-weighted image of the lower chest and upper abdomen that was obtained without a breath-hold. Respiratory gating was only partly successful in preventing the computer software from misinterpreting information from moving tissues. The bright bands across the image represent the resulting "misplacement" of structures when the image was reconstructed.

Both single-detector and multidetector spiral CT studies can image the entire chest in a single breath-hold, but multidetectors have the advantage of being able to do so using thinner CT sections and therefore creating more detailed pictures. Several new MRI imaging techniques also allow the entire chest to be imaged in a single breath-hold.

Because cardiac motion cannot be voluntarily suspended, other methods are needed to diminish motion artifact for cardiac imaging. Most of these methods involve cardiac "gating,"

that is, monitoring of the patient's electrocardiogram to determine when imaging data are acquired. For instance, multidetector CT scanners can create images from data acquired only during diastole when cardiac motion is least. Some MRI sequences acquire a fraction of each image at a specific point in several cardiac cycles. For instance, one eighth of the information for one slice might be acquired over 50 milliseconds in midsystole. After eight heartbeats, the image is complete. During the time remaining in those eight cardiac cycles, the MRI can obtain information to create additional slices at different locations in the heart. Alternatively, the MRI can obtain additional images of the *same* slice during multiple segments of the cardiac cycle. These images can be strung together to produce a "cine image" that contains functional information about the heart that is similar to that obtained from echocardiograms.

Metallic Artifacts

The presence of metal objects within or adjacent to the patient commonly causes artifacts on CT and MRI. These artifacts appear as white radiating streaks on CT. If the volume of metal is large, for example, a shoulder arthroplasty, the artifact can be severe enough to obscure most adjacent structures. Not all streak artifacts on CT, however, are caused by metal. Other high-attenuation structures, including catheters, and blood vessels containing high concentrations of contrast material (often the superior vena cava) also cause streak artifacts. The artifact may be more pronounced if the high-attenuation structure is moving during the scan (Fig. 2-11). The newest multidetector CT scanners use reconstruction algorithms that have reduced streak artifacts from metal.

Metal artifacts on MRI appear as a central signal void (blackened areas) with asymmetric surrounding areas of increased (brightened) signal intensity. These produce bizarre shapes that assume nonanatomic configurations. Such artifacts are commonly caused by surgical clips,

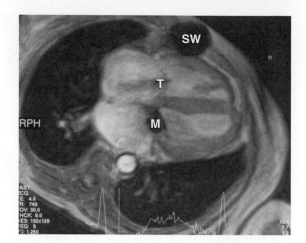

FIGURE 2-12 Metallic artifact on magnetic resonance imaging (MRI): gradient echo image from a cardiac MRI study. There is loss of signal (focal black areas) at the site of the patient's sternotomy wires (SW) and at the site of a prosthetic mitral valve (M). Currently manufactured mechanical valves are not a contraindication to MRI and produce relatively little artifact. Incidentally, note the black band originating from the tricuspid valve (T) caused by turbulent blood flow from tricuspid regurgitation.

prosthetic heart valves, electrodes, and other prosthetic devices (Fig. 2-12). Metallic objects that are not ferromagnetic (such as titanium) cause a lesser degree of artifact than ferromagnetic metallic (e.g., iron and nickel) objects. With nonferromagnetic substances, the size of the distortion (caused by the adjacent metal) seen on MR images may be smaller than that seen on CT images.

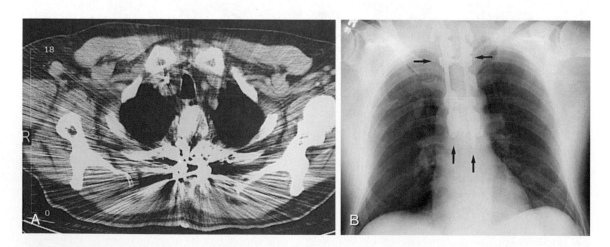

FIGURE 2-11 Metallic artifacts on computed tomography (CT).
  A, Upper thoracic CT cut using mediastinal windows shows marked radial streaking. This is typical of metallic artifact.
  B, A chest radiograph of the same patient shows the cause of the marked CT distortion: spinal fixation rods *(arrows)*.

Because of the differences in the magnetic properties of various metals, the gross amount of metal present often does not correlate with the size of the MR image artifact. Similarly, the health risk to the patient does not depend on the total amount of metal present in the body but rather depends on both the type of metal and its location. For instance, patients with pacemakers and cerebral aneurysm clips must not enter the MRI scanner, but patients harboring long-term orthopedic hardware are not at any increased risk for complications from the imaging procedure.

Partial Volume Artifacts

A common artifact seen with CT is the partial volume artifact. This artifact is caused by averaging of the x-ray attenuation of two tissues that are close together in space but very different in density—blood and lung alveoli (air), for example. The CT software merges the data from these two tissues and creates an image that shows an intermediate density at these locations. (A similar process can occur when MR images combine the radiofrequency signals from different tissues that are close together.) In this manner, partial volume artifacts can compromise the resolution of a small lesion or create a false-positive image, an abnormality where none is present (Fig. 2-13). In both instances, the problem is corrected by obtaining thinner sections.

☐ COMMON MIMICS OF INTRATHORACIC PATHOLOGY

Table 2-1 lists the more common variants and artifacts seen on radiographs, some of which have already been discussed. Others are described in the corresponding figure legends (Figs. 2-14 to 2-19). The previous and subsequent chapters, also referred to in the table, give specific information about various artifacts that can mimic pathologies.

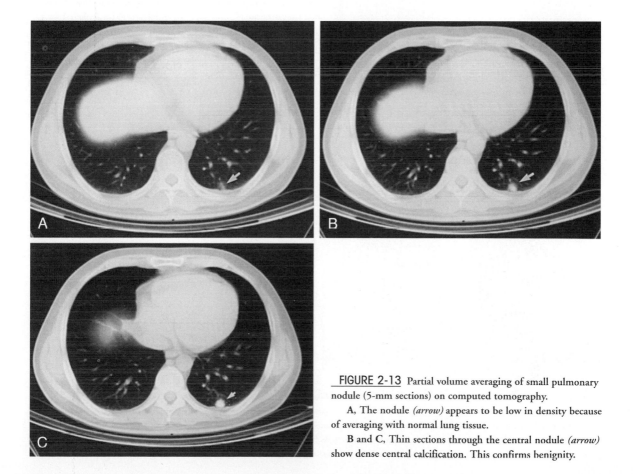

FIGURE 2-13 Partial volume averaging of small pulmonary nodule (5-mm sections) on computed tomography.

A, The nodule *(arrow)* appears to be low in density because of averaging with normal lung tissue.

B and C, Thin sections through the central nodule *(arrow)* show dense central calcification. This confirms benignity.

TABLE 2-1
Mimics of Intrathoracic Pathology

Structure	Mimicked Pathology
Rib companion shadows, skin folds	Pneumothorax (Fig. 2-7, Fig. 2-14)
Skin lesions (moles), nipples	Pulmonary nodule (Fig. 2-4, Fig. 1-6)
Breast prosthesis or asymmetry	Lung mass or pneumonia (Fig. 2-15)
Scapula osteochondroma or rib fusions	Lung mass or pneumonia (Fig. 2-16)
Costochondral calcification of the first rib	Apical mass (Fig. 2-17)
Rib fractures	Lung nodules (Fig. 2-18)
Diaphragmatic eventration	Diaphragmatic mass (Fig. 2-19)
Ectatic brachiocephalic vessels	Paratracheal mass (Fig. 2-3)
Azygous lobe	Paratracheal mass (Fig. 2-2)
Lateral vertebral body spur	Mediastinal mass or lung nodule (Fig. 2-1)
Pericardial fat pad	Mediastinal mass (Fig. 1-15)
Pectus excavatum	Cardiomegaly (Fig. 14-5)
Rotation	Mediastinal widening, unilateral pneumonia or effusion (Fig. 2-8)

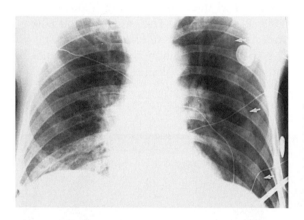

FIGURE 2-14 Posterior-anterior chest radiograph: skin fold mimicking pneumothorax. A curvilinear opacity parallels the left lateral rib margin *(arrows)*, resembling a visceral pleural line (pneumothorax). Note the gradual increase in lung opacity progressing medial to lateral up to the line. The diagnosis is made more difficult in this case because lung markings are difficult to see lateral to the line and the line does not extend beyond the thorax.

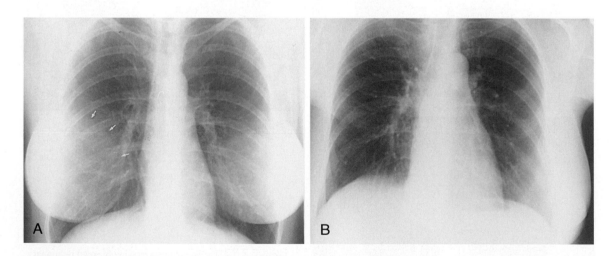

FIGURE 2-15 Posterior-anterior chest radiograph: breast prosthesis and unilateral mastectomy.

A, Note the difference in soft tissue opacity usually associated with breast implants *(arrows)*. Occasionally, this difference in opacities is very subtle. The homogeneous increased opacity and well-marginated contour are indicative of a breast prosthesis. Compare with part B.

B, This frontal radiograph demonstrates obvious asymmetry in breast shadows; in this instance, the right is absent. Sometimes the asymmetry is not as obvious. After lumpectomy, breast shadows are asymmetric but are still present bilaterally.

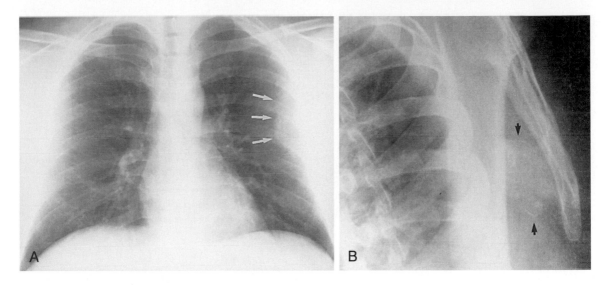

FIGURE 2-16 Chest radiograph: scapular lesion mimicking a lung mass.

A, Posterior-anterior chest radiograph reveals an opacity adjacent to the left rib margin *(arrows)*.

B, Tangential view of the scapula localizes the origin of the opacity to the scapula instead of the lung *(arrows)*. Scapular osteochondroma is diagnosed.

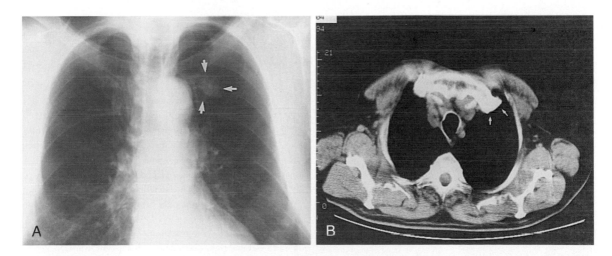

FIGURE 2-17 Posterior-anterior chest radiograph and computed tomography (CT): first rib calcifications mimicking lung tumor.

A, Routine chest radiograph of a 50-year-old man demonstrates an asymmetric opacity overlying the left first costochondral junction *(arrows)*. This can often be a normal variant but has been a frequent cause of error in diagnosis.

B, CT scan demonstrates the opacity to be an asymmetric, heavily calcified, costochondral junction calcification *(arrows)*. An apical lordotic view would have sufficed to demonstrate the same finding.

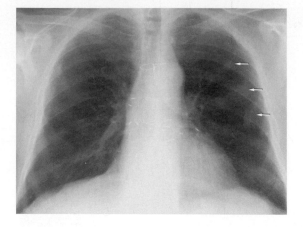

__FIGURE 2-18__ Posterior-anterior chest: multiple rib fractures. Multiple nodular opacities are seen in the left chest, caused by healed fractures of the anterior aspects of the ribs *(arrows)*. The orientation of these opacities along a line is characteristic of pseudonodules caused by rib fractures.

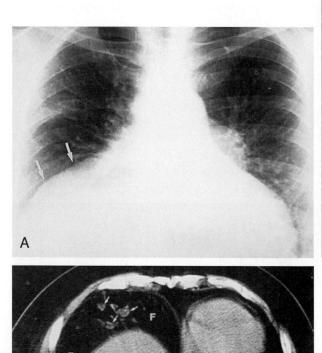

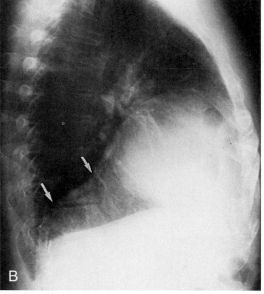

__FIGURE 2-19__ Posterior-anterior and lateral chest radiographs: diaphragmatic eventration.

A and B, Frontal radiograph demonstrates an abnormal contour of the right hemidiaphragm *(arrows)*. This contour is smooth, convex upward, and could be confused with loculated pleural fluid, a pleural mass, or possibly right heart enlargement. The lateral radiograph shows that the posterior aspect of the right hemidiaphragm is in a normal position *(arrows)*.

C, An axial computed tomography scan demonstrates an elevated right diaphragm with adjacent liver (D), abundant mesenteric fat (F), and a few small bowel loops *(arrows)* beneath it, consistent with diaphragmatic eventration. Eventrations are caused by thinning of the diaphragmatic muscle, without true herniation being present.

Pearls for Clinicians—Normal Variants and Artifacts

1. If the lungs look very much alike except that one is slightly whiter than the other, look for rotation, unilateral mastectomy, or a breast prosthesis before attributing the asymmetry to real disease.

2. If you suspect that an opacity is really within a rib or a vertebral body, see if it appears to be within that bone on multiple prior radiographs. Rib and vertebral body lesions appear within the bone on every radiograph, regardless of the degree of rotation or inspiration. Lung lesions usually do not.

3. Skin folds may mimic pneumothoraces and usually occur when portable radiographs are taken and the radiographic cassette is wedged behind the sitting patient. Consider this diagnosis if the "pneumothorax" border is not delineated by a discrete white line (see Chapter 11). Unless the patient is gravely ill, obtain another radiograph before opening the chest tube tray.

4. Many small lung nodules are often seen on only a single radiographic view. If a larger nodule (1 cm or greater), however, is seen on only one radiographic view, it may not lie within the lung. Reexamine the patient and if you discover a suspicious skin lesion, repeat the radiographs with a metallic marker in place. To be sure the skin lesion and nodule are one and the same, obtain two radiographic views.

5. The metallic artifact caused by sternotomy wires, prosthetic heart valves, and coronary artery stents is often sufficiently localized to allow diagnostic MRI. Patients in whom these metallic devices have been placed can usually undergo MRI safely; however, patients with pacemakers and defibrillators can not.

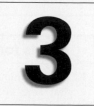

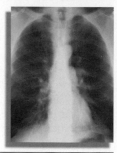

Large Airway Disease

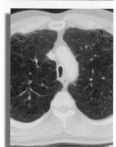

Diseases of the larynx, trachea, and bronchi, here termed the large airways, can be challenging problems. They are often difficult clinical diagnoses, and findings on routine posterior-anterior (PA) and lateral chest radiographs may be subtle or absent.

The most superior portion of the large airways, the *upper airway*, is usually defined as extending from the pharynx down to the tracheal carina. Diseases in this area cause dyspnea secondary to airway obstruction and are often overlooked because symptoms are attributed to pathology within the lung parenchyma. Disease occurring below the tracheal carina, in the bronchi, can present with signs of bronchiectasis (chronic cough and purulent sputum production) or first present with hemoptysis.

Bronchial pathology can also produce obstruction with secondary atelectasis and pneumonia. More distal airway disease, for example, in the terminal bronchioles, usually manifests as obstructive lung disease. Obstructive disease and patterns of atelectasis produced by bronchial obstruction are discussed in Chapters 4 and 5, respectively. In this chapter, we focus on the roentgenographic evaluation of upper airway obstruction, bronchiectasis, and hemoptysis.

☐ ANATOMY

A few anatomic points are important in guiding the roentgenographic evaluation of the upper airways. Soft tissue views of the neck are the best plain radiographs for evaluating the area extending from the hypopharynx to the subglottic trachea (Fig. 3-1). Key structures are the epiglottis, aryepiglottic folds, the larynx, and the retropharyngeal soft tissues seen just anterior to the cervical spine.

The hypopharynx is too superior to be visualized on most routine chest radiographs. Narrowing of the air column at the level of the larynx is often seen at the extreme upper margin on the PA chest radiograph. Below this level, the trachea is well visualized in the midline. Normally, there is slight deviation of the trachea to the right at the level of the aortic arch, deviation that is exaggerated in older patients.

The trachea bifurcates to form the carina at the level of the fifth to seventh thoracic vertebrae. The normal carinal angle is approximately 60 degrees, but there is much normal variation. Marked increase in the subcarinal angle (i.e., greater than 90 degrees) can be

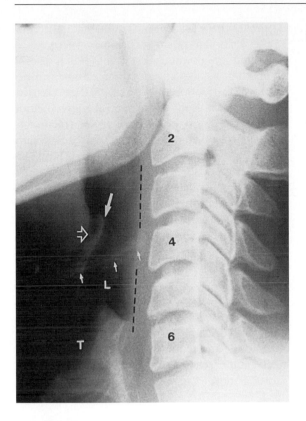

FIGURE 3-1 Normal anatomy: soft tissue structures of the neck, lateral view. Air outlines the key anatomic structures of the upper airways. The epiglottis is well defined *(large arrow)*, as are the anterior and posterior margins of the hypopharynx and the larynx (L). The vallecula *(open arrow)* lies anterior to the epiglottis. The hyoid bone *(small arrows)* overlies the base of the epiglottis. Note the width of the anterior cervical tissues, normally less than 7 mm at C2 and 21 mm at the C5-6 level *(dashed lines)*. T, trachea.

caused by pathology underneath the carina. This can range from metastatic adenopathy to an enlarged left atrium. Inferior to the carina, the right main stem bronchus travels a more vertical course than the left, making it a more common home for foreign bodies and errant endotracheal tube tips (Fig. 3-2).

To prevent right main bronchus intubation, the endotracheal tube tip is best positioned 2 to 5 cm above the carina. When checking tube placement, it is also important to note the position of the patient's chin. This is often visible along the superior margin of radiographs if the patient's neck is flexed. Neck flexion drives the endotracheal tube down, and extension pulls it up. Thus, a tube tip that looks high despite the flexion of the patient's neck is a real worry. The tube tip moves to a higher location if the

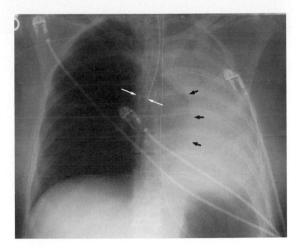

FIGURE 3-2 Anterior-posterior chest view: right main bronchus intubation with an endotracheal tube. Because of the vertical course of the right main bronchus, a distally placed endotracheal tube usually extends into this bronchus *(white arrows)*. Note the hyperaeration of the right lung with herniation of the lung across midlines *(black arrows)*. The collapse of the left lung has caused a mediastinal shift toward the left.

patient extends his or her neck, and the patient may be accidentally extubated. Endotracheal tube tips that project below the carina are always abnormal and lie either in a main stem bronchus or, if midline, within the esophagus (Fig. 3-3).

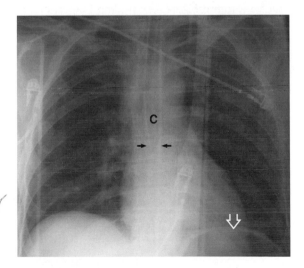

FIGURE 3-3 Portable chest radiograph of a trauma victim with aberrant placement of endotracheal tube. The endotracheal tube tip *(arrows)* lies inferior to the main carina (C), indicating that it is not in the trachea. There is also gaseous distention of the stomach *(arrow)* consistent with esophageal intubation.

☐ UPPER AIRWAYS OBSTRUCTION

The clinical diagnosis of upper airway obstruction is sometimes difficult because the acute respiratory distress caused by upper airway obstruction can be mistakenly attributed to asthma or other diseases. Once upper airway obstruction is suspected from the history, physical examination, pulmonary function testing, or a combination of these, the best imaging technique to evaluate the problem further depends on the suspected anatomic level of obstruction.

Larynx and Hypopharynx (Table 3-1)

If acute upper airway obstruction at the level of the pharynx or larynx is suspected, a lateral soft tissue view of the neck is often the first radiologic examination. One should make sure this view is ordered as a soft tissue examination rather than a lateral cervical spine examination because the latter is done with a technique that emphasizes bone structures. The borders of the soft tissues surrounding the airway may be harder to see on such radiographs.

Many disease processes in this area are infectious in origin. Head and neck infections (tonsillitis, dental disease) can extend into the retropharyngeal space through lymphatics or by direct extension, causing cellulitis, reactive adenopathy, or frank abscess. On the lateral neck radiograph, the key finding is an increase in the width of the retropharyngeal soft tissues (normally up to 7 mm at the C2 level and up to 21 mm at the C5-6 level). Gas may also be seen in the retropharyngeal soft tissues.

Acute epiglottitis, most commonly a disease of children, is also an infectious cause of upper airway obstruction in adults. The classical findings on a soft tissue lateral view include hyperaeration of the hypopharynx (related to obstruction during inspiration) and thickening of the epiglottis and aryepiglottic folds. This thickening causes the epiglottis, as seen on a lateral view, to be shaped like a thumb instead of having the normal thinner appearance similar to the fifth finger (Fig. 3-4).

Noninfectious inflammatory disease, such as angioneurotic edema and irritant inhalation, can cause more diffuse soft tissue swelling. Trauma, including that from difficult endotracheal intubations, can cause swelling and gas in the retropharyngeal soft tissues, simulating infection. Foreign bodies can also cause similar symptoms, and the lateral soft tissue view of the neck should be studied carefully for nonanatomic radiopacities.

TABLE 3-1
Causes of Airway Obstruction above the Trachea

Infection
Epiglottitis/abscesses
Trauma (e.g., laryngeal fracture)
Foreign body

Neoplasms
Squamous cell carcinoma
Lymphoma

Thyromegaly
Goiter

Miscellaneous
Vocal cord paralysis
Angioneurotic edema

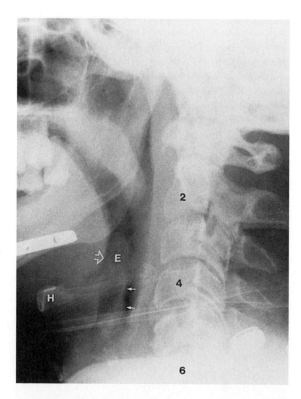

FIGURE 3-4 Lateral cervical soft tissue: acute epiglottitis. The bulbous epiglottis (thumb shape) is consistent with acute epiglottitis (compare with the normal epiglottis shown in Fig. 3-1). E, epiglottis; H, hyoid bone; *small arrows*, arytenoepiglottic folds; *open arrow*, vallecula.

Acute symptoms of obstruction in the hypopharynx and larynx may not be solely attributable to acute disease. Acute symptoms may occur with sudden decompensation after long-standing progressive narrowing of the airway lumen by neoplasm. Squamous cell carcinoma and, less commonly, non-Hodgkin's lymphoma can cause obstruction in this area (Fig. 3-5). Regardless of the suspected etiology of obstruction, further evaluation of hypopharynx and larynx is usually performed by laryngoscopy. In *no* case should a normal soft tissue lateral view of the neck preclude laryngoscopy in a patient with suspected upper airway obstruction.

If initial evaluation suggests obstruction of the hypopharynx or larynx by infection or tumor, a computed tomography (CT) study is usually performed. Because of the complex anatomy of the neck, CT is best done with intravenous contrast, which helps differentiate blood vessels from lymph nodes. Whenever infection is strongly suspected the study should also be extended to include the chest, particularly if the

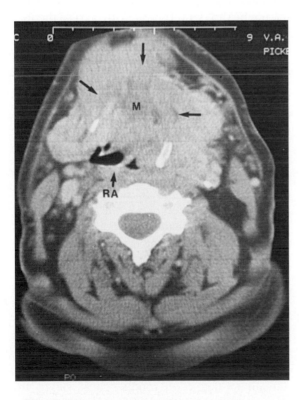

FIGURE 3-5 Axial computed tomography of the neck: squamous cell carcinoma of the hypopharynx. Extensive squamous cell carcinoma causing partial airway obstruction above the glottis *(arrows)*. M, mass; RA, residual airway.

infection appears to involve the retropharyngeal space. Neck infections in this area may spread inferiorly to the mediastinum through an ominously named potential space, the "danger space."

If the upper airway obstruction is chronic and the patient also complains of dysphagia or neuromuscular symptoms, a video swallowing study and esophagogram should be considered. These studies can document aspiration, swallowing dysfunction, or unsuspected esophageal masses. Vocal cord paralysis is best detected with a laryngoscope even though a video swallowing study may also demonstrate the problem. In patients with vocal cord paralysis, chest CT should also be considered to determine whether there is mediastinal pathology affecting the recurrent laryngeal nerves. This is more likely to occur on the left side because the left recurrent nerve has a longer intrathoracic course than the right, passing under the aortic arch. Figure 3-6 shows an algorithm for evaluating upper airway obstruction.

Magnetic resonance imaging (MRI) is widely used in the evaluation of oropharyngeal, hypopharyngeal, and laryngeal malignancies because of its ability to create images in the sagittal and coronal planes. CT can be performed more rapidly than MRI and the patient can be more easily monitored during the examination. For these reasons, CT is more commonly used in the setting of acute trauma or infectious disease, particularly if airway obstruction is questioned.

Tracheal Obstruction (Table 3-2)

Tracheal obstruction may be caused by extrinsic masses, intrinsic masses, post-traumatic stenosis, tracheomalacia, foreign bodies, and, rarely, by vascular rings, Wegener's granulomatosis, or amyloidosis. Unlike obstruction of the oropharynx and hypopharynx, acute tracheal obstruction from infectious disease is uncommon. Rarely, it can occur with staphylococcal tracheitis.

The presence of tracheal obstruction is suggested on chest radiographs by narrowing or deviation of the tracheal air column or by loss of a distinct air-tissue border along the wall of the inner trachea. The narrowing of the tracheal air column is normally seen at the level of the glottis, which projects over the sixth or seventh vertebral body on most chest radiographs. Pathologic tracheal deviation caused by

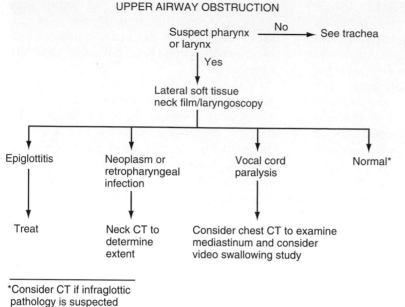

UPPER AIRWAY OBSTRUCTION

*Consider CT if infraglottic
pathology is suspected

FIGURE 3-6 Algorithm for the study
of an upper airway obstruction.

an extrinsic mass is usually focal. More diffuse apparent deviation of the trachea may be due not to tracheal pathology but to mediastinal shift from volume loss or to rotated positioning of the patient. The latter can be identified by unequal distances between the clavicular heads and their adjacent spinal pedicles (Fig. 3-7).

The most common extrinsic mass associated with tracheal deviation is an enlarged thyroid

TABLE 3-2
Causes of Tracheal Obstruction

Extrinsic masses
Thyroid masses
Esophageal carcinoma
Lymphoma

Intrinsic masses
Squamous carcinoma
Adenoid cystic carcinoma

Tracheomalacia
Postintubation
Relapsing polychondritis

Postintubation stenosis

Vascular anomalies (usually in children)
Right aortic arch with aberrant left subclavian artery

Miscellaneous
Wegener's granulomatosis
Amyloidosis
Mediastinal fibrosis

gland, usually from a goiter. Goiters normally arise from the lower pole or isthmus of the gland and usually (80% of cases) enter the mediastinum anterior to the trachea, causing the trachea to deviate posteriorly and to the left (Fig. 3-8). A clue on plain chest radiographs is the presence of coarse soft tissue calcifications within the mass. Thyroid malignancies, carcinomas of the upper portions of the esophagus, and more commonly lymphoma and bronchogenic carcinoma may also cause extrinsic compression of the trachea (Figs. 3-9 and 3-10). Compression from lymphomas can be severe and may narrow the trachea most severely front to back (sagittal plane). This is best seen on lateral views of the chest. Intrinsic tracheal masses are most often neoplasms, the two most common being squamous cell carcinoma and adenoid cystic carcinoma (Fig. 3-11).

Tracheal narrowing may also be caused by focal stenosis following prolonged endotracheal intubation or tracheostomy (Fig. 3-12). The incidence of this has fallen with the use of large-volume, low-pressure endotracheal tube balloons, but it is still seen. In postintubation stenosis, the area of narrowing is often 2 to 3 cm in length but may be a thin web that is very difficult to detect on routine chest views. In some instances, tracheal injury does not cause a fixed stenosis but instead produces tracheomalacia, a condition in which the trachea loses its structural rigidity. Airway obstruction from

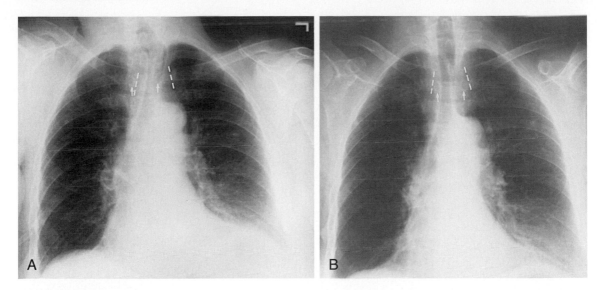

FIGURE 3-7 Serial posterior-anterior (PA) chest examination: minor chest obliquity simulating apparent trachea displacement.
A, PA radiograph demonstrates apparent shift of the trachea off midline (toward the left) caused by slight rotation of the patient toward the left, that is, the right chest closer to film. Note the slight asymmetry in the distance between the pedicle *(arrow)* and clavicle *(dashed lines)*: greater on the left.
B, A repeated PA film obtained within minutes of the study in part A. Tracheal position is normal and PA positioning is indicated by equidistant clavicle-to-pedicle measurements.

tracheomalacia may not be apparent on inspiratory plain radiographs or on CT when flaccid segments of the trachea distend as patients hold their breath. Tracheomalacia is best diagnosed when dynamic collapse of a tracheal

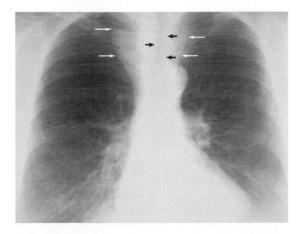

FIGURE 3-8 Routine frontal radiograph: substernal goiter.
A symmetric soft tissue mass is seen *(arrows)* at the level of the thoracic inlet, narrowing the trachea *(black arrows)*. The borders of the mass are sharply demarcated up to the level of the clavicle *(white arrows)* and become indistinct superiorly. This suggests that the mass is anterior in the mediastinum. Its border is sharply demarcated where it is adjacent to aerated lung tissue, but the border becomes indistinct where it lies adjacent to the soft tissues of the neck.

segment during expiration is seen with fluoroscopy, during bronchoscopy, or with CT. A normal trachea does not narrow more than a half of its diameter during expiration.

Fiberoptic bronchoscopy can be used to confirm the diagnosis of tracheal narrowing, but it may be difficult to determine the length of the stenosis endoscopically. This information is important if surgical resection or stenting is considered and can be obtained readily by the use of spiral CT using thin overlapping sections of the trachea. If the CT sections are very thin, data from these sections can be reformed into images oriented along the long axis of the trachea in the sagittal or coronal plane. These reformatted images allow accurate measurement of the stenosis.

Diffuse tracheomalacia is less common than focal tracheomalacia or stenosis and is usually not iatrogenic in origin. Acquired cases can be caused by chronic obstructive pulmonary disease (COPD) and less commonly by recurrent or chronic infection. Among patients with COPD, tracheomalacia is much less common than another tracheal abnormality, a "saber-sheath" trachea. A saber-sheath trachea is present when the coronal diameter of the trachea is less than half of its sagittal diameter. It may be caused by tracheal compression from the high

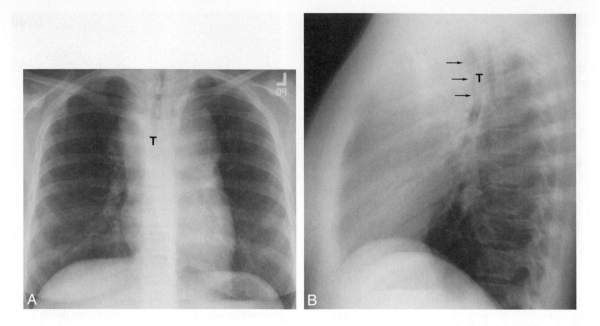

FIGURE 3-9 Posterior-anterior and lateral view radiographs and axial computed tomography section just below the carina of a patient with non-Hodgkin's lymphoma.

A, Frontal radiograph shows a large mediastinal mass. The trachea (T) is deviated to the right; however, its margins are poorly seen.

B, Lateral projection shows the tracheal margins more clearly. The trachea (T) is compressed and deviated posteriorly *(arrows)*.

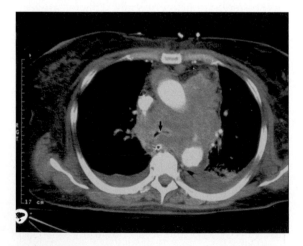

FIGURE 3-10 Computed tomography (CT) scan of a patient with small cell carcinoma. CT section at the level of the carina *(arrow)* shows nearly complete occlusion of the left and right main bronchi from extrinsic compression. This degree of airway obstruction is more common with aggressive tumors such as high-grade non-Hodgkin's lymphoma and bronchogenic carcinoma than in Hodgkin's disease.

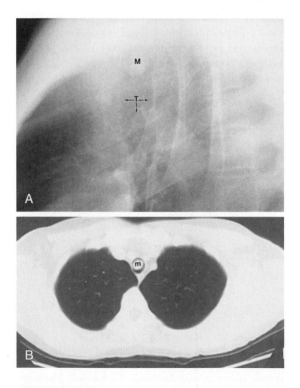

FIGURE 3-11 Posterior-anterior chest view and computed tomography (CT) scan: intratracheal tumor (cylindroma).

A, A lateral radiograph demonstrates a relatively smooth, sharply demarcated mass (M) projecting over the tracheal (T) air column.

B, An axial CT scan demonstrates a large intratracheal mass (m) with significant compromise in the overall luminal diameter.

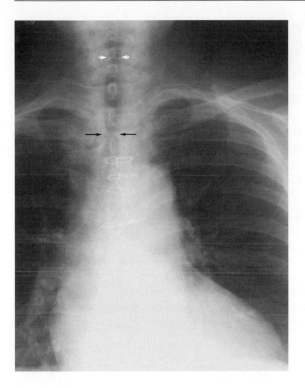

FIGURE 3-12 Anterior-posterior film of the neck: tracheal stenosis. Narrowing of the trachea is demonstrated at the thoracic inlet *(black arrows)*. Note that the normal narrowing of the air column at the glottis is considerably higher *(white arrows)*. This patient had developed tracheal stenosis following removal of a tracheostomy.

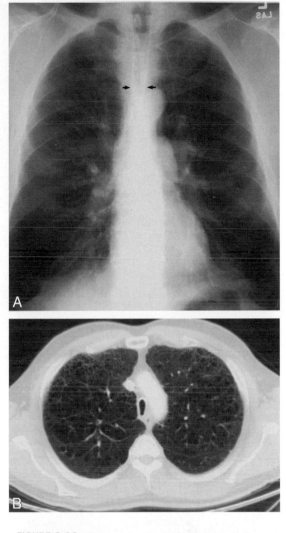

FIGURE 3-13 Posterior-anterior (PA) chest view and computed tomography (CT) scan: saber-sheath trachea.

A, AP chest view demonstrates narrowing of the transverse diameter of the intrathoracic trachea *(arrows)* in a saber-sheath trachea. The lungs are markedly hyperinflated.

B, An axial CT scan (lung windows) in the same patient shows that the trachea is narrowed in its coronal (right to left) dimensions but maintains a normal dimension in the sagittal (front to back) plane. Low-attenuation areas in the lung parenchyma represent marked centrilobular emphysema.

intrathoracic pressures generated in COPD and usually does not cause significant central airway obstruction (Fig. 3-13).

Rare etiologies of tracheomalacia include polychondritis and familial tracheobronchomegaly (Fig. 3-14). In tracheobronchomegaly, plain chest radiographs show increased diameter of the trachea (>2.5 cm) or main bronchi (>2.0 cm). Despite this apparent dilatation on inspiratory films, there can be significant narrowing with expiration.

Foreign bodies are an uncommon cause of tracheal obstruction in adults. Aspirated objects usually come to rest below the trachea at the level of the bronchi (main or segmental) (Fig. 3-15). Most of the foreign bodies aspirated are food products, such as peanuts. These objects are usually about the same density as soft tissue and therefore cannot be seen on plain radiographs. Indirect evidence of aspiration of a nonopaque object can be obtained with inspiratory and expiratory views of the chest or with fluoroscopy. If the foreign body is

causing a check-valve phenomenon, air trapping during expiration prevents obstructed lung from deflating normally and displaces the mediastinal structures away from the abnormal side (Fig. 3-16). Normal inspiratory and expiratory views should not preclude bronchoscopy if the clinical suspicion for a foreign body is high. Figure 3-17 shows an algorithm for evaluation of tracheal obstruction.

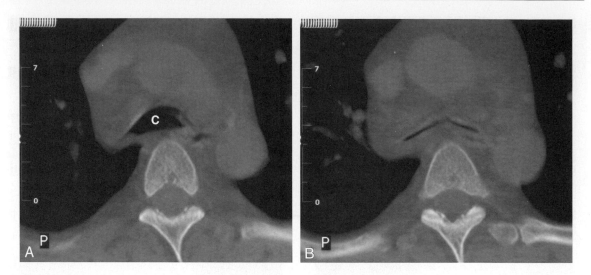

FIGURE 3-14 Computed tomography scan of the carina in a patient with bronchomalacia from polychondritis.
A, Detail of an axial image taken at the level of the carina (C) during inspiration does not show significant airway narrowing.
B, Detail from an axial image at the level of the carina during expiration in the same patient as pictured in A. The softened bronchial cartilage collapses, causing nearly complete airway obstruction.

☐ BRONCHIECTASIS

Bronchiectasis is an irreversible dilatation of the bronchial tree that can be diffuse or focal. The key symptoms of bronchiectasis are chronic cough and purulent sputum. Hemoptysis is also common and may be the presenting sign (see later discussion). In general, diseases cause bronchiectasis by exposing the bronchi to chronic inflammation that damages the cartilage within the bronchial tree. This leads to irreversible dilatation of the bronchial tree, which can be diffuse or focal in extent. These changes can be classified as cylindrical, varicose, and saccular types, roughly representing increasing degrees of bronchial wall destruction. (Saccular or cystic

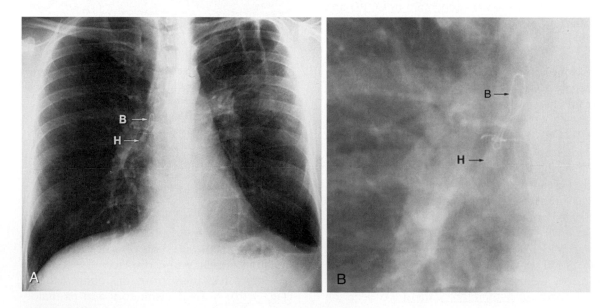

FIGURE 3-15 Posterior-anterior chest: foreign body at carina (kachina doll).
A, This film demonstrates the typical location of an aspirated foreign body (miniature kachina doll) in the right main stem bronchus. B, body; H, head.
B, Detail of the aspirated doll.

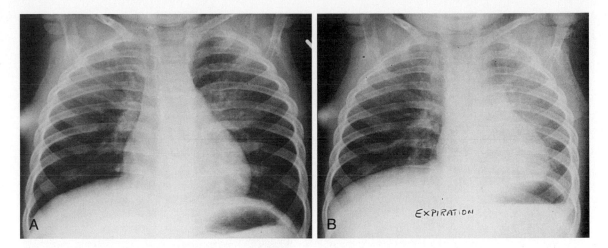

FIGURE 3-16 Serial posterior-anterior radiographs: foreign body in the right lower lobe with air trapping.

A, Inspiratory frontal film demonstrates normal position of the cardiomediastinum silhouette and symmetric aeration of the lungs.

B, With forced expiration, there is relative hyperlucency (air trapping) in the right lower lobe secondary to obstructed egress of air (ball-valve type of mechanism). There is a hazy appearance of the compressed normal left lung and associated mediastinal shift to the left.

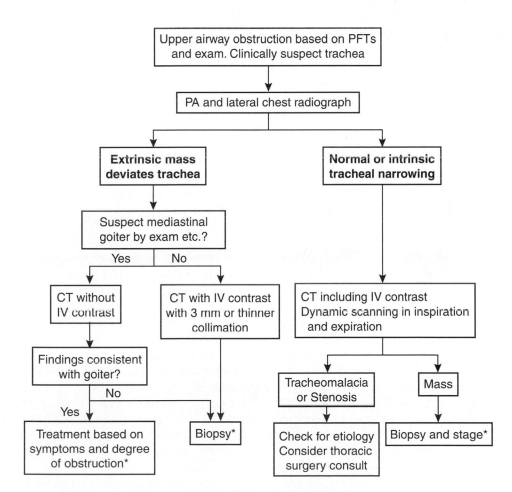

*If patient also complains of dysphagia consider esophogram

FIGURE 3-17 Algorithm for the study of a tracheal obstruction.

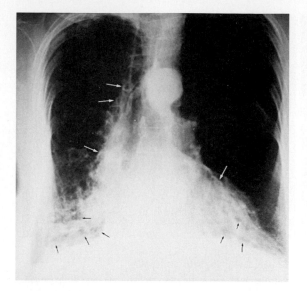

FIGURE 3-18 Posterior-anterior chest radiograph: bronchiectasis. Thickened bronchial walls are evident *(white arrows)*. Increased opacity at the lung bases is due to bronchial wall thickening and volume loss. A few cystic spaces caused by dilated bronchi are seen *(black arrows)*.

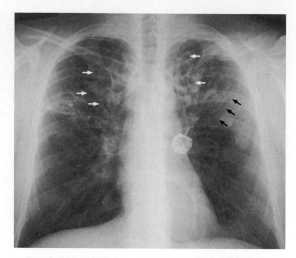

FIGURE 3-19 Posterior-anterior chest: upper lobe bronchiectasis in a patient with cystic fibrosis. Bilateral upper lobe cystic and varicose bronchiectasis is present. Thickened bronchial walls seen on end cause ring shadows *(white arrows)*. When thickened bronchi run parallel to the plane of the radiograph they cause "tram tracks," parallel white lines *(black arrows)*.

bronchiectasis indicates severe destruction of bronchial architecture.) Radiographic findings are typically nonspecific and include indistinctness and crowding of bronchovascular markings with accompanying volume loss in the affected area (Fig. 3-18). Occasionally, "tram tracks" (parallel white lines) can be identified. In patients with severe disease, radiographs show cystic spaces with or without air-fluid levels (Fig. 3-19). These can have a "honeycomb" look and may be mistaken for scarring from advanced pulmonary fibrosis.

Although routine chest radiographs may contain subtle findings that suggest bronchiectasis, CT scanning of the chest is the procedure of choice to confirm the diagnosis and determine the extent of the disease. The extent is particularly important if surgical resection of focal bronchiectasis is being considered. Most CT examinations for bronchiectasis are now performed with high-resolution CT (HRCT). HRCT uses thinner sections and a computer algorithm, providing finer spatial detail than standard CT (see Chapter 1). Bronchial dilatation is diagnosed on CT by visualizing bronchi in the peripheral lung fields (where they are normally too small to be seen) and by identifying bronchi with a greater diameter than their accompanying pulmonary artery (Figs. 3-20 and 3-21).

Conditions that cause bronchiectasis are listed in Table 3-3. Radiologic evaluation can provide helpful clues about the possible etiology of bronchiectasis. Bronchiectasis associated with excessive mucus production or impaction tends to be central. When filled with mucus, these dilated bronchi can form a glove-like shadow on routine chest films that can easily be mistaken for dilated blood vessels (Fig. 3-22). Careful evaluation of CT images shows that these opacities arise from the airways rather than from the pulmonary vasculature. Allergic bronchopulmonary aspergillosis (ABPA) produces bronchiectasis of this type. It is typically seen in adults and is the result of a hypersensitivity reaction to aspergillus that occurs in patients with asthma. It preferentially causes bronchiectasis in the proximal (central) upper lobes. Recognition of ABPA is important because treatment with steroids may prevent further bronchial damage. Occasionally, central bronchiectasis is caused by a slow-growing endobronchial tumor, and this possibility should be carefully looked for if the central bronchiectasis is confined to one lobe of the lung.

Traction bronchiectasis is caused by tension placed on the bronchi from adjacent scarring. When this is caused by diffuse fibrosis such as in idiopathic pulmonary fibrosis (see Chapter 6),

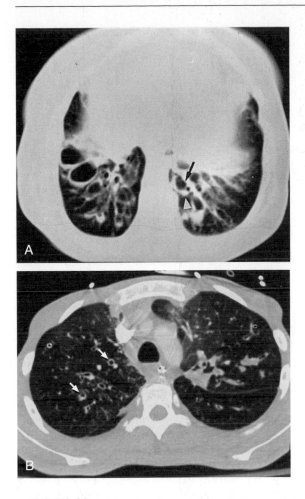

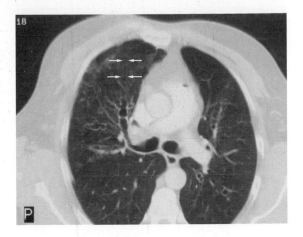

FIGURE 3-21 Axial image from a high-resolution computed tomography study in a patient with bronchiectasis. The enlarged bronchi do not taper normally as they approach the periphery of the lung. Some dilated bronchi can be seen within 1 to 2 cm of the pleural surface *(arrows)*.

FIGURE 3-20 Axial computed tomography (CT) images of bronchiectasis.

A, Image from conventional CT of cystic bronchiectasis. There are extensive cystic spaces at the lung bases. A grossly enlarged bronchus *(arrow)* is much larger than the adjacent pulmonary artery *(arrowhead)*. The combination of an enlarged bronchus (the "ring") and the smaller artery (the "stone") is sometimes referred to as the "signet ring" sign.

B, High-resolution CT image showing less dramatic signet ring signs *(arrows)*. This degree of bronchiectasis is more common than the bronchiectasis seen in image A.

Early in the course of the disease, patients develop bronchial wall thickening that is similar to that seen in patients with asthma or chronic bronchitis. The bronchial wall thickening is most marked in the upper lobes, where it produces increased linear markings. As a result, some radiologists include cystic fibrosis in the differential diagnosis for upper lung zone diffuse infiltrative lung disease (see Chapter 6). Cystic fibrosis, however, causes hyperinflation of the lungs instead of the diminished lung

the bronchiectasis is usually mild (cylindrical). Tuberculous destruction can cause more severe bronchiectasis that usually occurs in the upper lobes and is often asymmetric. Bronchiectasis caused by infections other than tuberculosis (or ABPA) is usually more severe in the lower lobes. It may be bilateral or localized to a specific lobe or segment. This is a classical sequela of pertussis infection but can occur after many other forms of pneumonia.

Cystic fibrosis is an increasingly common cause of bronchiectasis in adults and may also have characteristic radiographic findings.

TABLE 3-3
Causes of Bronchiectasis

Postinfectious
Granulomatous—most commonly mycobacterial
Pertussis
Recurrent pyogenic pneumonia
Immunoglobulin deficiency
Acquired immunodeficiency syndrome

Hereditary disorders
Cystic fibrosis
Kartagener's disease
Williams-Campbell syndrome
Mounier-Kuhn syndrome

Allergic bronchopulmonary aspergillosis

Chronic central airway obstruction
Foreign body or neoplasm

Pulmonary fibrosis
Traction bronchiectasis

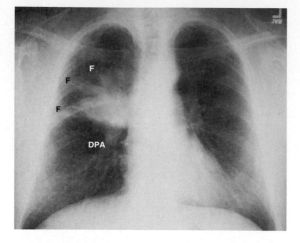

FIGURE 3-22 Posterior-anterior chest radiograph: allergic bronchopulmonary aspergillosis. Dilated central bronchi filled with impacted mucus are present on the right. This is sometimes termed a finger-in-glove appearance. The "fingers" (F) are caused by mucus-filled bronchi and may be mistaken for abnormal pulmonary blood vessels. The normal descending pulmonary artery (DPA) is evident.

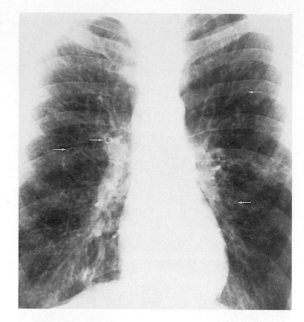

FIGURE 3-23 Posterior-anterior chest: cystic fibrosis in an adult. Frontal radiograph of a patient with more diffuse disease than seen in Figure 3-19. There is generalized hyperaeration and diffuse bronchial wall thickening. Some of the parenchymal opacities represent tram tracks and ring shadows *(arrows)* of the thickened bronchial walls. The hila are enlarged. In the setting of cystic fibrosis this can be caused by both enlarged pulmonary arteries and enlarged hilar lymph nodes.

volumes seen with most infiltrative diseases. By the time the disease is seen in adults, the process is often generalized (Fig. 3-23).

When a patient with cystic fibrosis presents with an acute exacerbation of symptoms, the radiograph is often unchanged, but it is important to look for signs of a secondary pneumothorax or superimposed pneumonia. Atelectasis of the right upper lobe is common but may be chronic. Chest films in advanced cases may show enlarged central pulmonary arteries, which is evidence of pulmonary arterial hypertension. If cardiac enlargement is also seen on the chest radiograph, right heart failure (cor pulmonale) is probably present. This predicts a poor long-term prognosis.

☐ HEMOPTYSIS

The first step in evaluating a patient with hemoptysis is the standard PA and lateral chest radiograph. If an abnormality is seen, this directs further evaluation. For example, the presence of upper lobe cavitary disease suggests tuberculosis and the need to collect sputum for mycobacterial culture. If the radiograph strongly suggests endobronchial obstruction, for example, lobar atelectasis without air bronchograms (see Chapter 5), clinicians may proceed directly to bronchoscopy. Otherwise, CT is usually performed with two diagnostic goals in mind:

(1) determine whether endobronchial lesions are likely to be present and (2) suggest alternative causes of hemoptysis (such as pulmonary emboli or diffuse pulmonary hemorrhage) if the bronchi appear normal.

If the initial chest radiograph is normal, the diagnostic decisions are more problematic. The most common cause of hemoptysis with a normal chest film is bronchitis. Hemoptysis is rarely the sentinel sign of an endobronchial neoplasm if the chest radiograph is normal. Despite the low yield, the possibility of neoplasm mandates further diagnostic evaluation in patients at risk for bronchogenic carcinoma. Occasionally, other clinically important but non-neoplastic diagnoses are made during the evaluation of patients with normal chest radiographs. Among patients with hemoptysis and a normal chest radiograph, bronchiectasis is more common than neoplasm. Pulmonary embolism can also produce hemoptysis, but when this occurs a pulmonary infarction is usually present and the chest radiograph is rarely normal (see Chapter 10).

Some clinicians still consider bronchoscopy the diagnostic procedure of choice in patients who experience hemoptysis despite a normal chest radiograph if the patient is at high risk for bronchogenic carcinoma (based on age, quantity of hemoptysis, smoking history, and so on). Spiral CT with thin sections, however, can identify the majority of neoplasms found by bronchoscopy in this setting. The sensitivity of CT is better if a multidetector scanner is used because it allows thin sections to be performed rapidly though a large area of the thorax. Unfortunately, nonspecific abnormalities or false-positive findings are also more common with this technique. CT scans may demonstrate small endobronchial "masses" caused by secretions in the central airways. If this is noticed while the patient is still in the CT scanner, the patient can be rescanned after voluntary coughing. Alternatively, the patient can be rescanned at a later date or bronchoscopy can be performed.

If the patient is at low risk for bronchogenic carcinoma (i.e., younger than 40 and a nonsmoker) or has symptoms suggestive of bronchiectasis, CT scanning is the most useful first diagnostic step. Evaluation should include a survey of the entire chest to evaluate the central airways and selected HRCT slices to look for peripheral bronchiectasis. Figure 3-24 shows an algorithm for the evaluation of nonmassive hemoptysis.

Evaluating patients with massive hemoptysis, defined as greater than 500 mL of blood in 24 hours, is a bit different. Prior to instituting any therapy, it is important to localize the source of bleeding to the right or left lung. Often the patient can sense the location of the bleeding when it starts. If not, spiral CT has proved accurate in identifying the correct lung as the source in most cases. Bronchoscopy can be performed, but unfortunately in this clinical situation the endoscopist can often see little but blood.

Once the site of bleeding is localized, radiology can play an important role in treatment of these patients. Most massive bleeding arises from the bronchial artery circulation, often related to bronchial artery hypertrophy in areas of bronchiectasis. This source of bleeding is particularly common in patients with cystic fibrosis. These abnormal bronchial arteries can be effectively occluded by catheter-directed embolization (Fig. 3-25).

DIAGNOSTIC ALGORITHM FOR HEMOPTYSIS (NON-MASSIVE)

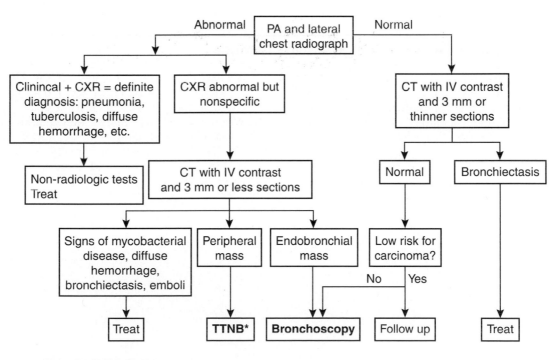

*Transthoracic needle biopsy

FIGURE 3-24 Algorithm for the evaluation of hemoptysis. CT, computed tomography; CXR, chest radiograph; IV, intravenous; PA, posterior-anterior.

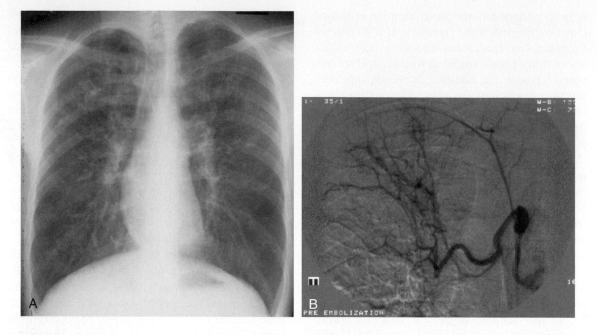

FIGURE 3-25 Posterior-anterior (PA) chest and bronchial artery angiogram of patient with cystic fibrosis and massive hemoptysis. A, PA chest radiograph shows extensive bronchiectasis related to cystic fibrosis. Bronchoscopy localized bleeding to the right lung. B, Right bronchial artery arteriogram. The bronchial artery is much larger than normal and has numerous tortuous branches. In this patient, as in most cases of hemoptysis caused by bronchiectasis, no focus of active extravasation is seen. The bronchial artery was empirically embolized and hemoptysis ceased.

Pearls for Clinicians—Large Airway Disease

1. Look carefully at the tracheal air column on both PA and lateral views in all dyspneic patients, particularly those with unremitting "asthma." Focal narrowing below the first thoracic vertebra is never normal.
2. In older patients the aortic arch often "pushes" the trachea to the right. If the trachea deviates to the left on the chest radiograph, look carefully for a mass and examine the patient's neck for a goiter.
3. When you see too many "lung markings" on a chest radiograph, think about the possibility that you are really looking at the ring shadows and tram tracks of bronchiectasis.

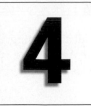

Obstructive Pulmonary Disease

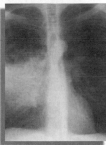

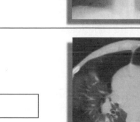

Obstructive lung disease is a heterogeneous group of clinical disorders with the common features of airflow obstruction and dyspnea. These disorders include emphysema, chronic bronchitis, asthma, bronchiectasis, and bronchiolitis. None of the conditions are mutually exclusive, and a single person may suffer from more than one obstructive disease simultaneously. (For example, a patient may have both asthma and chronic bronchitis.)

Although all obstructive lung diseases increase airway resistance and reduce (expiratory) airflow rates, asthma is the only one that is defined by its physiology. Asthma is diagnosed if there is evidence of increased airway reactivity and reversible bronchospasm. Chronic bronchitis is diagnosed by history. Affected patients have at least 3 consecutive months of productive cough for 2 consecutive years. The other obstructive diseases, emphysema, bronchiectasis, and bronchiolitis, are characterized anatomically. For instance, emphysema is defined as enlargement of air spaces distal to the terminal bronchiole. In general, radiology is best at identifying the anatomic components of these diagnoses. Accordingly, radiologic findings can make a specific diagnosis of

emphysema, bronchiectasis, or bronchiolitis but cannot make a specific diagnosis of chronic bronchitis or asthma.

☐ BRONCHIECTASIS

Bronchiectasis was discussed in Chapter 3 because of its involvement of more central airways. Its radiographic manifestations reflect this injury to larger, more easily visible structures. In postinfectious bronchiectasis, plain radiographs may show parallel lines ("tram tracks") and small ring-shaped opacities at the lung bases. These findings can be subtle and look similar to the prominent basilar lung markings seen in chronic bronchitis (see next section). High-resolution computed tomography (HRCT) is usually very accurate in establishing the diagnosis of bronchiectasis by showing dilated bronchi (see Chapter 3).

Among adults with cystic fibrosis, the severity of bronchiectasis may vary from mild (difficult to detect without CT) to very severe cases that can be easily diagnosed by chest radiography. In the latter patients the lungs are hyperinflated and there is marked bronchial wall thickening. Large air spaces may form in the upper lung zones, caused by bronchiectatic cysts or emphysematous bullae (see Chapter 3).

☐ CHRONIC BRONCHITIS

Some patients with chronic bronchitis have normal chest radiographs, whereas other patients' radiographs have been described as showing "dirty" lungs. In the latter cases, bronchial markings are increased, especially at the lung bases, where they may appear indistinct. This is caused in part by thickening of the bronchial walls. The thickened walls of large bronchi can cause tapering parallel shadows (tram tracks) similar in appearance to those seen in bronchiectasis. When seen end on, these thickened bronchial walls are wider than normal bronchi, which have walls about the thickness of a line drawn with a well-sharpened pencil. Because they are thickened, the bronchi may also appear to extend farther peripherally than normal. Bronchial shadows can be further accentuated at the lung bases if the upper lung zones contain severe emphysema and bullae. The damaged upper lung is more compliant than normal and allows the lower lung to contract, crowding bronchi and vessels into a smaller area. This combination of ill-defined crowded vessels and bronchial shadows is sometimes mistaken for basilar pneumonitis if old radiographs are not available for comparison. This is one of several possible errors in interpreting chest radiographs in patients with chronic obstructive pulmonary disease (COPD) (Table 4-1).

The radiographic findings seen in chronic bronchitis are neither sensitive nor specific. Patients with congestive heart failure or bronchiectasis have similar bronchial wall thickening, and heavy-set patients often appear to have increased bronchovascular markings at the lung bases. Much of the pathology in chronic bronchitis occurs in airways smaller than those involved by bronchiectasis and therefore cannot be seen on chest radiographs. Neither is chronic bronchitis readily diagnosed on HRCT.

☐ ASTHMA

Like those in chronic bronchitis, radiographic findings in asthma are nonspecific. During acute exacerbations, hyperinflation can be present. Chest radiographs of hyperinflated adult chests may show the anterior seventh costochondral junction to project above the diaphragm, and the retrosternal space may be increased. Some patients with long-standing asthma develop bronchial wall thickening like that seen in chronic bronchitis (Fig. 4-1). Although these radiographic findings may be present, chest radiography's principal utility in caring for asthmatics (as in most obstructive lung disease) is to detect new acute disease (e.g., pneumonia, atelectasis, and pneumothoraces) superimposed upon chronic findings (see section on complications). Because "all that wheezes is not asthma," it is also important to look for other potential causes of wheezing such as central airway obstruction by a mass or foreign body or for unsuspected heart disease such as mitral stenosis. Even when used for these purposes,

TABLE 4-1
Potential Errors in Interpretation of the Chest Radiographs of Patients with Chronic Obstructive Pulmonary Disease

Error	Signs to Look For
Chronic bronchitis mistaken for CHF	No Kerley's B lines or vascular redistribution; pleural effusions uncommon
Cardiac enlargement unrecognized	Increasing cardiac silhouette compared with prior radiographs (cardiothoracic ratio may still be normal)
Bullae mistaken for pneumothorax	Walls of bullae convex toward the mediastinum, visible only for short segments
Flattened diaphragm mistaken for posterior pleural effusion on lateral view	Lateral decubitus films do not show free-flowing fluid
Chronic bronchitis mistaken for lower lobe pneumonitis	Appearance unchanged from prior radiographs; bilateral bronchial wall thickening present; no air bronchograms

CHF, congestive heart failure.

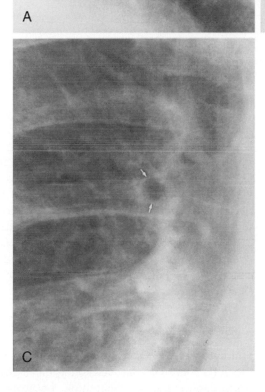

FIGURE 4-1 Serial posterior-anterior chest examinations: progressive bronchial wall thickening in chronic asthma.

A, Frontal close-up radiograph shows prominent peribronchial cuffing *(arrows)* on a background of increased lung markings, a frequent appearance for chronic asthma or bronchitis.

B, Follow-up radiograph of same patient demonstrates a further increase in the thickness of the bronchial wall.

C, This normal (segmental) bronchus *(arrows)*, in a different patient has a pencil-point thin wall.

however, radiographs are usually of low yield in young asthmatics who are otherwise healthy.

☐ EMPHYSEMA

Emphysema is an obstructive lung disease characterized by abnormal permanent enlargement of air spaces distal to the terminal bronchioles (acini). There are four types of emphysema: (1) central lobular emphysema, (2) panlobular emphysema, (3) paraseptal emphysema, and (4) paracicatricial emphysema. Central lobular emphysema (CLE) is associated with cigarette smoking and is by far the most common type. CLE is caused by progressive destruction of the alveolar walls. It begins in the center of the lobule but in advanced stages involves all the

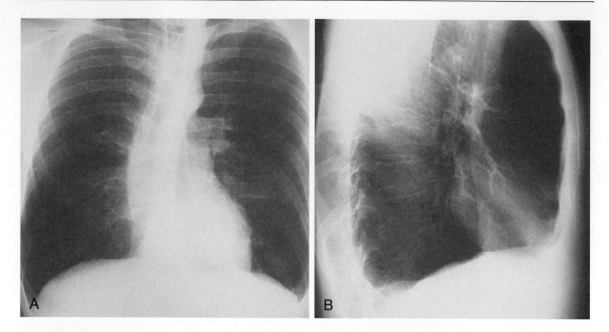

FIGURE 4-2 Posterior-anterior and lateral chest views: alpha₁-antitrypsin deficiency.

A, Hyperinflation is present. There is marked flattening of the hemidiaphragms; the paucity of vessels is most marked at the lung bases. Features of basilar predominance and early age of onset (second and third decades) suggest alpha₁-antitrypsin deficiency.

B, The marked flattening of the diaphragms and widening of the retrosternal clear space (well over 2.5 cm in this radiograph) are signs of hyperinflation. Note that the flattening of the diaphragms is more evident on the lateral view than on the frontal projection.

alveoli in the lobule. (See Chapter 6 for a description of a secondary lobule.)

The other three types of emphysema are uncommon but not rare. Panlobular emphysema involves the entire acinus and is associated with alpha₁-antitrypsin deficiency. The latter is responsible for about 1% of all emphysema and should be considered in young adults with rapidly progressive disease. Radiographic changes seen in patients with this disease are usually more pronounced at the lung bases, which is the opposite of the pattern seen with CLE (Fig. 4-2).

Paraseptal emphysema occurs in the lung periphery and occasionally along the lobar fissures, causing subpleural blebs or bullae. These are both bubble-like air collections, free of internal airways and alveoli. A bulla is a collection within the peripheral lung parenchyma that has a diameter greater than 1 cm. Blebs are also peripheral, usually described as occurring within the visceral pleura. Although any type of emphysema can cause bullae, paraseptal emphysema differs from other types of emphysema because the bullae formed are often bounded by normal lung. Because of this, patients may have well-preserved lung function. Most morbidity is caused by pneumothoraces,

which occur following rupture of one of the peripheral blebs or bullae. Occasionally, very large isolated bullae can form (Fig. 4-3).

Paracicatricial emphysema also differs from CLE. It is caused not by destruction of alveolar walls but by scarring in the adjacent lung parenchyma. This scarring stretches and distorts the surrounding lung, forming open spaces in the parenchyma by traction. Silicosis complicated by progressive massive fibrosis can cause localized emphysema in this manner (see Chapter 6).

Radiographic Findings

Emphysema commonly causes overinflation of the lung parenchyma. Radiographic signs of overinflation include flattening or inversion of the hemidiaphragmatic domes, increases in retrosternal clear space (>2.5 cm), accentuation of the thoracic kyphosis, and horizontally inclined, widely spaced ribs. Flattening of the hemidiaphragms is the most specific sign of hyperinflation (Fig. 4-4). Sometimes this effaces the posterior costophrenic sulcus (the posterior costophrenic angle exceeds 90 degrees) and mimics a small posterior pleural effusion.

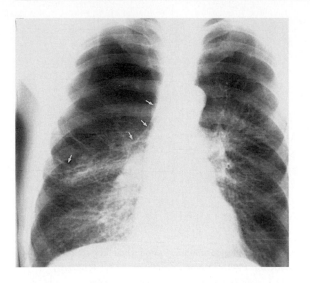

FIGURE 4-3 Posterior-anterior chest radiography: apical bullae. Frontal chest view shows a paucity of lung markings in the right upper lobe because of a large bulla *(arrows)* that displaces the upper lobe bronchi and blood vessels inferiorly toward the hilum. Similar but less severe involvement is seen on the left side.

Peripheral oligemia is also seen on chest radiographs of some patients with emphysema. The pulmonary vessels in the peripheral lung are thinner and fewer in number than in normal lungs. On angiography, the pulmonary vasculature looks like a pruned tree. A radionuclide perfusion lung scan can show similar findings (Fig. 4-5). In CLE, this peripheral oligemia is usually more pronounced in the upper lobes. This finding is usually not seen in other types of nonemphysematous obstructive lung disease, such as asthma.

Although the combination of hyperinflation and peripheral oligemia is fairly specific for uncomplicated emphysema, it is not sensitive, especially early in the course of the disease. These findings are more common in advanced disease, and even then a radiograph is able to establish a diagnosis in only two thirds of cases. Many patients with significant emphysema may have normal or minimally abnormal chest radiographs. Furthermore, the classical appearance

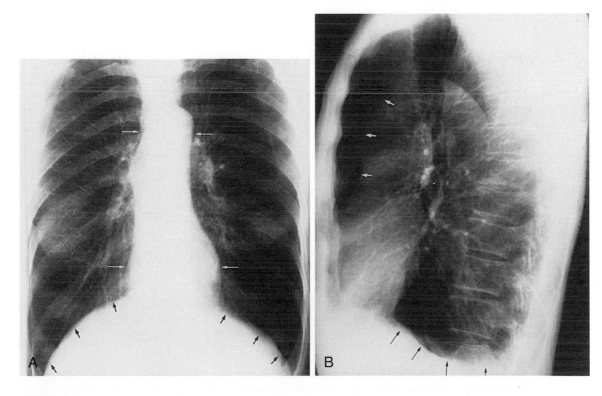

FIGURE 4-4 Posterior-anterior and lateral chest examination: severe emphysema with diaphragmatic inversion.

A, Frontal radiograph shows marked overinflation, oligemia, and markedly depressed diaphragms *(black arrows)*, common radiographic features of severe emphysema. Note the narrowed cardiomediastinal silhouette *(white arrows)*.

B, Lateral radiograph demonstrates increased retrosternal clear space *(white arrows)* with anterior bowing of the sternum, increased anterior-posterior thoracic diameter, and hyperaeration so severe that the diaphragms are actually inverted *(black arrows)*. Plain radiographs are only 65% to 75% sensitive for emphysema even if the disease is severe.

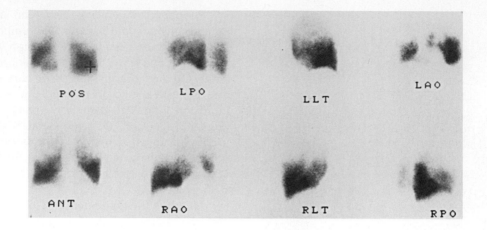

FIGURE 4-5 Pulmonary perfusion scan: centrilobular emphysema (CLE). Perfusion portion of a radionuclide lung scan in a patient with CLE. Perfusion to the upper lobes is markedly diminished. POS, posterior; LPO, left posterior oblique; LLT, left lateral; LAO, left anterior oblique; ANT, anterior; RAO, right anterior oblique; RLT, right lateral; RPO, right posterior oblique.

of emphysema can be distorted by coexistent disease. For example, peripheral oligemia can be obscured by vascular engorgement from concurrent congestive heart failure (Fig. 4-6).

Both CT and HRCT have limited clinical roles in the evaluation of emphysema. Spiral CT can be used to quantify the extent and heterogeneity of emphysema prior to lung reduction surgery. This is a procedure in which the most severely emphysematous portions of lung are excised in the hope of decreasing the hyperinflation of the chest and thereby improving the mechanical advantage of the respiratory muscles. HRCT is also useful in identifying

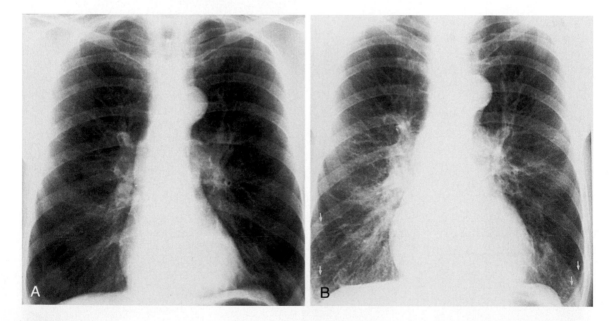

FIGURE 4-6 Serial posterior-anterior chest radiographs: congestive heart failure with chronic obstructive pulmonary disease.

A, A narrowed cardiomediastinal silhouette with large central pulmonary arteries and moderate peripheral tapering are apparent, consistent with pulmonary arterial hypertension. Parenchymal fields are hyperaerated but otherwise unremarkable. No Kerley's B lines are evident.

B, Frontal chest view obtained a few weeks later in the now symptomatic patient demonstrates a significant increase in generalized lung markings (interstitial pulmonary edema), especially bibasilar, obscuring the peripheral oligemia evident in part A. Many prominent Kerley's B lines are present (*arrows* indicate only some), and there is an increase in cardiac size, hilar vascular opacity, and hilar indistinctness (central edema).

emphysema as a cause of dyspnea in patients who have an impaired diffusing capacity on pulmonary function testing but normal or near normal spirometry and chest radiographs. These patients are sometimes referred to as having "mystery" dyspnea, and many are ultimately found to suffer from emphysema, pulmonary vascular disease, or early infiltrative disease. Although HRCT may not always detect primary pulmonary vascular disease, it can detect emphysema or infiltrative disease that is not visible on routine radiographs. On HRCT images, mild to moderate CLE appears as multiple focal areas of low attenuation within otherwise normal-appearing lung parenchyma. These low-attenuation areas occur in the center of the "lobule" and are differentiated from bullae and bronchiectasis because they do not have definable walls (Fig. 4-7). Unlike the findings in CLE, focal lucencies are not characteristic of HRCT images of panlobular emphysema. Instead of well-defined low-attenuation areas, there may be a more generalized decrease in attenuation throughout the lower lobes, sometimes called "simplification" of the lung structure (Fig. 4-8). Severe cases of CLE can look very much like panlobular emphysema because as the disease progresses it extends beyond the center to involve the entire lobule.

Bullous Disease

Bullae are air-containing spaces within the lung greater than 1 cm in diameter. Located in the lung, bullae walls are formed by pleura,

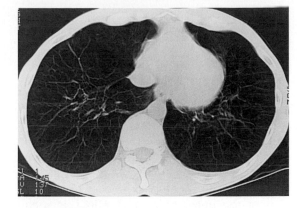

FIGURE 4-8 High-resolution computed tomography: panlobular emphysema. An axial image at the level of the lung bases in a 45-year-old male patient with alpha$_1$-antitrypsin deficiency shows confluence of low-attenuation areas without demarcated walls. Lung vascular markings are uniformly sparse. No normal, higher density lung is seen between areas of emphysema, as seen in Figure 4-7.

connective tissue septa, or compressed lung parenchyma. Bullae can be solitary or multiple. They should not be confused with pneumatoceles, which are focal intraparenchymal air collections that occur in an area of lung injured by infection or trauma. Unlike bullae, pneumatoceles are not permanent and usually resolve over several months. Before 1981, pneumatoceles were most commonly seen following staphylococcal pneumonia and in chronic adult respiratory distress syndrome. Today, *Pneumocystis carinii* pneumonia in patients with acquired immunodeficiency syndrome (AIDS) is a frequent

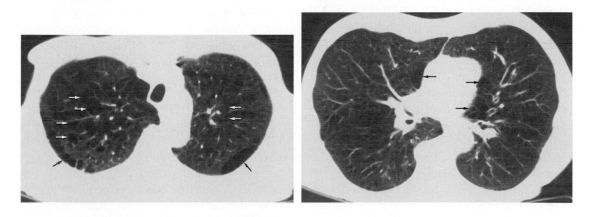

FIGURE 4-7 Computed tomography (CT): centrilobular emphysema (CLE).

A, CT image through the upper lobe shows many focal areas of emphysema that appear as very low attenuation *(white arrows)* surrounded by higher density normal lung. These areas of low attenuation are not demarcated by discernible walls (as are bullae and lung cysts).

B, CT image in same patient inferior to A. Note CLE's predilection for upper lung zones. Paraseptal emphysema is also present, as seen in the small bullae along the pleural surfaces in A and B *(black arrows)*.

cause of pneumatoceles (see Chapter 7). Some AIDS patients also develop premature emphysema and therefore could have both bullae and pneumatoceles.

Occasionally, patients develop extensive bullous disease that compresses a significant amount of adjacent lung tissue (e.g., greater than a third of the hemithorax). This characteristically occurs in the upper lobes of young men who smoke and have emphysema elsewhere. If the compressed lung tissue is relatively normal, these patients may benefit from resection of the bullae (Fig. 4-9). HRCT is useful in assessing the disease within the compressed lung. If extensive emphysema is present within the lung adjacent to the bullae, a bullectomy is unlikely to improve the patient's symptoms. Other uses of HRCT in obstructive lung disease are listed in Table 4-2.

☐ UNILATERAL HYPERLUCENT LUNG

Emphysema and bullous disease may be markedly asymmetric, causing one lung to appear more lucent than the other. There is a long list of other diseases that can cause one lung to appear hyperlucent, usually by causing unilateral air trapping or a unilateral decrease in pulmonary blood flow. Swyer-James syndrome is one abnormality in which air trapping causes a unilateral hyperlucent lung. In most cases it is thought to be the sequela of constrictive bronchiolitis early in childhood (see next section). The peripheral bronchial anatomy is deformed, with diffuse pruning of peripheral bronchi and bronchioles. Chest radiographs taken during inspiration (as routine radiographs are) show the abnormal lung to be more lucent and smaller than the normal lung (Fig. 4-10). During exhalation, however, air is trapped within the abnormal lung so that it is larger than the contralateral normal lung on radiographs taken at end expiration. The same appearance can also be seen with bronchial obstruction by a foreign body or much less commonly by an endobronchial tumor.

Obstruction of blood flow to most of one lung by mediastinal fibrosis, tumor, or a huge pulmonary embolism can also cause relative hyperlucency of one lung. When this occurs secondary to an embolism, it is termed the Westermark sign (see Chapter 10). Unilateral aplasia of a pulmonary artery (usually the right) also causes marked asymmetry of pulmonary blood flow but has a much different appearance. Unlike the appearance in Westermark's sign, the abnormal lung is small and because it is less well aerated than the normal side, it may be more opaque. More important, unlike patients with Westermark's sign, patients with pulmonary artery aplasia are asymptomatic.

Although it is important to consider the preceding diseases when confronted with marked asymmetry in the opacity of one side of the chest, it should be remembered that the cause of the asymmetry is often not within the lungs. Asymmetric lucency of the thorax is usually not caused by Swyer-James syndrome, a radiolucent foreign body, or an embolism. The most common cause is either rotation of the patient or mastectomy, both of which affect overlying soft tissue shadows (Table 4-3).

☐ BRONCHIOLITIS OBLITERANS

Bronchiolitis obliterans (BO) causes obstruction of the small airways (bronchioles) proximal to the alveoli by fibrosis that surrounds the bronchioles. BO, in the past referred to as "constrictive" bronchiolitis, can be the result of early childhood infection, leaving one lung hyperlucent owing to chronic air trapping. This results in the Swyer-James syndrome described earlier. Adults can develop BO following exposure to toxic fumes, after bone marrow transplantation, and following viral infections.

Although the diagnosis of BO cannot be made on the basis of the chest radiograph, CT imaging can be useful. CT images may show direct evidence of damage to the airways, such as bronchial wall thickening or bronchiolar dilatation. More commonly, however, CT shows only evidence of air trapping that is caused by patchy bronchiolar obstruction. On CT these areas of air trapping appear as lung of decreased attenuation ("blacker" lung) that contains lower than expected numbers of blood vessels (Fig. 4-11). These areas of low attenuation are patchy and often have geographic (clearly demarcated) borders. Unlike that in CLE, this low-attenuation lung is not confined to the center of lobules. If air trapping is suspected as the cause of heterogeneous lung parenchyma on CT, it can be verified with images performed during both full inspiration and full expiration.

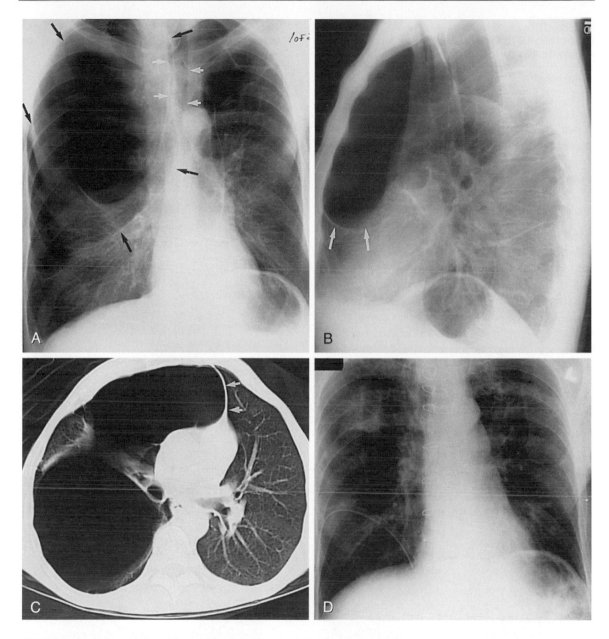

FIGURE 4-9 Serial radiographs and computed tomography (CT): before and after bullectomy.

A, Primary bullous disease is present bilaterally but more notably on the right *(black arrows)*, with marked displacement of bronchovascular markings inferiorly. The large bulla on the right has displaced the trachea *(white arrows)* and cardiomediastinal structures toward the left.

B, Lateral chest view shows the larger right bulla herniating across the midline *(arrows)* through a widened retrosternal clear space.

C, Axial CT scan (lung windows) shows virtual absence of all lung markings on the right and the anterior herniation of the right lung. This causes displacement of the "anterior junction line" *(arrows)*, the confluence of the right and left pleural surfaces.

D, Radiograph taken after right bullectomy demonstrates excellent results: the compressed lung has reexpanded to fill the space previously occupied by the large bulla.

The expiratory images accentuate focal areas of air trapping because these areas remain the same density (measured in Hounsfield units, HU) during expiration while the remainder of the lung becomes more opaque (Fig. 4-12).

Bronchiolitis obliterans with organizing pneumonia (BOOP) was previously termed "proliferative" bronchiolitis and is a much different disease than BO. BOOP is classified as a diffuse infiltrative lung disease and results in a

TABLE 4-2
Uses of High-Resolution Computed Tomography in Obstructive Lung Disease

Detection of emphysema in patient with impaired diffusing capacity but normal spirometry and chest radiograph

Prior to consideration for bullectomy or lung reduction surgery

Detection of bronchiolitis obliterans

Differentiation of bullae from pneumothorax

Detection of coexisting disease (e.g., interstitial fibrosis)

TABLE 4-3
Causes of Asymmetric Lucency of One Hemithorax

Soft tissue abnormality
Breast (mastectomy with or without prosthesis)
Rotation or other technical factors

Pleural disease
Asymmetric pleural thickening
Posterior layering pleural effusion

Airway obstruction (with air trapping)
Central airway
Neoplasm
Foreign body (primarily in children)
Peripheral (small) airway obstruction
Bullous emphysema
Bronchiolitis obliterans (Swyer-James syndrome)

Decreased blood flow
Pulmonary embolism
Central tumor or fibrosis obstructing pulmonary artery
Pulmonary artery hypoplasia

Compensatory hyperinflation adjacent to atelectatic or resected lung

restrictive rather than an obstructive physiologic defect. Chest radiographs are usually abnormal (see Chapter 6).

There are also several other type of bronchiolitis. Respiratory bronchiolitis occurs in smokers, is usually not detectable on the chest radiograph, and appears as ill-defined nodules in the upper lung zone on HRCT scans (see Chapter 6). The disease is not accompanied by severe airflow obstruction and usually has a benign course. Infectious bronchiolitis is probably the most common form of bronchiolitis and characteristically causes plugging of the

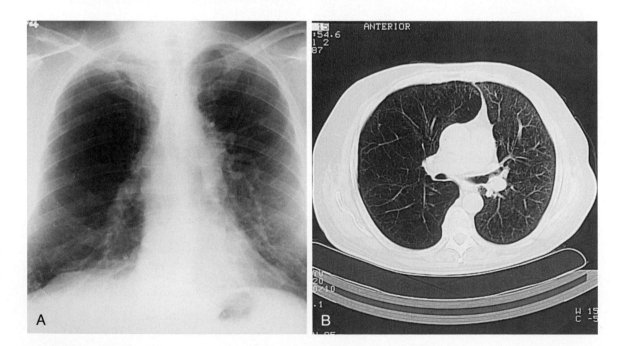

FIGURE 4-10 Posterior-anterior chest radiograph and computed tomography (CT) scan: Swyer-James syndrome—right lung.

A, Frontal radiograph demonstrates generalized hyperlucent right (affected) lung, with diminutive hilar vessels.

B, CT of the same patient shows increased aeration on expiration in the right lung, with marked loss in the number of vessels (compare with normal left lung). Swyer-James syndrome is also known as unilateral lobar emphysema and idiopathic unilateral hyperlucent lung.

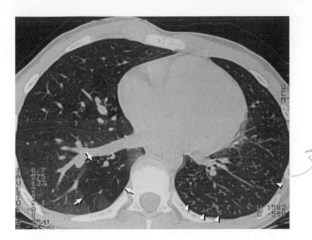

FIGURE 4-11 Computed tomography scan of a patient with postinfectious bronchiolitis. In the right lung there is a well-circumscribed area of low attenuation ("blacker") lung *(arrows)*. This is caused by air trapping related to obstructed bronchioles. On the left there is more diffuse air trapping. Bronchioles filled with secretions appear as small branching structures *(arrowheads)*, sometimes referred to as "tree in bud."

small bronchioles with secretions. Sometimes these small airways filled with secretions cause a micronodular appearance on chest radiography (Fig. 4-13). On CT the abnormal airways are seen as small branching structures, each "branch" a centimeter or less in length and ending in a tiny nodule. This branch and nodule appearance on CT, called a "tree in bud" pattern, is almost always related to acute or chronic infection.

COMPLICATIONS

During acute exacerbations of obstructive lung disease, chest radiographs cannot assess the degree of airflow obstruction but are useful in determining a possible cause for the exacerbation, such as atelectasis, pneumothoraces, and pneumonias. Atelectasis, either segmental or lobar, is caused by mucus plugging and is most commonly seen in asthmatic patients, particularly children. Whenever a new lung opacity is present in an asthmatic with an acute attack, atelectasis should be considered before antibiotics are prescribed for a presumed infection.

Pneumothoraces are probably more common in patients with emphysema and asthma than in patients with chronic bronchitis or bronchiolitis. A pneumothorax can be the primary cause of increasing symptoms or can occur during therapy, particularly when mechanical ventilation is used. Pneumothoraces may be caused by the rupture of a bulla. If the bullous disease is extensive, the lack of peripheral vascular markings may make the radiographic recognition of the pneumothorax difficult, and a chest CT scan may be needed. In other cases, bullous disease may be mistaken for a pneumothorax when no pneumothorax is present. On chest radiographs, both pneumothorax and bullae cause oligemia, and both have pencil-thin curvilinear lines along their margins. In a pneumothorax, however, the visceral pleural

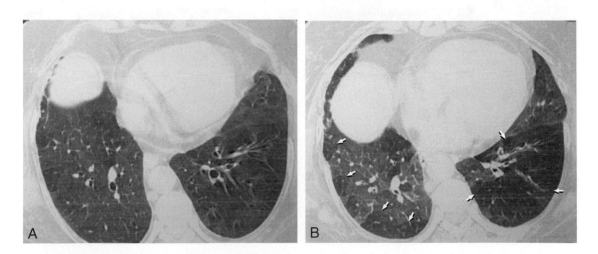

FIGURE 4-12 Computed tomography (CT) mosaic pattern.

A, CT section during inspiration shows portions of lung that appear to be lower in attenuation (blacker) than others, particularly in the left lower lobe.

B, CT section during expiration accentuates the differences between the normal and the low-attenuation lung *(arrows)*. Note that many areas of low attenuation have sharp margins, termed geographic borders. These areas of low attenuation are caused by air trapping.

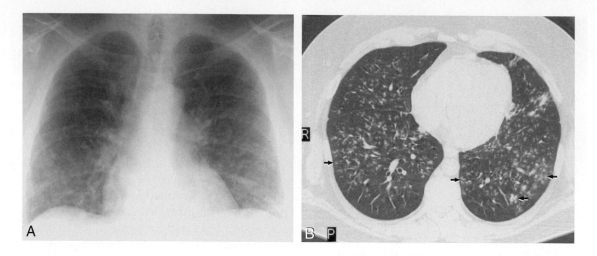

FIGURE 4-13 Posterior-anterior chest radiograph and computed tomography (CT) of patient with infectious bronchiolitis.

A, There are diffuse tiny nodular opacities in the parenchyma. The lungs do not appear hyperinflated.

B, CT section from the same patient shows multiple tiny branching structures that end in micronodules *(arrows)*. This appearance has been likened to a tree in bud. Although this pattern is caused by the filling of bronchioles with secretions, no signs of air trapping are seen in this case.

line is convex toward the rib cages. The thin wall of the bullae appears differently. It is convex toward the mediastinum and is usually seen in short segments instead of as a continuous line (Fig. 4-14). Pneumomediastinum can also occur but by itself is not harmful (see Chapter 8).

Pneumonias in patients with moderate to severe COPD may have a heterogeneous, "bubbly" appearance on chest radiographs (Fig. 4-15).

This is because of air trapping in areas of emphysema interspersed between parts of the lung that are filled with purulent secretions. Larger areas of apparently "clear" lung may be caused by the presence of a large bullae.

Sometimes in the setting of pneumonia or bronchitis, air-fluid levels may form within these bullae. The bulla walls then become thicker, and the process may be mistaken for a

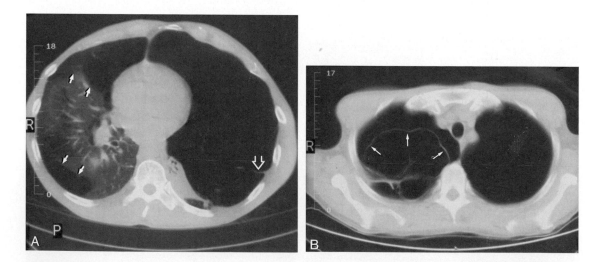

FIGURE 4-14 Computed tomography (CT) scans of two different patients with severe bullous disease, one with a pneumothorax.

A, The small amount of remaining lung parenchyma seen on the right contains foci of centrilobular and paraseptal emphysema *(arrows)*. On the left the lung is entirely replaced by bullae. A few bands of connective tissue, the walls of bullae, are present in the posterior chest *(open arrow)*. No pleural line is seen.

B, CT section from another patient with severe bullous disease and a right-sided pneumothorax. A white pleural line is seen *(arrows)* dividing the bullae from the pleural space in the right upper chest. The left lung apex is entirely filled by a large bulla.

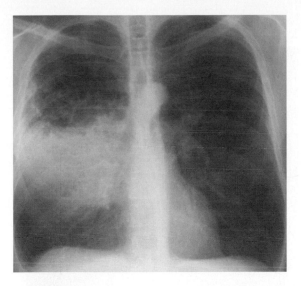

FIGURE 4-15 Posterior-anterior chest radiograph of patient with right upper lobe pneumonia and underlying emphysema. The pneumonia appears to be very heterogenous, containing small lucent (dark) areas that could be mistaken for areas of necrosis and cavitation.

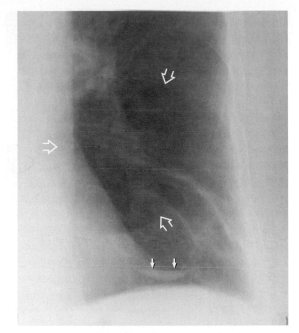

FIGURE 4-16 Posterior-anterior chest examinations: air-fluid level in infected bulla. Multiple bullae are present at the left lung base, one of which does not have a discernible wall on the radiograph *(open arrows)*. One bulla contains a small amount of fluid *(solid arrows)*. The wall of the bulla is only slightly thickened and the adjacent lung appears free of pneumonia.

lung abscess. Unlike the case of a lung abscess, however, there is no acute destruction of lung parenchyma. The accumulation of fluid in the bullae is probably related to impaired drainage from inflammatory narrowing of the neck of the bullae. Accordingly, infected bullae generally have thinner walls and less surrounding parenchymal opacity than do abscesses (Fig. 4-16). Despite adequate antibiotic treatment, the air-fluid levels in the bullae may take weeks to clear.

Right-sided heart disease is another complication of obstructive lung disease that is frequently detected on chest radiography. Signs of cor pulmonale and pulmonary hypertension are frequently seen. These findings are discussed in Chapters 10 and 12.

Patients with COPD often have coexistent left-sided heart disease such as dilated cardiomyopathy and congestive heart failure. The radiographic diagnosis of congestive heart failure can be difficult in patients with COPD (see Table 4-1). Prior radiographs are often essential. For example, these radiographs may show that when the patient is at baseline condition the cardiac silhouette is small owing to pulmonary hyperinflation. Subsequent development of a "normal-sized" cardiac silhouette on a radiograph actually represents pathologic enlargement of the heart. Congestive heart failure also decreases the apparent degree of hyperinflation seen on radiographs of patients with COPD (Fig. 4-17). In patients with COPD and congestive heart failure, Kerley's B lines and effusions are often detected, but the emphysematous lung may cause pulmonary edema to be markedly asymmetric in appearance.

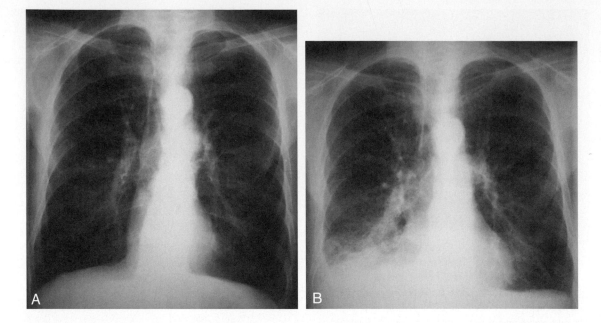

FIGURE 4-17 Posterior-anterior chest: baseline and acute congestive heart failure.

A, Patient with emphysema on initial examination.

B, The patient later developed heart failure. In addition to right-sided effusion and air space disease, the radiograph shows a marked decrease in hyperinflation. Underlying emphysema could be overlooked.

Pearls for Clinicians—Obstructive Pulmonary Disease

1. Pulmonary function tests diagnose obstructive lung disease. Radiographic diagnosis is neither sensitive nor specific for these disorders. Use the chest radiographic to look for central airway obstruction or a complicating condition (e.g., pneumothorax).

2. Emphysema and bronchiolitis obliterans are the only obstructive lung diseases that CT scanning can definitely diagnose, and the latter is rare.

3. Patients with chronic bronchitis may have "increased lung markings" that can be mistaken for congestive heart failure or basilar pneumonia. Always look (hard) for old radiographs to determine whether the increased markings are a chronic finding before using the radiograph as evidence of acute disease.

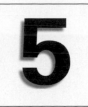

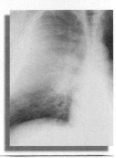

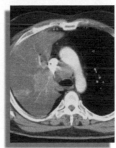

Lung Parenchyma: Basic Terminology

The range of parenchymal lung disease is vast. To make this book useful to clinicians, we have categorized these diseases according to etiology rather than according to their radiographic appearance. On occasion, however, clinicians also need to create a differential diagnosis for a specific radiographic pattern. To generate this differential, it is helpful to recognize three common radiographic patterns of parenchymal lung pathology: (1) air space disease, (2) interstitial disease, and (3) atelectasis.

Our ability to differentiate between air space and interstitial disease on chest radiographs is imprecise. Pathologic specimens often show evidence of both processes. Nevertheless, these terms remain a useful starting point for creating a differential diagnosis and selecting further diagnostic studies.

□ AIR SPACE DISEASE

Lung disease that primarily affects the alveoli and respiratory bronchioles is called air space disease. Air bronchograms are the key radiographic finding of air space disease. Air bronchograms occur when airless alveoli outline air-filled bronchi, seen on chest radiographs as a dark branching pattern within the opaque (white) homogeneous lung parenchyma (Fig. 5-1).

Some air space disease may not uniformly affect the lung parenchyma. In such instances, small radiolucencies are visible within the opacified lung where normal air-containing alveoli have yet to be affected. These normal areas interspersed between opacified acini are known as air alveolograms (Fig. 5-2). The identification of air alveolograms is not as straightforward as the identification of air bronchograms. The small radiolucencies that make up the alveolograms can look very similar to the small spaces between the "strands" of the mesh like (reticular) pattern seen with interstitial diseases (see later). Air bronchograms are a much more reliable sign.

Air bronchograms are usually produced when the alveoli are filled with blood (from contusion or hemorrhage), pus (from pneumonia), water (from pulmonary edema), or cells (from lymphoma or alveolar cell carcinoma) (Table 5-1). Because the alveolar spaces are filled with some material in these diseases, the volume of the lung is usually preserved. Atelectasis can also produce air bronchograms. In this situation, the alveoli are not filled but are airless and collapsed. When air bronchograms

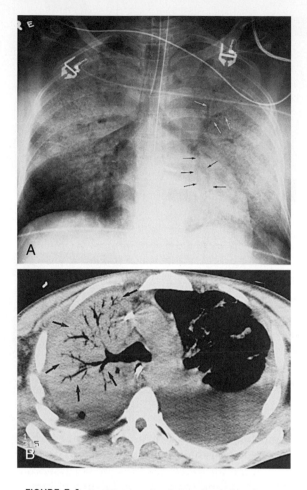

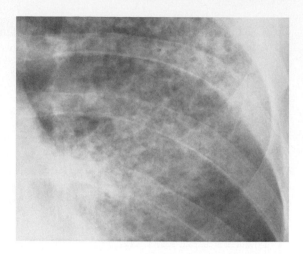

<u>FIGURE 5-2</u> Posterior-anterior (PA) chest view with close-up: air alveolograms. The close-up from a PA chest radiograph demonstrates the small radiolucencies (air alveolograms) within the opacified lung.

<u>FIGURE 5-1</u> Anterior-posterior chest radiograph and computed tomography (CT) scan: air bronchograms.

A, Radiograph of the typical branching pattern of air bronchograms *(arrows)*: the air-filled bronchi are outlined by the exudative process filling the alveoli.

B, CT shows multiple air (black bronchi) bronchograms *(arrows)* throughout an area of consolidation.

are caused by atelectasis, there is always accompanying volume loss (see later discussion).

There must be air within the bronchi for an air bronchogram to be present. Therefore, chest radiographs of air space disease may not show air bronchograms if the proximal bronchus is completely occluded with mucus or a tumor. In this case, the chest radiograph shows a homogeneous opacity, an appearance identical to that of a pleural effusion (Fig. 5-3). Unfortunately, the physical examination of a patient with parenchymal lung disease and an occluded bronchus and that of a patient with a large pleural effusion can yield similar findings (e.g., dullness to percussion, diminished breath sounds). Endobronchial obstruction is more

likely than effusion if there is decreased volume on the opacified side, but sometimes the chest radiograph findings are ambiguous. Differentiating bronchial obstruction from effusion is clinically important, and further evaluation with lateral decubitus radiographs, ultrasonography, or computed tomography (CT) of the thorax should be considered. Ultrasonography can easily detect a massive effusion because the very large fluid collections are almost always in contact with a large segment of the chest wall. Because sound is poorly transmitted through an aerated lung, however, ultrasonography usually gives little information about the lung tissue adjacent to the pleura. CT is preferable if there is a need to examine both the pleura and the lung

<u>TABLE 5-1</u>
Substances That Fill Alveoli and Cause Air Bronchograms

Water	Acute respiratory distress syndrome (ARDS), congestive heart failure, volume overload/renal failure, drowning
Pus	Pyogenic infections, less commonly mycobacterial or fungal infections
Blood	Chest trauma, vasculitis (e.g., microscopic polyarteritis, lupus), severe thrombocytopenia (usually with coexistent infection)
Cells	Bronchoalveolar cell carcinoma, lymphoma

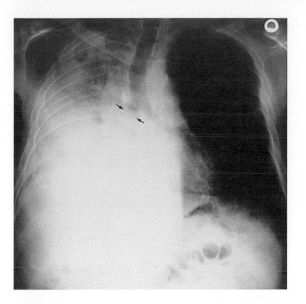

FIGURE 5-3 Posterior-anterior chest view: air space disease with obstructive bronchus. Frontal chest radiograph shows opacification of the right lower lobe caused by proximal bronchial obstruction *(arrows)*. Distal air bronchograms are absent. There is ipsilateral mediastinal shift, a sign of volume loss inconsistent with a massive effusion.

parenchyma or airways. For example, CT imaging is preferable to ultrasonography if a bronchogenic malignancy is the suspected cause of a large pleural effusion (see Chapter 11).

☐ INTERSTITIAL DISEASE

Diseases that affect the tissue surrounding the alveoli and capillaries within the lung, but do not fill the alveoli, are called interstitial diseases. Interstitial disease can usually be distinguished from air space disease on chest radiographs because air remains in the alveoli. Therefore, the opacities do not form a homogeneous white background. When interstitial disease is severe, the small amounts of air scattered between the coarse interstitial thickening can look like the alveolograms caused by air space disease (Fig. 5-4). Air bronchograms are formed only if the interstitial disease is very severe.

The most easily recognized radiographic sign of interstitial disease is the presence of Kerley's B lines. Kerley's B lines are small septations in the lung that contain lymphatics and venules and are visible on chest radiographs only when abnormally thickened. These septations form short (1 to 2 cm), horizontal lines

that connect with the pleura along the lateral margins of the lung (on the posterior-anterior [PA] view of the chest) (Fig. 5-5). Kerley's B lines have a different appearance than lung blood vessels because normal vessels do not extend all the way to the pleura. Although Kerley's B lines are often discussed with reference to congestive heart failure, they can also be seen in other interstitial processes (e.g., lymphangitic carcinoma). Kerley's A lines are less commonly seen than Kerley's B lines. They are longer lines that radiate from right and left pulmonary hilum, the central areas where the pulmonary vessels arising from the heart enter the lungs. When Kerley's lines are the dominant finding seen on chest radiographs, the pattern is described as "linear." When interstitial edema is the cause of the linear pattern, subpleural fluid is also commonly seen. This is fluid inside the lung just under the pleura, not within the pleural space, and it is often most apparent on the lateral projections (Fig. 5-6).

It is also helpful to categorize the other types of opacities produced by interstitial disease. These opacities can appear mesh-like (reticular pattern) or as uncountable minute nodules (Fig. 5-4 and Fig. 5-7, respectively). Some radiologists further divide reticular opacities into fine reticular and coarse reticular patterns (Fig. 5-8). The "mesh" seen in a coarse reticular pattern appears to be made of thicker, more distinct strands. This pattern is more commonly present in chronic diseases, particularly those that cause fibrosis. If the spaces between the strands in a coarse reticular pattern become large (e.g., >5 mm) and distinct, the pattern looks less like a mesh than a collection of cysts. It is important to remember that although this cystic pattern may represent fibrosis, it may instead represent thickened bronchial walls caused by bronchiectasis (Fig. 5-9). Fortunately, the distribution of these coarse or cystic changes on the chest radiograph helps differentiate bronchiectasis from fibrosis; cystic changes of bronchiectasis are often easiest to see in the central lung and changes of diffuse fibrosis are easiest to see in the lung periphery (Fig. 5-10).

In addition to the preceding patterns, some physicians use the term "reticulonodular." This can be more confusing than helpful. The problem is that where two lines intersect on a radiograph their opacities can sum together and can look like a small nodule. Moreover, a line can look like a nodule if seen end on. Accordingly the jumble of lines that make up

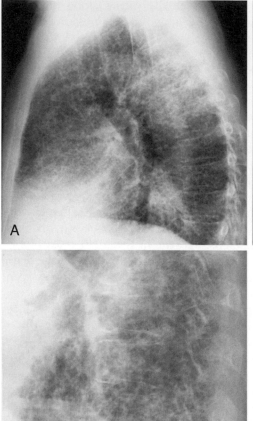

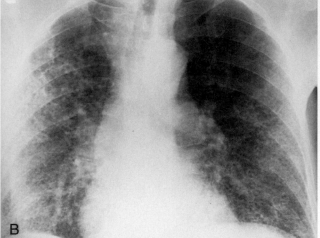

FIGURE 5-4 Lateral, posterior-anterior (PA), and lateral close-up views of the chest: coarse reticular pattern.

Lateral (A) and PA (B) views: The net or mesh-like markings within the lung are referred to as a reticular pattern. The individual strands of the mesh are formed by irregular opacities that obscure Kerley's A or B lines.

C, The close-up lateral view shows that lung opacities in this coarse reticular pattern are relatively thick and irregular. In places the small lucent (dark) areas between the strands of the mesh appear similar to air alveolograms.

any reticular pattern is bound to have some apparent "nodules" within it (Fig. 5-11).

In order to generate a differential diagnosis, it is best if the observer chooses the predominant pattern present on the plain radiograph from the menu of three patterns: (1) nodular, (2) linear, or (3) reticular. This can be very difficult and often represents an educated guess. Refining the differential diagnosis further usually depends on the distribution of the pattern (peripheral or central), the presence of ancillary findings such as lymphadenopathy, and, of course, the patient's history. This analysis and the use of CT to evaluate diffuse infiltrative lung disease are discussed briefly in Chapter 6.

☐ GROUND GLASS OPACITIES

The term "Ground glass" is often used in interpreting high-resolution CT (HRCT), where it is defined as increased opacity of the lung parenchyma that is not dense enough to obscure underlying pulmonary vessels. Some radiologists also apply the term to opacities on the chest radiograph. These ground glass opacities are hazy areas of increased lung opacity that have the same translucent appearance as glass that has been mechanically ground. Diseases that cause ground glass opacities on chest radiographs may involve the interstitium, the alveolar spaces, or both. The increase in opacity is subtle and, like ground glass seen on HRCT, usually does not obscure the pulmonary vasculature (the vasculature may appear more indistinct). Unfortunately, on chest radiographs, ground glass parenchymal opacities can be difficult to distinguish from images that are underexposed or from opacities caused by pleural fluid that overlies the lung parenchyma. Because the nuances of ground glass opacities on chest radiographs might be misleading for the novice observer, we have chosen to apply the term only to HRCT images in this book.

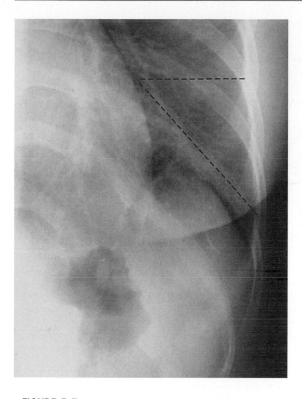

FIGURE 5-5 Posterior-anterior chest view: Kerley's B lines. A close-up of the left lower lung field shows multiple short white horizontal lines extending to the lateral pleural surface (within area defined by *dashed lines*), indicative of interstitial disease. Normal vessels do not extend to the pleural surface.

☐ **ATELECTASIS**

Atelectasis is incomplete expansion of a portion of the lung. It is similar to air space disease in that both processes produce airless alveoli. However, atelectasis occurs when the air in the alveoli is absorbed and not replaced by fluid or cells. This causes a loss of volume, which is the key radiographic finding. Atelectasis may be caused by extrinsic compression on the lung (passive atelectasis), fibrosis of the parenchyma (cicatrization), increased surface tension within the alveoli (adhesive atelectasis, e.g., from surfactant deficiency), or obstruction of the bronchus (resorptive atelectasis) (Table 5-2).

The central airway is usually patent if the atelectasis is caused by any of the first three conditions. Passive atelectasis occurs when intrapleural fluid or air collections squeeze the air out of the lung (Fig. 5-12). The adjacent atelectatic lung is often more opaque than normal, and a mass or pneumonia can be camouflaged by this opacity. When there are clinical indications of malignancy, a CT scan sometimes demonstrates a mass hidden by surrounding atelectatic lung (Fig. 5-13). In cicatricial atelectasis, the primary pathologic process is fibrosis. Typical examples are the postinflammatory

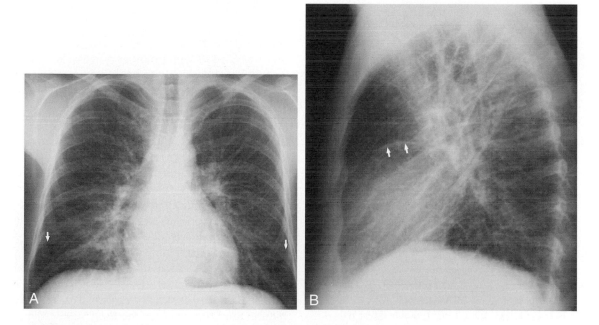

FIGURE 5-6 Posterior-anterior and lateral view of linear interstitial pattern from acute interstitial edema.

A, Frontal projection: Kerley's B lines *(arrows)* and Kerley's A lines radiating from the hilum are present.

B, On the lateral view, some Kerley's B lines are present just behind the sternum, but the thickening of the minor fissure *(arrows)* that is caused by the same disease process is more conspicuous. The major fissures are also thickened.

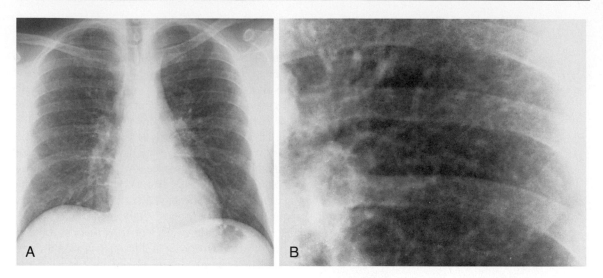

FIGURE 5-7 Posterior-anterior chest view: miliary pattern—disseminated coccidiomycosis.

A, Innumerable small nodules are scattered throughout the lung. They are relatively uniform in size, 2 to 4 mm, resembling millet seeds, hence the name of this pattern (see Figs. 6-3 and 7-21).

B, Typical appearance on close-up.

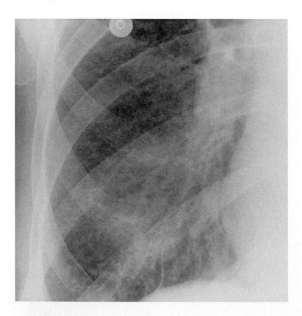

FIGURE 5-8 Detail from posterior-anterior (PA) chest showing fine reticular pattern. Detail of PA radiograph shows a mesh-like pattern that is finer than that seen in Figure 5-4. This fine reticular pattern is more commonly associated with early or acute disease. The coarse pattern shown in Figure 5-4 is more commonly seen with chronic diseases that cause fibrosis.

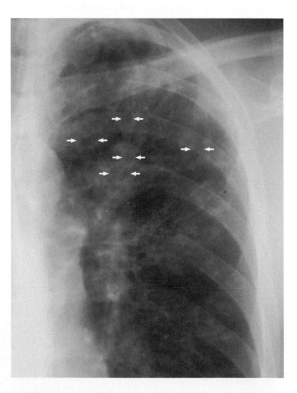

FIGURE 5-9 Detail from posterior-anterior (PA) chest: bronchiectasis. Detail from PA radiograph from patient with cystic fibrosis. Note that the ring shadows caused by dilated, thick-walled bronchi are more evident centrally (arrows). This is the opposite of the pattern usually seen with honeycombing (Fig. 5-10).

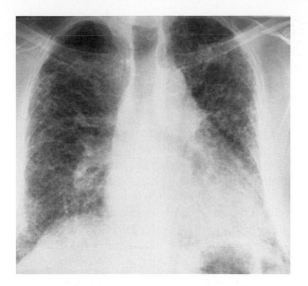

FIGURE 5-10 Posterior-anterior chest view: honeycombing. Innumerable small cysts are seen diffusely throughout the lungs, particularly in the middle and basilar peripheral lung fields. This end-stage interstitial fibrotic pattern can evolve from many different causes. Note that unlike the bronchiectasis in Figure 5-9, the cystic changes are most prominent peripherally.

changes of tuberculosis or changes of progressive massive fibrosis in advanced silicosis (Fig. 5-14). Rounded atelectasis is a special localized form of cicatricial atelectasis that can mimic a lung nodule. In rounded atelectasis, focal scarring of the pleura folds a portion of the peripheral lung in on itself, creating a mass adjacent to the pleura. Asbestos-related pleural disease is frequently associated with such scarring. The presence of pleural plaques or diffuse pleural thickening should be a clue that an apparent lung nodule may actually represent rounded atelectasis. The diagnosis is best made by CT, which shows bronchi and vessels spiraling into a juxtapleural mass that is usually at the lung base. This is described as the "comet tail" sign (see Chapter 9, Fig. 9-6).

The third type of atelectasis, adhesive atelectasis, also occurs with an open airway. Because the airway is open, peripheral air bronchograms can be present. The condition is associated with inactivation of surfactant. Classical examples are hyaline membrane disease and acute radiation pneumonitis. Pulmonary emboli may also cause atelectasis by this mechanism.

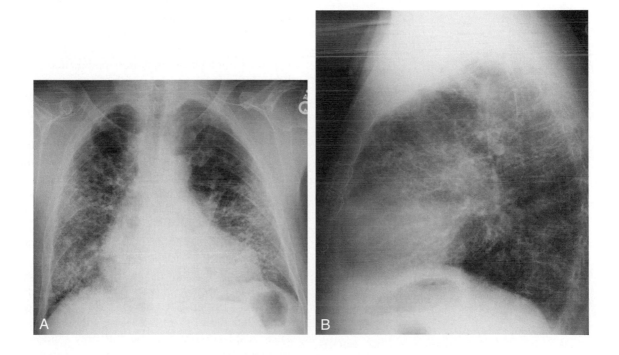

FIGURE 5-11 Posterior-anterior and lateral view of patient with idiopathic pulmonary fibrosis.

A, Frontal projection shows a coarse reticular pattern that is most prominent peripherally. Some observers might describe this pattern as reticular, others as reticulonodular; however, the distinction does not change the differential diagnosis. It is more important to note that the reticular shadows are peripheral, which makes bronchiectasis or eosinophilic granuloma less likely (see Chapter 6).

B, Lateral projection also shows the reticular changes; however, the peripheral predominance is less evident.

TABLE 5-2

Major Types of Atelectasis and Associated Common Etiologies

Obstructive	Mucous plugs, foreign bodies, neoplasms, and bronchial stenosis
Adhesive	Surfactant deficiency, radiation pneumonitis
Cicatrization	Postinflammatory scarring (tuberculosis), silicosis
Passive (compressive)	Pneumothorax, bullae, hydrothorax

Unlike the other types of atelectasis, resorptive atelectasis occurs because of obstruction of a bronchus; examples include obstruction by a bronchogenic carcinoma, a large mucous plug, or a foreign body (Fig. 5-15). Many foreign bodies are made up of vegetable matter and therefore not radiopaque and cannot be seen on conventional chest radiographs. This organic material can produce an intense inflammatory reaction and cause a long-standing, high-grade obstruction.

After a central bronchus is completely obstructed, gas distal to the obstruction is

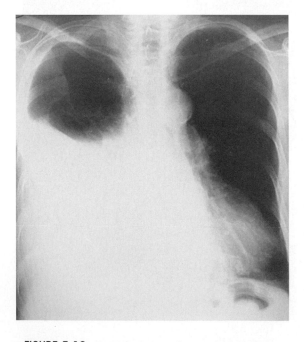

FIGURE 5-12 Anterior-posterior chest view: large effusion with compressed adjacent lung (passive atelectasis). Large right effusion with complete opacification of the lower two thirds of the right hemithorax. Instead of volume loss on the right, there is expansion of the right hemithorax and a slight mediastinal shift to the left.

reabsorbed over 18 to 24 hours (more rapidly in children). Occasionally, in the case of high-grade central obstruction, there can be sufficient accumulation of fluid and cells within the alveoli to limit volume loss. This condition is called a "drowned lung" (Fig. 5-16).

Sometimes bronchial obstruction occurs peripherally rather than centrally. Peripheral obstruction (small bronchi and bronchioles) can be caused by the accumulation of secretions, such as during an asthma exacerbation or following surgery when diaphragmatic excursion is impaired by pain. Air loss in these peripheral lesions is rapid, and radiographic changes can occur within several hours.

Radiographic Signs of Atelectasis

As the atelectatic lung loses volume, structures within the lung change position; the fissures shift position and intrapulmonary vessels and bronchi may become crowded together. These are sometimes called the direct signs of atelectasis. The easiest direct sign to detect is a shift in the interlobar fissures. Occasionally, this may be the only sign of collapse. If this shift in the fissures is overlooked, atelectasis may be mistaken for other pathology (Table 5-3). The decreasing volume of the atelectatic lung can also affect adjacent structures. These "secondary" signs of atelectasis include mediastinal and hilar shift, elevation of the hemidiaphragm, and compensatory hyperaeration of the adjacent lung parenchyma. If atelectasis persists, the mediastinal shift and diaphragmatic elevation lessen, and overinflation of the adjacent lung becomes more marked. The overinflated lung appears less opaque than normal. In cases of extensive unilateral atelectasis, the opposite lung may even enlarge enough to "herniate" across the midline.

Often, hilar shift is the easiest secondary sign of atelectasis to detect. The left hilum is normally higher than the right. If it is not, possible causes include elevation of the right hilum from right upper lobe collapse and depression of the left hilum from left lower lobe collapse. Hilar displacement may be the only evidence of atelectasis if collapse is so advanced that the entire lobe is hidden by the mediastinal structures (Fig. 5-17). When there is advanced collapse of the upper lobes, the pulmonary vessels travel almost vertically, creating the waterfall sign (see Chapter 13).

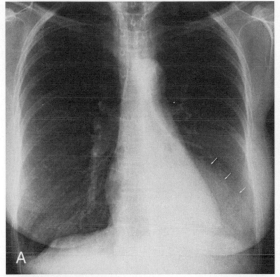

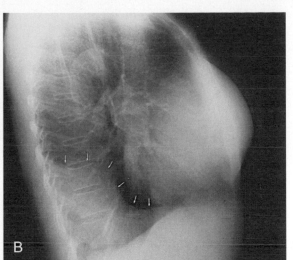

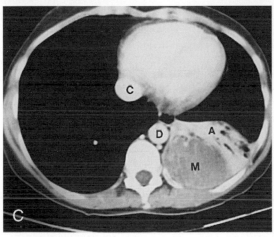

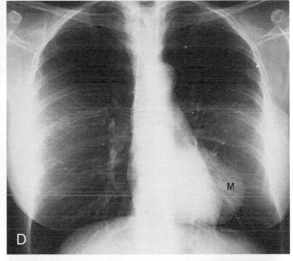

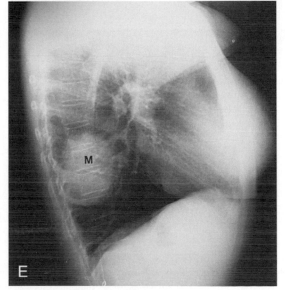

FIGURE 5-13 Posterior-anterior and lateral chest views and conventional computed tomography (CT): mass hidden by atelectasis.

A, Frontal radiograph demonstrates the typical appearance of left lower lobe atelectasis/consolidation *(arrows).* The mass is obscured.

B, Left lateral chest view demonstrates the left lower lobe atelectasis *(arrows)*; this retrocardiac opacity is associated with the spine sign (apparent increased opacity of lower thoracic vertebrae).

C, Axial CT scan at the level of atelectasis demonstrates that a mass (M) is contained within the collapsed lobe (A). The mass is conspicuous because intravenous contrast material has been used. If CT is done without intravenous contrast, tumors may be at the same density as atelectatic lung. C, inferior vena cava; D, descending aorta.

D and E, Follow-up posterior-anterior and lateral radiographs taken 2 weeks later demonstrate resolution of the atelectasis and reveal the mass (M) in the superior segment of the left lower lobe.

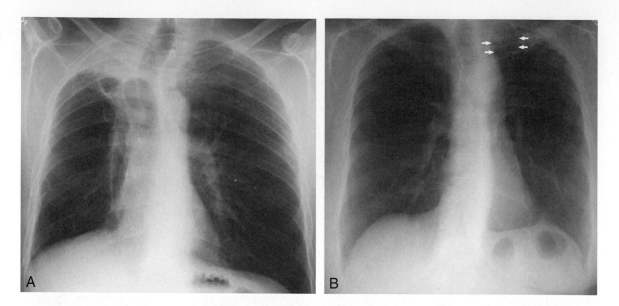

FIGURE 5-14 Posterior-anterior chest examination: upper lobe cicatricial atelectasis.

A, Frontal chest view demonstrates right upper lobe volume loss caused by postprimary tuberculosis. Although not seen in this case, air bronchograms are sometimes visible in cicatricial atelectasis.

B, Frontal chest radiograph from a different patient with a history of tuberculosis. Surrounding fibrosis has "pulled open" the bronchi in the left apex *(arrows)*, causing traction bronchiectasis.

Although volume loss may be the only radiographic evidence of atelectasis, there is often increased opacity in the airless lung. When the atelectasis is localized it may appear as horizontal or oblique linear opacities that are 1 to 3 mm thick. These changes are called discoid, subsegmental, or plate-like atelectasis (Fig. 5-18). Parenchymal scarring from previous inflammatory conditions can have a similar appearance and often can be differentiated from discoid atelectasis if the scarring can be shown to be unchanged from prior studies or on follow-up chest radiographs.

Atelectasis can also cause larger pulmonary opacities, involving segments or entire lobes of the lung. If the degree of volume loss is relatively

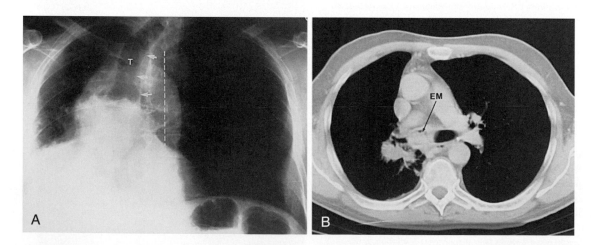

FIGURE 5-15 Chest radiograph and contrast-enhanced computed tomography (CT): right main bronchus obstruction.

A, Posterior-anterior chest radiograph shows right lower lobe atelectasis with mediastinal shift *(arrows;* midline is indicated with *dashed lines).* T, trachea.

B, CT shows right main obstruction by bronchogenic carcinoma *(arrow)* with resulting right lung atelectasis and mediastinal shift. EM, endobronchial mass.

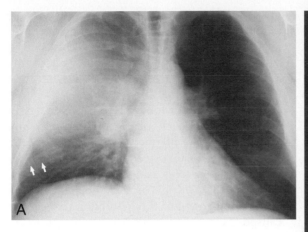

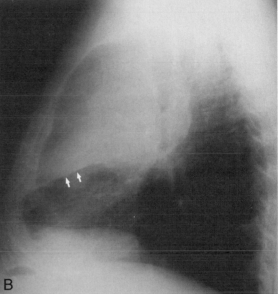

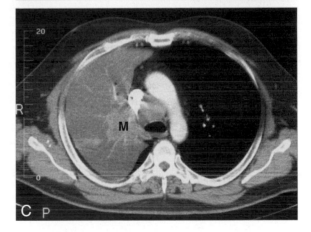

FIGURE 5-16 Posterior-anterior (PA), lateral chest view, and computed tomography (CT): endobronchial obstruction with limited volume loss (drowned lobe).

A and B, PA and lateral radiographs show diffuse increased opacity of the right upper lobe. The lobe is not significantly decreased in size and the minor fissure *(arrows)* is not shifted.

C, CT shows the central mass (M) surrounded by low-attenuation lung. No air bronchograms are seen within the lung; however, pulmonary vessels are clearly seen against the low-attenuation background. These findings are consistent with a "drowned lobe." Gradually progressive obstruction has allowed accumulation of secretions that replace absorbed alveolar air with fluid. Note that the accumulation of secretions makes the lung much lower in attenuation than in other kinds of atelectasis, in which the lung enhances markedly after intravenous contrast (see Fig. 5-13).

small, radiographs alone cannot distinguish these opacities from pneumonia. If the degree of collapse is marked or if the clinical setting is most consistent with atelectasis, a diagnosis of atelectasis can be made more confidently. It is important to recognize these patterns of lobar collapse since atelectasis of an entire lobe can be a presenting sign of endobronchial obstruction from carcinoma (resorptive atelectasis).

Patterns of Lobar Atelectasis

When the right upper lobe collapses, the minor fissure and upper half of the major fissure shift

TABLE 5-3
Potential Pitfalls in the Diagnosis of Atelectasis

Misperception	Radiographic Clue
Combined right middle and lower lobe mistaken for pleural effusion	Downward displacement of both the minor and right major fissure. Opacity more extensive medially than laterally
Right middle lobe collapse missed	On lateral view minor and major fissures converge and triangular opacity overlies the heart
Right upper lobe atelectasis mistaken for paratracheal mass	Elevation of minor fissure and right hilum
Left upper lobe atelectasis mistaken for pneumonia or mass	Left upper lobe "pancaked" against anterior chest wall on lateral view and major fissure displaced forward

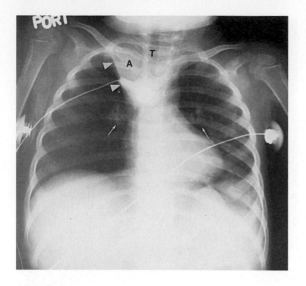

FIGURE 5-17 Posterior-anterior chest view: advanced right upper lobe atelectasis. The minor fissure is shifted superomedially *(arrowheads)* and the atelectatic upper lobe (A) is almost flat against the right paravertebral margin. The right hilum is slightly higher than the left *(arrows)*. T, trachea.

progressively upward. In complete collapse, the upper lobe lies flat against the superior mediastinum and becomes almost imperceptible on a PA chest radiograph. The lateral projection shows an indistinct upside-down triangle, with its apex at the hilum and its base in the extreme apex of the lung. If a right hilar

mass is also present, the combined contour of the mass and the atelectatic lung form an S-shaped curve on the PA view. This sign is called Golden's S sign and is usually caused by a malignant hilar mass obstructing the right upper lobe bronchus (Fig. 5-19).

The left upper lobe differs from the right because of the lack of a left minor fissure. Because of this, all the lung anterior to the major fissure is involved when the left upper lobe collapses. This can be mimicked in the right lung if *both* right upper and right middle lobes collapse together, a condition that can be caused by a right upper lobe tumor growing downward into the middle lobe bronchus. As the left upper lobe collapses, the major fissure moves forward in a plane roughly parallel to the anterior chest wall and is best seen on the lateral view (Fig. 5-20). In the PA projection, there may be obliteration of the left cardiac border. Some observers are confused by the presence of aerated lung above or medial to the atelectatic lung on this view. This is common and represents compensatory overinflation of the left lower lobe.

When the right middle lobe collapses, the diagnosis is easiest to make on the lateral projection. In this projection, the minor fissure and lower half of the major fissure become progressively closer together until, with complete collapse, they approximate each other (Fig. 5-21).

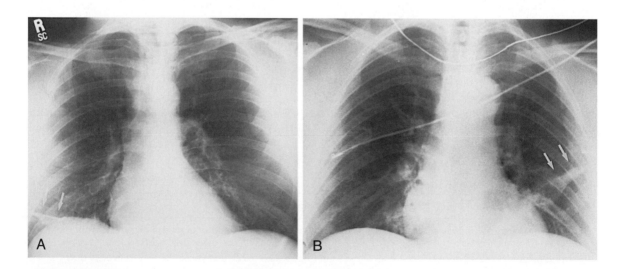

FIGURE 5-18 Posterior-anterior chest view: discoid (plate-like) atelectasis.
A and B, Linear basilar opacities *(arrows)* are often seen in conditions that diminish the diaphragmatic excursion, such as in patients who are postoperative, confined to bed, or obese. These linear opacities vary from 1 to 3 mm in thickness and 4 to 10 cm in length. They may be almost indiscernible when superimposed on the diaphragm.

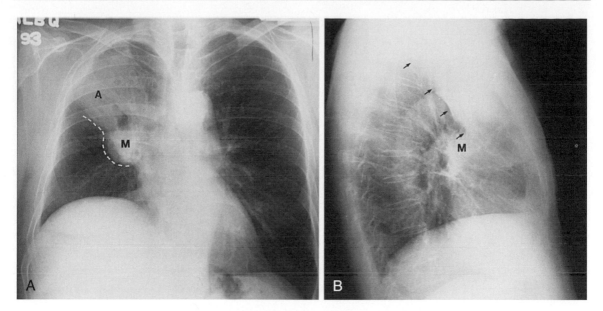

FIGURE 5-19 Posterior-anterior and lateral radiographs: right upper lobe collapse secondary to a hilar mass (Golden's S sign).

A, Frontal radiograph shows a large right hilar mass (M). Occlusion of the right upper lobe bronchus results in opacification (atelectasis) of the right upper lobe (A). The outer contour of the right upper lobe is a combination of a convex border (medially) and a concave border (laterally), termed Golden's S sign *(dashed lines)*.

B, Lateral radiograph shows the hilar mass (M) and upper lobe collapse outlined by the upper margin of the major fissure *(arrows)*. The fissure is farther forward than normal because of loss of volume in the upper lobe.

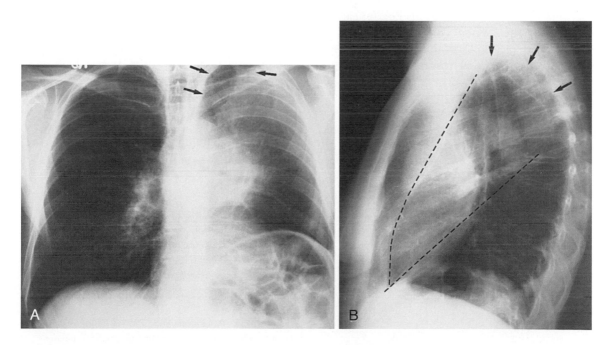

FIGURE 5-20 Posterior-anterior and lateral chest examinations: left upper lobe collapse caused by proximal mass.

A, Frontal view shows loss of the left-sided cardiac and mediastinal silhouette related to the adjacent mass and atelectatic upper lobe. As the degree of the atelectasis increases, the upper lung field becomes opacified except for the apex *(arrow)* (compensatory hyperaeration of superior segment of the lower lobe).

B, Lateral radiograph demonstrates anterior shift of the major fissure *(anterior dashed lines)* with a pancake of opacified lung in the retrosternal clear space. *Posterior dashed lines* mark the normal position of the oblique fissure.

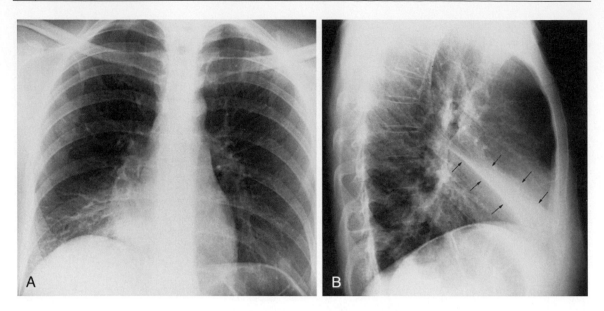

FIGURE 5-21 Posterior-anterior and lateral chest views: right middle lobe collapse.

A, Frontal radiograph shows ill-defined parenchymal opacity above the level of the hemidiaphragm, obscuring the silhouette of the right cardiac border.

B, Lateral chest radiograph demonstrates a homogeneous triangular (almost linear) opacity extending from hilum to anterior costophrenic angle. The lower margin *(arrows)* of the opacity is the major fissure and the upper margin *(arrows)* the horizontal (minor) fissure, respectively.

On a PA view, the atelectatic lobe can obscure the right cardiac border, but this finding can be difficult to see. When combined with lower lobe collapse, collapse of the right middle lobe causes an opacity that extends from the right heart border to the costophrenic angle on frontal projection and from the sternum to the spine on lateral projection. This can mimic elevation of the hemidiaphragm or a subpulmonic effusion (loculated medially). More than once, this condition has been the reason for a "failed" thoracentesis of the right chest (Fig. 5-22).

Collapse of either lower lobe is also best seen on lateral view. The upper half of the major fissure swings inferiorly and the lower half posteriorly (as if folding around the hilum). With progressive atelectasis, the lobe moves posteromedially to occupy a position in the

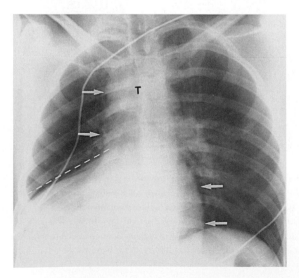

FIGURE 5-22 Posterior-anterior (PA) view: right middle and lower lobe collapse. On a PA upright radiograph the inferior aspect of the right hemithorax is opaque, a finding that could be mistaken for elevation of the right hemidiaphragm or for a pleural effusion. The shape of the opacity (higher medially than laterally), however, is atypical for either effusion or elevated diaphragm. The homogeneous opacity paralleling the *dashed lines* is collapsed middle and lower lobes. Note the ipsilateral mediastinal shift *(arrows)*. T, trachea.

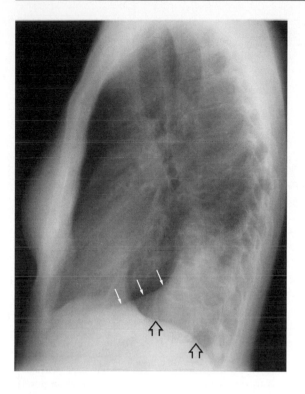

FIGURE 5-23 Lateral chest radiograph: lower lobe collapse secondary to endobronchial carcinoid. A lateral chest view demonstrates the typical triangular opacity in the posterior sulcus (A). The anterolateral border of the lower lobe, that is, the major fissure, is concave *(arrows)* because of the decreased volume taken up by the lower lobe. The left hemidiaphragm silhouette is obliterated, and the spine sign is obvious.

medial posterior costophrenic gutter (Fig. 5-23). There, the collapsed lung tissue makes the lower thoracic vertebral bodies appear just as dense as the upper thoracic spine. (Normally, the lower thoracic vertebral bodies appear more lucent than the upper thoracic spine.) This "spine sign" is another example of a summation sign (see Chapter 1).

Instances of both right and left lower lobe atelectasis appear similar on lateral chest radiographs. Left lower lobe atelectasis, however, is more common. It is present in virtually all patients following coronary artery bypass surgery. The anterior-posterior (AP) view shows a triangular opacity in the retrocardiac region that often obliterates the silhouette of the descending aorta (Fig. 5-24). Opacity in this area immediately after surgery almost always represents atelectasis rather than pneumonia.

As noted earlier, lobar obstruction can affect more than one lobe. The likelihood of an obstructing malignancy decreases, however, if the collapse of both lobes (or segments within the lobes) cannot be explained by obstruction at a single site. For example, collapse of the right upper and the right lower lobe, with sparing of the middle lobe, suggests two discrete endobronchial obstructions. This is more often caused by multiple mucous plugs than by synchronous carcinomas (Fig. 5-25).

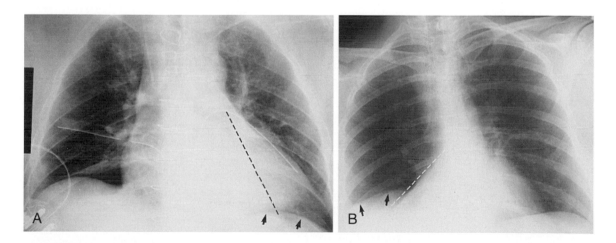

FIGURE 5-24 Anterior-posterior (AP) chest view: left and right lower lobe collapse.

A, AP chest radiograph obtained after coronary artery bypass graft surgery shows retrocardiac opacity caused by left lower lobe atelectasis *(dashed line* is the lateral border of the lobe). Left lower lobe atelectasis is almost universal following cardiac surgery. Because of the overlying cardiac shadow, left lower lobe collapse is often not as evident as right lower lobe collapse. In this case the diaphragm silhouette is obscured medially but preserved laterally *(arrows)*.

B, Right lower lobe collapse. Right lower lobe atelectasis obscures the silhouette of the medial border of the hemidiaphragm. Laterally, the right middle lobe now lies adjacent to the diaphragm and preserves its silhouette *(arrows)*.

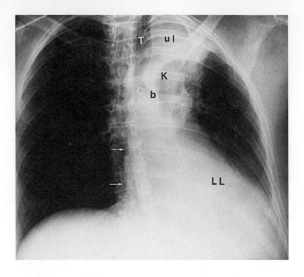

<u>FIGURE 5-25</u> Posterior-anterior radiograph: Atelectasis in different lobes. Volume loss in the left lung with atelectasis of the upper division of the left upper lobe (ul) and the left lower lobe (LL). Because the intervening lingula is not involved, a single endobronchial obstruction is less likely. The heart border is displaced because of midline shift *(arrows)*. b, left main bronchus; C, carina; K, aortic knob; T, trachea.

Pearls for Clinicians—Lung Parenchyma: Basic Terminology

1. Air bronchograms are proof that something is wrong in the lung parenchyma. That "something" is either atelectasis or filling of the alveoli with water, blood, pus, or cells.

2. It is often difficult to differentiate pneumonia from focal atelectasis. The presence of focal volume loss favors the latter, and the most reliable sign of focal volume loss is shift of a pleural fissure.

3. Kerley's B lines are also proof that something is wrong in the lung parenchyma, more specifically something within the lung interstitium.

4. The absence of both air bronchograms and Kerley's lines does not mean the lung is normal. Reticular, micronodular, or ground glass opacities can also indicate important lung disease, but these findings may be subtle on chest radiographs.

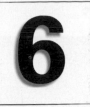

Pneumoconioses, Immunologic and Proliferative Disorders: Chronic Diffuse Infiltrative Lung Disease

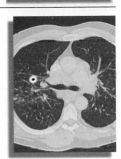

It is important to have some kind of system, even an imperfect one, to organize a differential diagnosis when confronted by a patient with chronic diffuse lung disease. Many diseases need to be considered. They vary widely in etiology and radiologic appearance but share the ability to affect the lung parenchyma diffusely. In this chapter, we have chosen to classify the diseases according to etiology, dividing diffuse infiltrative lung diseases into those that are definitely linked to inhalation of a inorganic material (pneumoconioses), diseases with strong evidence of an immunologic origin, those characterized by abnormal proliferation of cells (e.g., granulomas, histiocytes, eosinophils), and diseases best described as the idiopathic pneumonias.

The terms "air space disease" and "interstitial disease" have long served as a practical means of categorizing disease on plain radiography. This is especially true of infectious diseases (see Chapter 7). Many of the diffuse lung diseases discussed in this chapter are referred to as interstitial lung diseases even if this is not entirely accurate. We understand that many of these processes may have an intra-alveolar component as well as an interstitial component,

and we acknowledge that our ability to differentiate interstitial from air space disease radiographically is imperfect.

High-resolution computed tomography (HRCT) can better determine the location of lung pathology, but even it is not foolproof. For instance, ground glass is a term used to describe a portion of an HRCT image where there is hazy increased density of the lung parenchyma. The increased opacity must be subtle and not dense enough to obscure the pulmonary vessels (Fig. 6-1). This pattern was initially thought to be caused by early air space disease. It is now understood that ground glass opacities may also be caused by interstitial disease below the resolution of HRCT.

☐ RADIOGRAPHIC INTERPRETATION

The coexistence of interstitial and air space components in many diffuse lung diseases has led some physicians to refer to these disorders as diffuse "infiltrative" lung disease rather than diffuse "interstitial" lung disease. Regardless of whether diffuse lung disease is truly interstitial,

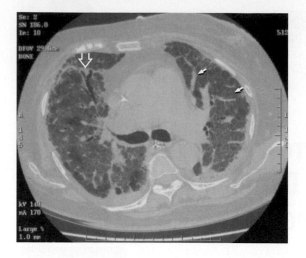

FIGURE 6-1 High-resolution computed tomography scan: ground glass opacities. A single axial scan (lung windows) shows extensive bilateral areas of increased density in the lung parenchyma. Note that the pulmonary vessels are not obscured as they traverse this abnormal area *(arrows)*. There is also evidence of fibrosis, including traction bronchiectasis *(open arrow)*.

it is helpful to use some of the same terms introduced in Chapter 5 to describe its appearance on chest radiographs. By using the term infiltrative instead of interstitial lung disease we can add an additional radiographic pattern, "chronic air space disease." The four morphologic patterns are then (1) chronic air space disease, (2) linear disease (interlacing Kerley's lines), (3) nodular disease, and (4) reticular disease (including reticulonodular pattern). Notice that patterns 2 to 4 are the same morphologic patterns used to describe interstitial opacities in Chapter 5.)

This method is not exact, but it is a practical way to think about chest radiographs that show evidence of chronic diffuse disease. A practical goal would be to remember two or three of the most common diseases in each of these four patterns. This may sound simple, but it accelerates work-up of the patient (and you will be well ahead of most of your colleagues) (Table 6-1).

Chronic air space disease describes the appearance of some chronic infiltrative disease on chest radiographs. Air bronchograms are present, the opacity is homogeneous, and there may be little or no linear or reticular component. Bronchoalveolar carcinoma and bronchiolitis obliterans with organizing pneumonia (BOOP) are two typical causes of this pattern (Fig. 6-2). Other causes include sarcoid, lymphoma, chronic eosinophilic pneumonia, lipoid pneumonia, and, rarely, alveolar proteinosis.

The linear pattern resulting from congestive heart failure is one of the most commonly encountered causes of diffuse parenchymal abnormalities on chest radiographs. Radiographic changes can include thickening of the interlobar fissures, presence of Kerley's A and B lines, and peribronchial cuffing. Kerley's B lines are short linear opacities seen adjacent to the pleural surfaces (see Chapter 5), whereas A lines are several centimeters long and radiate from the hilum. Peribronchial cuffing is present if the bronchial wall is thicker than the tracing of a well-sharpened pencil (see Fig. 4-1).

Heart failure should always be considered in the differential diagnosis of this linear interstitial pattern. "Diurese and then diagnose" remains a pragmatic dictum. It should be remembered, however, that similar interstitial changes can occur with lymphangitic carcinoma and less commonly with acute hypersensitivity (drug) reactions and a handful of less common diseases. Chronic bronchitis can cause thickening of tissues in the bronchoarterial bundles (seen as peribronchial cuffing) but does not cause Kerley's A and B lines.

TABLE 6-1
Categorization of Diffuse Infiltrative Lung Disease on Chest Radiograph—Common Diseases

Nodules	Reticular	Linear	Air Space Disease
Sarcoidosis	IPF*	Lymphangitic carcinoma	Bronchoalveolar carcinoma
Silicosis	Asbestosis	CHF	BOOP
Miliary infections	CVD*		Sarcoid
Metastases			Chronic eosinophilic pneumonia

*Pathologic findings of UIP and NSIP.
BOOP, bronchiolitis obliterans with organizing pneumonia; CHF, congestive heart failure; CVD, collagen vascular disease; IPF, idiopathic pulmonary fibrosis; NSIP, nonspecific interstitial pneumonitis; UIP, usual interstitial pneumonia.

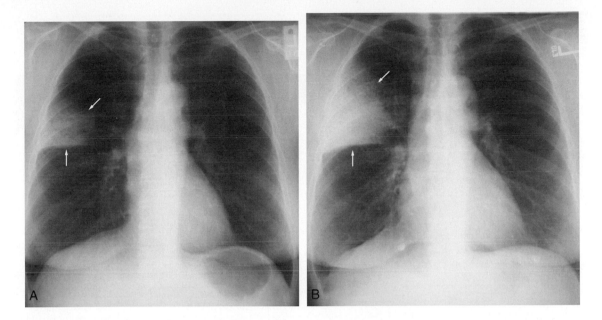

FIGURE 6-2 Serial posterior-anterior (PA) chest radiographs: bronchoalveolar carcinoma (BAC).

A, Frontal radiograph shows a homogeneous opacity in the anterior segment of the right upper lobe *(arrows)*. In an acutely ill patient this would very likely represent a community-acquired pneumonia.

B, PA radiograph of the same patient taken several months later shows expansion of the area of consolidation. Although BAC more commonly manifests as a solitary nodule, presentation of BAC as focal or diffuse air space disease is important to recognize since it can be mistaken for chronic pneumonia. Careful inspection of the radiograph reveals small nodules along the superior margin of the consolidation, a common finding in air space disease caused by bronchoalveolar cell carcinoma.

The nodular pattern of interstitial disease is formed by discrete, punctate opacities ranging from 1 mm in diameter (barely visible radiographically) to 5 mm in diameter. Although discernible on radiographs, the pattern is accentuated on HRCT (Fig. 6-3). There are only a few common causes: hematogenously spread infections, pneumoconioses, sarcoidosis, and occasionally metastatic disease (e.g., thyroid carcinoma) (Fig. 6-4). Miliary tuberculosis is the prototypical infectious disease that causes this type of chest radiographic pattern. Histoplasmosis and other fungal disease can cause an identical picture.

Silicosis and coal workers' pneumoconioses are the most common inhalation diseases. These diseases show upper lobe predominance, in contradistinction to the predilection of metastatic disease to affect the lower lobes. Sarcoidosis can also cause striking micronodular disease and can be difficult to differentiate from other diseases with a nodular pattern when intrathoracic adenopathy is absent (stage 3 disease; see later). Histiocytosis and allergic alveolitis can also have a nodular component on radiographs, but the nodularity is usually

not as striking. Although the appearance of sarcoid, silicosis, miliary infections, metastases, and so forth may appear similar on chest radiographs, HRCT has proved particularly useful in differentiating these diseases. For instance, HRCT of miliary infections shows the nodules to be randomly distributed through the lungs whereas sarcoid granulomas are concentrated around bronchovascular bundles and along pleural surfaces (see later). Algorithms for using HRCT to sort out nodular diseases are available in many in-depth pulmonary radiology texts.

Radiographs of patients with reticular or reticulonodular disease show varying combinations of mesh-like opacities, sometimes mixed with tiny nodules. The fact that occasional nodules are seen in most reticular opacities should not be a surprise. If one imagines sticks (lines) thrown randomly into a pile, a few of the sticks are bound to be seen end on and appear as nodules. Radiographs with a very coarse reticular or reticulonodular pattern are also referred to as demonstrating "honeycombing." When this pattern is present, the strands in the mesh-like pattern may be so coarse that there appear

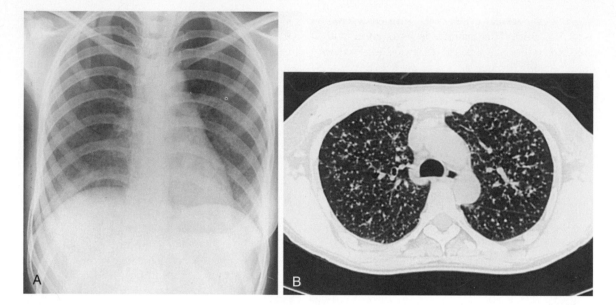

FIGURE 6-3 Posterior-anterior (PA) chest radiograph and high-resolution computed tomography (HRCT): miliary disease (tuberculosis).

A, Too-numerous-to-count 2- to 5-mm nodules are scattered throughout the pulmonary parenchymal fields, sparing the apices.

B, An HRCT single axial slice at the level of the carina demonstrates innumerable small nodules randomly distributed (not grouped around the bronchovascular structures).

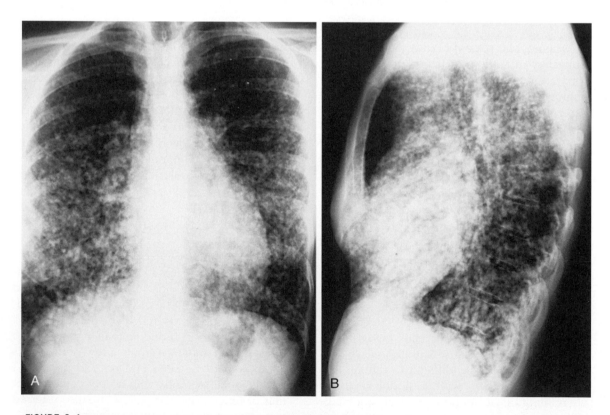

FIGURE 6-4 Posterior-anterior and lateral chest radiographs: metastatic thyroid carcinoma.

A and B, The nodules seen here are larger and appear more opaque than those seen with infectious and inflammatory miliary patterns. There is basilar predominance, as is usual with hematogenous metastases. Melanoma metastases can also present with this appearance.

to be individual cysts, or "ring shadows" (see Fig. 5-4). This pattern is associated with the late stages of several diseases and is an earlier manifestation of a few conditions (e.g., histiocytosis). Cystic bronchiectasis may have a similar appearance on a chest radiograph but, unlike most cases of honeycombing, is usually most evident centrally in the lung. Cystic bronchiectasis is also easily differentiated from honeycombing on HRCT, where the small cysts can be seen to connect with the bronchial tree.

Unfortunately, the last category of radiographic patterns, reticulonodular or "everything else," contains scores of diseases. This makes the differential diagnosis difficult to limit by using the chest radiograph alone. When confronted with this pattern it is crucial to look for other findings that might help limit the diagnosis. For instance, if pleural disease is apparent, one should think about the possibility of rheumatoid arthritis or asbestosis. If the patient is undergoing chemotherapy, the patients' medications should be reviewed and possible drug toxicity considered as a cause for the reticular pattern.

Evaluation of the spatial distribution of disease on a plain radiograph also helps direct the differential diagnosis, although not as much as observations about the pattern of opacities. The most common chronic infiltrative diseases that preferentially affect the upper lobes are silicosis, sarcoidosis, and eosinophilic granuloma. Hypersensitivity pneumonitis is much more common than eosinophilic granuloma, and although it can preferentially affect the upper lobes, differential involvement between upper and lower lobe is often not striking on chest radiographs. When looking for upper lobe predominance it is important to think about the shape of the thorax. Viewed from the front, the lung is much thicker at the bases than at the apices. The extra lung tissue at the bases can trick the observer into thinking that a disease is evenly distributed through the lung even if in reality the upper zones are more severely affected (Fig. 6-5). Looking at the lateral radiograph can help to determine whether the upper lung zone is really preferentially involved. Aside from the diseases already mentioned, most chronic infiltrative diseases involve the lung bases more extensively than the upper lung. These include usual interstitial pneumonitis (UIP) and asbestosis (Table 6-2).

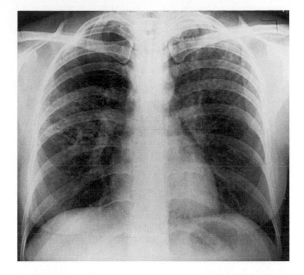

FIGURE 6-5 Posterior-anterior chest radiograph: sarcoidosis. The radiograph of a patient with sarcoidosis shows a nodular interstitial pattern with an upper lobe predominance. (In light of this lung parenchymal disease and the absence of definite hilar adenopathy, this case would represent stage 3 sarcoidosis; see text.)

Lastly, it is important to remember that most infiltrative diseases make the lung stiffer than usual, and therefore the lungs appear small, or "hypoinflated" on chest radiographs. It can be difficult to differentiate hypoinflation caused by stiff lungs from hypoinflation related to poor effort. It is important to look for extrapulmonary causes of hypoinflation (e.g., obesity, ascites). After that, review of serial radiographs helps to determine whether an infiltrative disease is truly present. Patients with lungs that remain "small" on multiple radiographs (in both frontal

TABLE 6-2
Distribution of Diffuse Infiltrative Diseases on Chest Radiograph

Upper lobes > lower lobes
Sarcoidosis
Silicosis
Eosinophilic granuloma

Diffuse
Hypersensitivity pneumonitis
Miliary tuberculosis, miliary metastases

Lower lobes > upper lobes
Usual interstitial pneumonitis
Asbestosis
Infiltrative disease associated with collagen
   vascular disease

and lateral projections) are more likely to harbor true pathology. As noted earlier, true basilar lung disease is often most visible along the lateral chest wall.

☐ HIGH-RESOLUTION COMPUTED TOMOGRAPHY

HRCT is key to the evaluation of chronic infiltrative lung disease. An in-depth description of the parenchymal abnormalities seen on HRCT is beyond the scope of this text. In general terms, HRCT can be thought of as a method of detecting fibrosis, micronodules (nodules <1 cm in size), thickening of tissues around lymphatics (see later), and small areas of ground glass or consolidation. Just as with chest radiographs, once abnormalities are detected, it is important to characterize their spatial distribution.

Infiltrative diseases can be divided into those that mainly affect the periphery (cortex) of the lung and those that affect the central portions (medulla) of the lung. The axial distribution of disease can sometimes be determined by evaluating the chest radiograph, but the pattern is often more obvious on either conventional CT or HRCT. Infiltrative diseases such as idiopathic pulmonary fibrosis and asbestosis result in fibrosis that is predominantly peripheral in distribution (Fig. 6-6). Chronic eosinophilic pneumonia, BOOP, and some vasculitides cause peripheral ground glass and consolidation. In contrast, sarcoidosis and lymphoma are more likely to involve nodules that are clustered along the bronchovascular bundles.

In addition to defining the distribution of disease as either central or peripheral, HRCT is used to localize parenchymal abnormalities by their relationship to a lung structure called the "secondary pulmonary lobule." Understanding the architecture of the secondary pulmonary lobule helps explain the distribution and appearance of disease on CT scans. The secondary lobule is the smallest discrete portion of the lung surrounded by connective tissue septa. The lobules are polyhedral structures about 1 to 2 cm in diameter and are best defined at the lung periphery and lung bases. A lobular bronchiole and lobular artery run in the center of the lobule and veins run peripherally in the septum. Lymphatics travel in the pleura, in the septum, and centrally along the bronchi (Fig. 6-7).

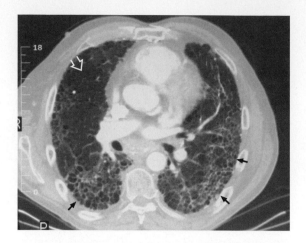

FIGURE 6-6 High-resolution computed tomography scan: usual interstitial pneumonia/interstitial pulmonary fibrosis. Axial HRCT demonstrates the peripheral predominance of severe fibrosis manifest as multiple rows of small peripheral cysts, termed honeycombing *(arrows)*. Note that a portion of the lung *(open arrow)* appears relatively normal. This heterogeneity of fibrosis is characteristic of usual interstitial pneumonia.

In light of this lung architecture, it makes sense that diseases that are caused by damage to the small airways affect the center of the lobule, around the bronchiole This is where hypersensitivity pneumonitis forms nodules caused by immunologic reaction to inhaled antigens. It is also where chronic inhalation of cigarette smoke first affects the lung, causing *centrilobular* emphysema and respiratory bronchiolitis (see later). Similarly, the distribution of lymphatics in the secondary lobule explains why lymphangitic carcinoma causes thickening of the lobular septa. Because sarcoid also involves the lymphatic system, it forms nodules that cluster along the lymphatics in the septa, pleura, and along the bronchi (Fig. 6-8). Lymphoproliferative diseases in the lung parenchyma may have a similar distribution in the lung parenchyma. Diseases that are spread through the blood stream, such as miliary tuberculosis, are not confined to the airways in the center of the lobule or to the lymphatics. As these organisms spread through the blood stream, these foci of infection are randomly distributed in the secondary lobule, against the pleura, near the central bronchiole, or anywhere in between. Some describe this distribution as random. Like blood-borne disease, fibrosis often affects multiple parts of the secondary lobule. Fibrosis may thicken the interlobular septa,

SCHEMATIC OF LUNG SECONDARY LOBULE

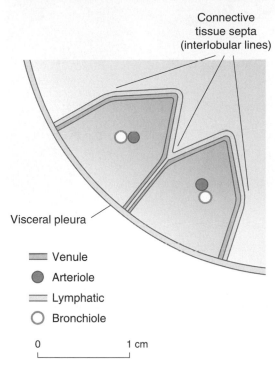

Connective
tissue septa
(interlobular lines)

Visceral pleura

▭ Venule
● Arteriole
▭ Lymphatic
○ Bronchiole

0 _____ 1 cm

FIGURE 6-7 Diagram of secondary lobule. The connective tissue septa that divide the lobules are seen well only if thickened pathologically, such as in lymphangitic carcinoma. They are most evident in the peripheral lung and at the lung bases.

distort centrilobular bronchioles, and fill the lobule with tiny net-like lines (termed irregular lines) (Table 6-3). Because the entire lobule may be involved, this distribution is also described as "panlobular."

TABLE 6-3

Distribution of Infiltrative Disease as Seen on High-Resolution Computed Tomography

Distribution of disease with respect to the entire lung

Peripheral—examples: usual interstitial pneumonitis, bronchiolitis obliterans with organizing pneumonia

Central (bronchovascular)—examples: sarcoid, lymphoproliferative diseases

Diffuse—examples: miliary infections, hypersensitivity pneumonitis

Distribution of disease with respect to the secondary lobule

Centrilobular (center of the lobule)—example: hypersensitivity pneumonitis

Perilymphatic (periphery of lobule)— examples: lymphangitic carcinoma, sarcoid

Panlobular or random—examples: fibrosis, miliary infection

Used together with the patient's history, these plain film and HRCT findings refine the differential diagnosis enough to guide important clinical decisions. For instance, if the history, chest radiograph, and HRCT all suggest silicosis, a biopsy is usually unnecessary. If the same indicators point toward sarcoidosis or lymphangitic carcinoma, a bronchoscopic biopsy is very likely to be diagnostic and should be performed instead of a surgical procedure (see the section on sarcoidosis and Fig. 6-8). When an open biopsy is indicated, HRCT may be helpful in selecting the optimal biopsy site.

The remainder of this chapter describes a few of the more common diffuse infiltrative

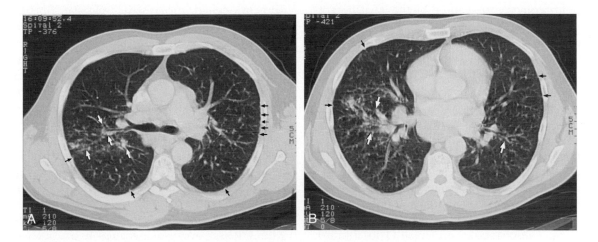

FIGURE 6-8 High-resolution computed tomography: sarcoidosis.

A and **B**, Axial HRCT sections at the level of the carina and upper lobes. Images show innumerable tiny nodules. Most nodules are clumped around bronchi and blood vessels *(white arrows)* and many are visible adjacent to the pleural surface *(black arrows)*. This is the characteristic distribution of diseases that involve the lung lymphatics.

lung diseases mentioned earlier. Diffuse infectious disease is discussed in Chapter 7 and neoplastic lung is discussed in more depth in Chapter 9.

☐ SPECIFIC DISEASES

Most classification systems have an arbitrary component, and categorization schemes for chronic diffuse lung disease are not exceptions. Nevertheless, a classification system is an indispensable aid in grappling with the large number of diseases that have in common the ability to affect the lung parenchyma diffusely. In this chapter, we divide diffuse infiltrative lung diseases into those that have a proven link to inhalation of a specific mineral (pneumoconiosis), those for which there is strong evidence of an immunologic origin (collagen vascular diseases and allergic alveolitis), and those that are characterized by abnormal proliferations of cells (chronic eosinophilic pneumonia and BOOP). We have included sarcoid, the eosinophilic pneumonias, and eosinophilic granuloma in the latter category because their pathogenesis is closely linked to the abnormal proliferation of granulomas, eosinophils, or histiocytes, respectively. Idiopathic pneumonias are considered separately.

☐ PNEUMOCONIOSES

Silicosis

Pneumoconioses are caused by the inhalation of inorganic dusts and differ from many of the diseases associated with toxic inhalants discussed in Chapter 8 in that the pathologic process occurs over many years. Most pneumoconioses are caused by inorganic dusts with which patients come in contact during occupational exposure.

Silicosis is a common pneumoconiosis produced by the inhalation of silica or silicon dioxide. Diffuse air space disease can occur in response to a massive exposure, for example, after unprotected sandblasting. More commonly, chronic silicosis (from mining, foundry work, and so on) produces a nodular pattern on radiographs. These nodules are small (1 to 10 mm) and have an upper lobe predominance. Sometimes there is an associated reticular pattern. Rarely, peripherally calcified hilar nodes ("egg shell calcifications") are present. The last

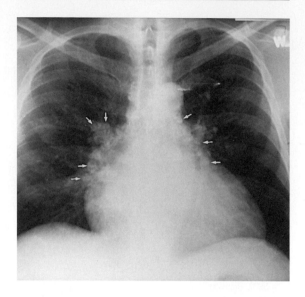

FIGURE 6-9 Posterior-anterior chest radiograph: silicosis with eggshell (lymph node) calcification. This frontal radiograph demonstrates easily seen bilateral hilar adenopathy, some nodes showing peripheral eggshell calcification *(arrows)*. The middle and upper lung reticulonodular interstitial pattern is difficult to see on this image.

finding is nearly pathognomonic for silicosis (Fig. 6-9). Sarcoidosis, granulomatous disease, or lymphoma that has been treated can occasionally mimic these findings.

Patients with multiple small parenchymal nodules have simple silicosis and rarely suffer from significant physiologic impairment. In a minority of patients, the disease progresses, and these smaller nodules coalesce to form parenchymal masses. Patients with this development, called progressive massive fibrosis (PMF), are often symptomatic and have diminished pulmonary function (Fig. 6-10).

The masses formed by PMF usually occur in the upper lobes and gradually extend toward the hilum, placing traction on the remainder of the lung. Unlike carcinoma, masses from PMF are usually bilateral and often oblong (rather than spherical). The radiographic findings are characteristic but by themselves are inadequate to differentiate PMF from a bronchogenic neoplasm. A good occupational history and prior radiographs are crucial to avoid unnecessary biopsy.

Chest CT is useful for evaluation of patients with silicosis because it makes it possible to see small masses that represent PMF before they become apparent on plain radiographs. CT is also more sensitive in identifying traction-related emphysema, the finding that most

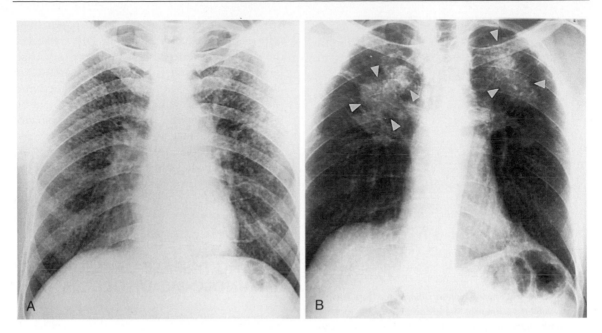

__FIGURE 6-10__ Serial posterior-anterior chest views: silicosis with progressive massive fibrosis (PMF).

A, Radiograph demonstrates the typical diffuse nodular pattern of simple silicosis with characteristic upper lung predominance.

B, Progression in simple silicosis with bilateral coalescence of silica nodules forming irregular masses *(arrowheads)* in the upper lobes. PMF masses are usually in the midlung zone and their outer margins may parallel the chest wall. Note that the number of visible small nodules has decreased as they have been incorporated into the large masses. The lung surrounding the masses is very low in attenuation because of traction emphysema.

closely correlates with physiologic impairment (Fig. 6-11). Although no treatment for silicosis is available, radiography is helpful in determining prognosis and evaluating the extent of disability. Unfortunately, CT (like plain radiographs) cannot unequivocally differentiate masses of PMF from bronchogenic carcinoma (Fig. 6-12). Neither can it exclude the possibility of concomitant tuberculous infection, for which these patients are at increased risk.

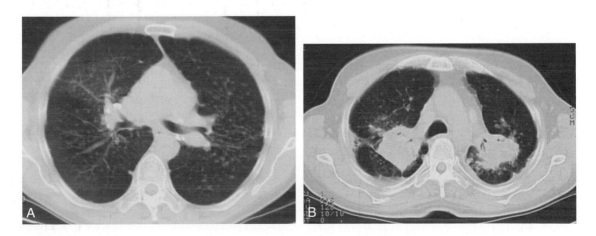

__FIGURE 6-11__ High-resolution computed tomography: simple silicosis and silicosis with progressive massive fibrosis and emphysema.

A, Single axial scan through the upper lung fields shows diffuse nodules, 2 to 5 mm in diameter. Nodules are seen adjacent to the pleura and on the left nodules coalesce and appear similar to a pleural plaque (pseudoplaque). Lymph node calcifications are also evident.

B, Single axial HRCT section in a different patient. Large bilateral upper lobe masses and a few scattered micronodules are present. In the adjacent lung there are areas of decreased lung markings caused by traction emphysema. This occurs as lung tissue is stretched as it is drawn toward the fibrotic masses.

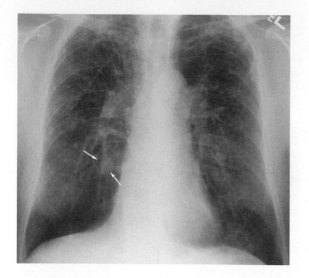

FIGURE 6-12 Posterior-anterior radiograph of patient with silicosis and lung carcinoma. Multiple small lung nodules are seen in the upper and midlung zones. There is early coalescence of nodules to form progressive massive fibrosis (PMF) in the right upper lobe with upward retraction of the hilum. A 2-cm nodule *(arrows)* caused by non-small cancer is also seen below the right hilum. A round nodule in the lower lung is unlikely to represent PMF.

Coal workers' pneumoconiosis is very similar to silicosis and produces a nodular pattern that can progress to PMF. Caplan's syndrome, the occurrence of necrobiotic lung nodules in patients with both rheumatoid arthritis and coal workers' pneumoconiosis, is often mentioned but rarely seen.

Asbestosis

Asbestos-related lung disease is also a common diffuse lung disease caused by inhaled inorganic material. The combined incidence of pleural disease caused by asbestos exposure (plaques, benign effusions, or diffuse fibrosis), however, is probably 5 to 10 times greater than the incidence of parenchymal disease (Fig. 6-13). Only the parenchymal lung disease is correctly called "asbestosis." This parenchymal disease produces a reticulonodular pattern on chest radiographs that is often indistinguishable from UIP. These changes are initially more prominent at the lung bases, causing a "shaggy heart" appearance. They become more generalized as the disease progresses.

HRCT has been shown to be more sensitive than plain film radiography in detecting the infiltrative disease caused by asbestosis (Fig. 6-14).

This includes findings of lung parenchyma fibrosis that look very much like UIP. (Detecting the subtle differences between the two diseases is very challenging for the authors.) HRCT is also better than radiography at the detection of pleural plaques, which are present in about 90% of patients with asbestosis. The combination of chronic interstitial and pleural disease suggests a differential diagnosis of rheumatoid lung, asbestosis, or talc inhalation. (Intravascular talc exposure from drug abuse produces a different, diffuse nodular pattern without accompanying pleural disease.)

☐ LUNG DISEASE CAUSED BY IMMUNOLOGIC DISORDERS

Collagen Vascular Disease

Rheumatoid arthritis is the collagen vascular disease most likely to affect the chest, usually resulting in pleural disease, which is discussed in Chapter 11. Interstitial disease is less common, but the reported incidence varies widely (ranging from 1% to 50%). This variation is probably influenced by the technique used for detection. Linear and reticular markings are most common at the lung bases and may progress to honeycombing (Fig. 6-15). Lung biopsy specimens and HRCT images usually show findings consistent with UIP or nonspecific interstitial pneumonitis (NSIP). Extensive fibrosis can lead to pulmonary hypertension and right-sided heart failure. Rarely, primary vasculitis can also cause pulmonary hypertension.

Several less common lung manifestations of rheumatoid arthritis (including Caplan's syndrome) occur. It is also worth remembering that a few patients with rheumatoid arthritis can develop bronchiolitis obliterans. The resulting airway obstruction causes hyperinflation that can be seen on chest radiographs.

Like rheumatoid arthritis, systemic lupus erythematosus (SLE) causes pleural disease more commonly than it affects lung parenchyma. Isolated diffuse infiltrative disease is relatively rare in patients with SLE. Patchy air space disease (lupus pneumonitis) and discoid atelectasis are more common. It is difficult to make a definite radiographic diagnosis of lupus pneumonitis because patchy air space disease and pleural effusions can also be caused by pneumonia and pulmonary embolism. Many patients with SLE

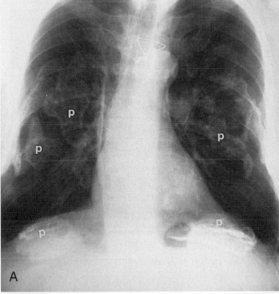

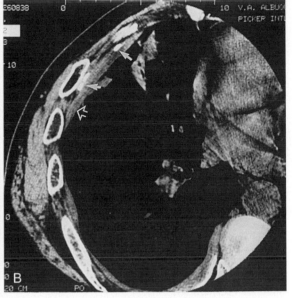

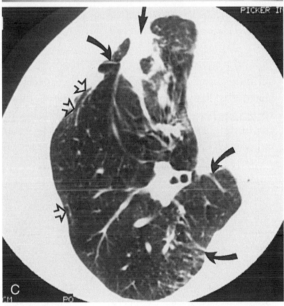

FIGURE 6-13 Posterior-anterior (PA) chest radiograph, conventional computed tomography (CT), and high-resolution CT (HRCT): asbestos pleural disease and early asbestosis.

A, PA chest view demonstrates multiple calcified pleural plaques (p) involving the diaphragm and the midhemithoraces bilaterally.

B, Conventional CT (different patient) with mediastinal windows highlights a parietal pleural plaque *(open arrow)* with focal areas of calcification *(solid arrows)*.

C, HRCT image of the right lower lobe (same patient as in part B) demonstrates parenchymal bands *(curved arrows)* and subpleural lines *(open arrows)*, both seen with asbestosis. No other signs of fibrosis, however, are seen. Rounded atelectasis, associated with asbestos pleural disease *(straight arrow)*, is also present.

are at increased risk for pneumonia because of their use of immunosuppressive agents. Patients with SLE may also be hypercoagulable owing to circulating lupus anticoagulants, nephrotic syndrome, or both and therefore are also at increased risk for pulmonary embolism.

Progressive systemic sclerosis (PSS or scleroderma) causes infiltrative lung disease that is reticular and predominantly basilar on radiographs and may progress to honeycombing. Esophageal disease is also frequent in patients with PSS, and a dilated air-filled esophagus may be seen on chest radiographs (Fig. 6-16). Abnormal esophageal motility and gastroesophageal sphincter function can lead to

chronic aspiration, and recurrent aspiration pneumonitis can contribute to the basilar lung opacities.

Interstitial disease is usually less severe in CREST syndrome (Calcinosis cutis, Raynaud's phenomenon, Esophageal dysfunction, Sclerodactyly, and Telangiectasia) than in PSS. Patients with CREST, however, more commonly develop pulmonary vasculitis and pulmonary hypertension. The latter diagnosis should be considered in the CREST syndrome patient who is breathless despite radiologically normal lung parenchyma.

Dermatomyositis and polymyositis may also cause interstitial lung disease. Respiratory muscle

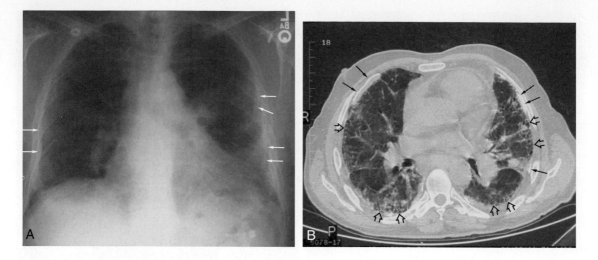

FIGURE 6-14 Posterior-anterior (PA) chest and computed tomography (CT) of patient with asbestosis.

A, PA chest shows bilateral pleural plaques that spare the costophrenic angles. The reticular opacities are more evident in the peripheral lower lung fields.

B, High-resolution CT images through the lung bases. The very short, irregular lines seen peripherally are intralobular lines *(open arrows)* and are a sign of fibrosis in the lung parenchyma. Calcified pleural plaques are also present *(solid arrows)*.

weakness can secondarily affect the lung by causing decreased lung volumes and atelectasis. Pharyngeal weakness can lead to aspiration. A summary of the more common manifestations of collagen vascular diseases is listed in Table 6-4.

Extrinsic Allergic Alveolitis

Extrinsic allergic alveolitis (EAA) or hypersensitivity pneumonitis is a hypersensitivity reaction within the lung parenchyma that can be caused by a variety of organic antigens, including

actinomycetes in moldy hay and avian proteins (farmer's lung and pigeon breeder's lung, respectively). The radiographic findings vary depending on the stage of the disease. Acute exposures can cause ground glass opacities or,

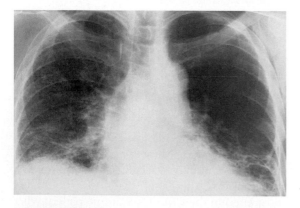

FIGURE 6-15 Posterior-anterior chest view: rheumatoid lung disease. Prominent reticular opacities are present with obvious lower lobe bias. Blunting of the right costophrenic angle may represent associated pleural disease.

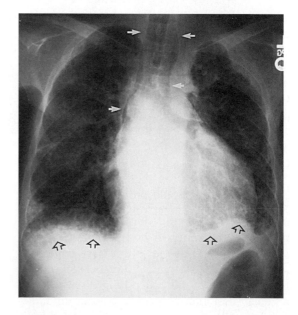

FIGURE 6-16 Posterior-anterior chest radiograph: progressive systemic sclerosis (scleroderma). Frontal radiograph shows widened air-filled esophagus *(solid arrowheads)*, termed an air esophagogram. Bibasilar coarse reticular opacities with honeycomb pattern *(open arrowheads)* are seen at the lung bases, caused by advanced fibrosis.

TABLE 6-4
Pulmonary Manifestations of Collagen Vascular Disease

Disease	Most Common Manifestation	Other Manifestations
Rheumatoid arthritis	Pleural disease	Interstitial fibrosis
Systemic lupus erythematosus	Pleural disease	Patchy air space disease, atelectasis, pericardial effusion
Progressive systemic sclerosis	Interstitial fibrosis	Aspiration pneumonitis, pulmonary hypertension
CREST syndrome	Pulmonary hypertension	Interstitial fibrosis, aspiration
Polymyositis	Interstitial fibrosis	Decreased lung volumes from muscular weakness

CREST, calcinosis cutis, Raynaud's phenomenon, esophageal dysfunction, sclerodactyly, and telangiectasia.

if the exposure is more intense, patchy air space disease. In the subacute stage, these opacities may evolve into an ill-defined nodular pattern. Continued, chronic exposure leads to a diffuse reticulonodular pattern and eventually to honeycombing. This stage can appear very similar to usual interstitial pneumonia (see later). Occasionally, acute findings can be superimposed on chronic interstitial changes. This radiographic pattern, acute air space disease superimposed on chronic reticulonodular changes, can also be caused by recurrent pulmonary hemorrhages (see discussion of vascular diseases, Chapter 10).

In patients with acute or subacute EAA, HRCT may show both nodules and patchy ground glass opacities. These ill-defined nodules are much easier to see on HRCT than on chest radiographs, and in some cases the nodules can be widespread and striking (Fig. 6-17). Although these findings are not diagnostic, they very strongly suggest the presence of EAA, particularly if there is evidence of air trapping caused by the obstruction of small airways. At times the history of an exposure to a significant antigen is initially overlooked. The presence of typical HRCT changes despite a negative exposure history should prompt a return to the bedside for a more detailed history.

☐ LUNG DISEASE CAUSED BY PROLIFERATION OF CELLS

Bronchiolitis Obliterans with Organizing Pneumonia (BOOP)

Bronchiolitis obliterans with organizing pneumonia is an infiltrative parenchymal disease that can cause chronic bilateral air space disease. The disease is caused by the proliferation of granulation tissue in bronchioles and alveoli. It can occur as part of a graft-versus-host reaction and following viral infections or noxious gas exposures but often is idiopathic (referred to as cryptogenic organizing pneumonia). Patients with BOOP develop symptoms over months. Findings on the chest radiograph are pleomorphic and include both focal nodules and patchy bilateral infiltrates that can be migratory (Fig. 6-18). If the air space disease occurs at the bases, the appearance can be similar to that of recurrent aspiration.

HRCT demonstrates bronchial wall thickening, small nodules, consolidation, and ground glass opacities. In immunocompetent hosts, there may be a peripheral distribution of air space

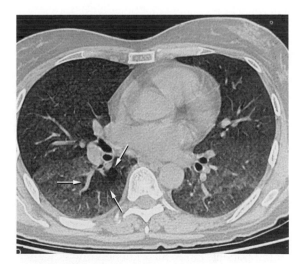

FIGURE 6-17 High-resolution computed tomography: extrinsic allergic alveolitis (EAA). Diffuse, poorly defined ground glass nodules are scattered evenly throughout the lung. This pattern, combined with proper clinical history, strongly suggests EAA. The low-attenuation (blacker) lung seen at the right base *(arrows)* represents air trapping caused by obstruction of small airways. This is also a common finding in EAA.

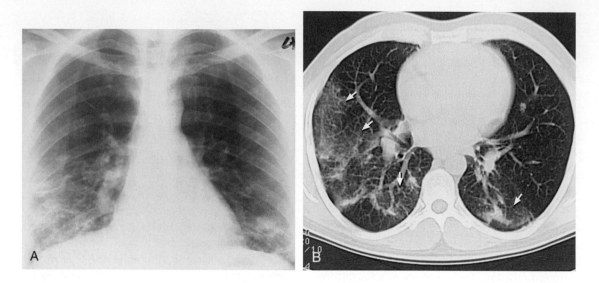

FIGURE 6-18 Posterior-anterior (PA) chest radiograph and computed tomography (CT): bronchiolitis obliterans with organizing pneumonia (BOOP). PA chest radiograph (A) and high-resolution CT (B) show bibasilar opacities. The peripheral distribution of opacities is typical of BOOP in a normal host.

disease very similar to that in chronic eosinophilic pneumonia. (Bone marrow transplant recipients may be less likely to manifest this peripheral distribution.) Alternatively, there can be a bronchovascular distribution. Like eosinophilic pneumonia, bronchiolitis obliterans with organizing pneumonia also readily responds to systemic steroids.

Sarcoidosis

Although the pathologic changes of sarcoidosis are immune mediated, the initiating agent or event for the disease remains elusive. Pathologically sarcoidosis is characterized by granuloma formation. The disease is pleomorphic and is commonly graded as stage 1, hilar and mediastinal nodal involvement (Fig. 6-19); stage 2, nodal and parenchymal involvement (Fig. 6-20); stage 3, parenchymal involvement alone (Fig. 6-21); and stage 4, pulmonary fibrosis (Fig. 6-22).

Stage 1 disease is often an incidental finding in an asymptomatic or minimally symptomatic young patient. Once hilar adenopathy is identified, the diagnoses of sarcoidosis and lymphoma (usually Hodgkin's) are both considered. Lymphoma involves predominantly the mediastinal nodes and, if it is Hodgkin's disease, almost always the anterior compartment (see Chapter 13). If hilar involvement is also present, it is often asymmetric. In contrast, hilar adenopathy in sarcoidosis is more pronounced than mediastinal involvement and is usually symmetric. Chest CT can delineate the distribution of adenopathy better than standard posterior-anterior and lateral chest radiographs (Fig. 6-23).

Stages 2 through 4 figure prominently in the differential diagnosis of chronic infiltrative lung disease. Parenchymal involvement by sarcoidosis can be nodular, reticulonodular, or, rarely, acinar (see earlier discussion of chronic air space disease). The nodular pattern is often diffuse but can show upper lobe predominance. Scarring with marked distortion of the parenchyma, including cavity formation, can occur in stage 4 disease.

In patients with parenchymal involvement, HRCT can suggest the diagnosis of sarcoidosis by showing that many of the nodular opacities cluster about the bronchovascular bundles and, to a lesser extent, about the pleura and fissures. This bronchocentric pattern of sarcoid probably accounts for the fact that transbronchial biopsy often yields a histologic diagnosis and that thoracotomy or thoracoscopy can usually be avoided.

The presence of acute onset of constitutional symptoms, erythema nodosum, and asymptomatic adenopathy is referred to as Löfgren's syndrome (no relation to the author). This and most other cases of stage 1 sarcoid regress spontaneously, but the course of the other stages is more difficult to predict. If imaging could be

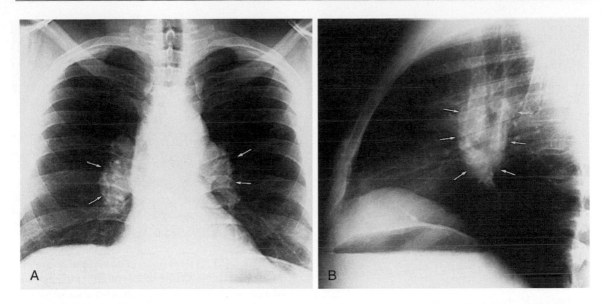

FIGURE 6-19 Posterior-anterior and lateral chest views: stage 1 sarcoidosis.

A, The enlarged bilateral perihilar lymph nodes *(arrows)* are not accompanied by parenchymal disease, consistent with stage 1 sarcoid, in this asymptomatic patient.

B, Lateral radiograph of the same patient shows enlarged lymph nodes *(arrows)* surrounding the hilar vessels and bronchi. No parenchymal abnormalities are seen.

used to identify the cases of sarcoid most likely to progress, these patients might warrant early treatment with steroids or other medications. Unfortunately, the role of imaging in predicting the course of sarcoid remains inconclusive.

Eosinophilic Lung Disease

A variety of drugs and infectious agents (usually parasitic) have been associated with peripheral blood eosinophilia and pulmonary infiltrates. Löffler's syndrome consists of idiopathic

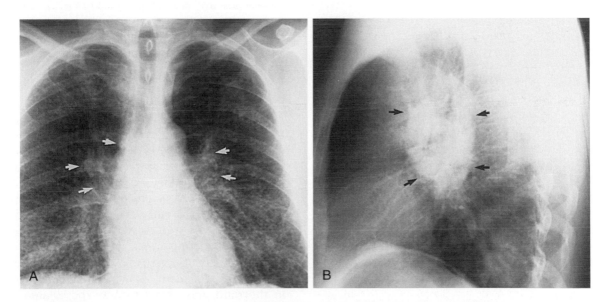

FIGURE 6-20 Posterior-anterior and lateral chest views: stage 2 sarcoidosis.

A, A diffuse reticulonodular disease pattern is present (without upper lobe bias in this case) (see Fig. 6-5). Bilateral hilar and right paratracheal adenopathy is present *(arrows)*.

B, Lateral chest radiograph demonstrates perihilar enlarged lymph nodes *(arrows)*.

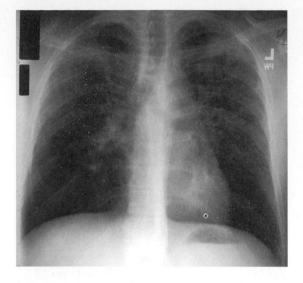

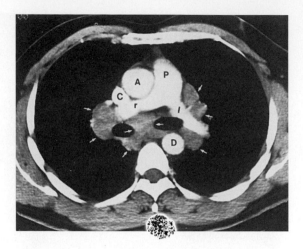

FIGURE 6-21 Posterior-anterior chest view: stage 3 sarcoidosis. A reticulonodular pattern is seen, predominating in the middle and upper lung fields. No definite lymph node enlargement is visible.

FIGURE 6-23 Contrast-enhanced conventional computed tomography: sarcoidosis with mediastinal and hilar lymph node enlargement. A single axial slice at the subcarinal level with contrast enhancement demonstrates extensive hilar and mediastinal adenopathy *(arrows)* associated with stage 2 sarcoidosis (same patient as in Fig. 6-20). Note the superior vena cava (C), ascending aorta (A), main pulmonary artery (P), descending aorta (D), and right (r) and left (l) pulmonary arteries.

eosinophilia accompanied by pulmonary infiltrates that change position over days. Symptoms are usually minimal and chest radiographs are often not obtained.

Chronic eosinophilic lung disease is also an idiopathic process. It characteristically affects women aged 20 to 50, causing ill-defined air space disease. Classically, these infiltrates are located peripherally, most prominently in the upper lobes (Fig. 6-24). Most patients with chronic eosinophilic pneumonia, however, do not have these classical findings on chest radiographs. HRCT can demonstrate peripheral distribution in cases in which it is not evident on a plain chest radiograph. Alternatively, the diagnosis can be suggested if the chest radiographs show a rapid response to corticosteroids.

Eosinophilic Granuloma

Eosinophilic granuloma, or pulmonary Langerhans cell histiocytosis, is an uncommon cause of infiltrative lung disease. The disease is caused by abnormal proliferation of a specific subgroup of histiocytes (Langerhans cells) within the lungs. More generalized proliferation of Langerhans cells can cause severe disease in children, and focal disease can affect bones in children and young adults.

Pulmonary Langerhans cell histiocytosis, eosinophilic granuloma, is most often diagnosed in the third and fourth decade and is almost always free of involvement of other organs. Almost all patients with the disease are cigarette smokers. Radiographs typically show a coarse reticular pattern that is more prominent

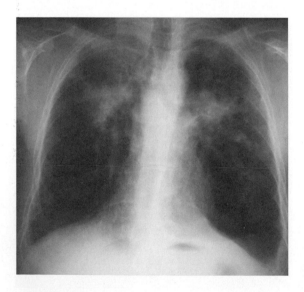

FIGURE 6-22 Posterior-anterior chest view: stage 4 sarcoidosis. A few nodular opacities are present. The lung parenchyma is distorted by fibrotic masses in the upper lobes, producing a similar radiographic appearance to that of silicosis with progressive massive fibrosis.

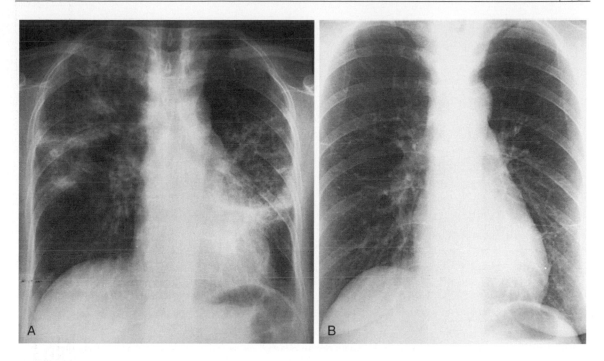

FIGURE 6-24 Posterior-anterior chest films: chronic eosinophilic pneumonia.

A, Frontal radiograph demonstrates patchy middle and upper lobe air space disease that is more peripheral than central. Had high-resolution computed tomography been performed, it might have shown more convincing "mantle" peripheral predominance.

B, Frontal radiograph of the same patient following steroid treatment shows dramatic resolution of the infiltrates.

in the upper lung zones, tends to involve the central lung parenchyma more than the peripheral lung, and often spares the costophrenic angles (Fig. 6-25).

Most diffuse infiltrative lung diseases make the lung parenchyma stiffer and therefore more difficult for the lungs to expand. The patient's lungs therefore appear smaller than normal on chest radiographs. Eosinophilic granuloma is one of the few diffuse infiltrative lung diseases in which lung volumes usually appear normal. Lung volumes are also normal or increased in lymphangiomyomatosis (which is very rare). More commonly, if a patient's lungs appear normally expanded despite the presence of infiltrative lung disease, chronic obstructive pulmonary disease (COPD) is also present. COPD causes overexpansion of portions of the lung that compensates for decreased expansion of lung tissue stiffened by infiltrative disease.

HRCT of eosinophilic granuloma shows that the coarse reticular markings seen on radiographs actually represent cyst walls. Nodules and ground glass opacities can also be seen.

Taken together with the patient's history, these findings strongly suggest the diagnosis.

Lymphangitic Carcinoma

Lymphangitic carcinoma is also discussed in Chapter 9. It is a form of lung metastasis in which tumor cells spread along the lymphatics adjacent to the bronchi and within the lobular septa. Radiographs show Kerley's B lines, which may be unilateral or bilateral, often accompanied by pleural effusions (Fig. 6-26). HRCT images show thickening of the lobular septa and thickening of the tissues along the bronchovascular bundles. The distribution of disease is similar to that of sarcoid, but usually the two diseases can be told apart. In cases of lymphangitic spread, lobular septa are usually even thicker than seen with sarcoid but the nodules are usually smaller and less numerous. As with sarcoid, transbronchial biopsy is usually successful in making a diagnosis because disease travels along the bronchovascular bundles. If HRCT and the clinical setting strongly

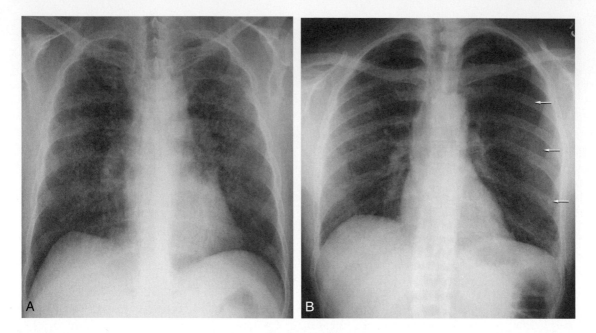

FIGURE 6-25 Posterior-anterior (PA) chest radiographs: two patients with eosinophilic granuloma (pulmonary Langerhans histiocytosis).

A, A symmetric, coarse reticulonodular pattern with upper lobe predominance and sparing of the costophrenic angles is present. Note the lack of peripheral predominance, usually seen in cases of fibrosis from other disease.

B, PA radiograph of a different patient shows a faintly seen reticular pattern and normal lung volumes. A pneumothorax is also present *(arrows)*. Although many infiltrative lung diseases predispose patients to pneumothoraces, a coarse reticulonodular disease accompanied by a pneumothorax is a classical presentation for eosinophilic pneumonia.

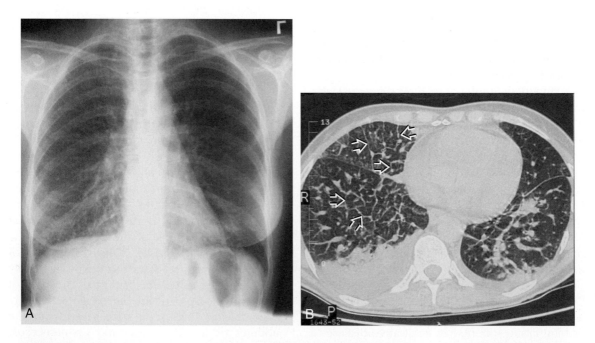

FIGURE 6-26 Posterior-anterior chest radiograph and high-resolution computed tomography: lymphangitic carcinoma.

A, Frontal radiograph shows linear interstitial opacities most apparent in the right lung.

B, HRCT. There is marked thickening of the septa between the secondary lobules at the lung bases, more widespread on the right *(arrows)*, caused by infiltration with malignant cells. A posterior pleural effusion is present.

suggest the diagnosis, however, biopsy is unnecessary.

☐ THE IDIOPATHIC PNEUMONIAS

It is hard for physicians to develop a systematic approach to idiopathic pneumonias. It is made particularly difficult by the use of both nomenclature based on pathology and nomenclature based on clinical presentation to categorize these diseases. In addition to bronchiolitis obliterans with organizing pneumonia (described earlier), there are six recognized pathologic types of idiopathic interstitial pneumonia (Table 6-5). In some cases the pathologic diagnosis can be related to specific causes; in other cases the etiology of the pathologic changes is unknown. For instance, UIP is a pathologic diagnosis that describes a heterogeneous fibrosing process in the lung. When the patient is free of underlying diseases that might produce similar pathologic changes in the lung (e.g., rheumatoid arthritis), the patient is diagnosed as having idiopathic pulmonary fibrosis (or, in Britain, cryptogenic fibrosing alveolitis).

Idiopathic pulmonary fibrosis is a disease of unknown etiology that results in pulmonary fibrosis that has the pathologic pattern of UIP (see earlier). In the past, this disease was thought to have an inflammatory component, but it is now recognized to be a fibrogenic disorder in which there is abnormal proliferation of fibrous tissue in the lung without a prior inflammatory stimulus. The disease characteristically affects lung in an inhomogeneous pattern, some portions of the lungs showing end-stage fibrosis, other portions appearing nearly normal. If a biopsy is needed, samples from multiple locations are required because of the

inhomogeneity of the disease. Currently, the diagnosis is often made by history and HRCT pattern.

Radiographs show a reticular pattern, most extensive in the lung periphery and at the lung bases (Fig. 6-27; see Figs. 5-10 and 5-11). Lung volumes are diminished. In fact, the fall in lung volumes over time can be the most obvious radiographic finding, even in cases of moderately severe disease. In patients with both interstitial fibrosis and COPD, the opposing effects of the two diseases may balance each other, and the lung volume can remain normal (Fig. 6-28). HRCT demonstrates that the changes of fibrosis are mainly peripheral in location (see Figs. 6-6 and 6-27). These changes include multiple small cysts that are arranged in layers (honeycombing) and mild bronchiectasis caused by the fibrotic lung "pulling open" the distal bronchi (traction bronchiectasis) (see Fig. 6-1). Thickened interlobular septa (about 1 to 1.5 cm long) and shorter interlobular ("irregular") lines are also visible in the lung periphery.

A type of idiopathic pneumonia called nonspecific interstitial pneumonitis has been described. This infiltrative disease tends to be more homogeneous than UIP and often has a better prognosis. Also unlike the findings in UIP, at least some cases of NSIP do not show evidence of much fibrotic tissue. This disease is still incompletely understood and will probably turn out to be several different diseases that we currently lump together.

Desquamative interstitial pneumonitis (DIP), another idiopathic pneumonia, was once considered a precursor of UIP but now is recognized as a separate entity. DIP and respiratory bronchiolitis with interstitial lung disease (RBILD) are both caused by the abnormal deposition of macrophages in the alveoli, and both

TABLE 6-5
Pathologic Types of Idiopathic Interstitial Pneumonia

Pathologic Diagnosis	Incidence	Common Etiologies
Usual interstitial pneumonitis (UIP)	Common	Idiopathic pulmonary fibrosis
Nonspecific interstitial pneumonitis (NSIP)	Common	Drug-induced lung toxicity, CVD-associated lung disease
Acute interstitial pneumonitis (AIP)	Uncommon	Idiopathic (viral?)
Respiratory bronchiolitis and interstitial lung disease	Uncommon	Smoking related
Desquamative interstitial pneumonitis	Rare	Smoking related
Lymphoid interstitial pneumonitis	Rare	Sjögren's syndrome, HIV infection

CVD, collagen vascular disease; HIV, human immunodeficiency virus.

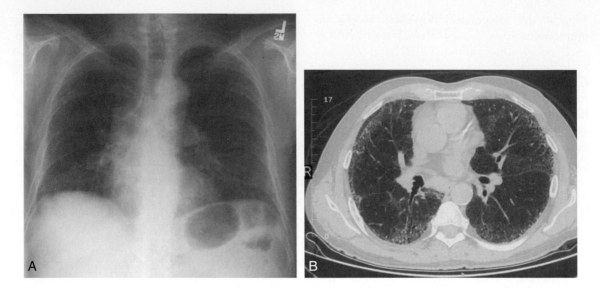

FIGURE 6-27 Posterior-anterior (PA) radiograph and high-resolution computed tomography: early usual interstitial pneumonia.

A, PA chest radiograph in a patient with early UIP shows diminished lung volumes and a faint reticular pattern that is better seen at the lung periphery.

B, HRCT section in the same patient. Intralobular (irregular) lines are seen in the periphery of the lower lung. Early traction bronchiectasis is present in the right lower lobe.

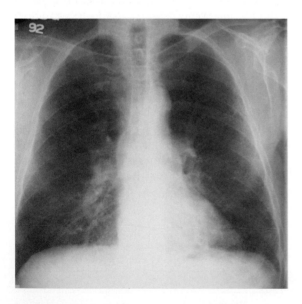

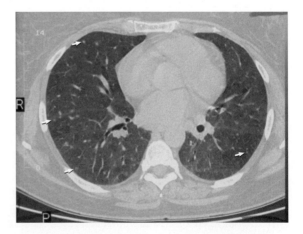

FIGURE 6-28 Posterior-anterior chest view: chronic obstructive pulmonary disease and diffuse interstitial fibrosis. PA chest radiograph shows reticular opacities in the peripheral lung caused by fibrosis. Because chronic obstructive pulmonary disease is also present, the lung volumes have remained normal. Note the enlargement of the right descending pulmonary artery, caused by mild pulmonary hypertension.

FIGURE 6-29 High-resolution computed tomography: respiratory bronchiolitis with interstitial lung disease (RBILD). HRCT through the lower lungs in a patient with RBILD shows patchy ground glass opacity and scattered small nodules *(arrows)*. RBILD usually shows an upper lobe predilection. Lower lobe disease in this case is more commonly seen with desquamative interstitial pneumonitis (DIP). RBILD and DIP are similar pathologically, and both are associated with cigarette smoking.

are related to smoking. Both cause ground glass opacities on HRCT rather than fibrosis. RBILD is more common than DIP, but neither is common and the radiologic findings are subtle (Fig. 6-29). Radiologic diagnosis of either requires consultation with an experienced thoracic radiologist.

Although the mortality associated with DIP and RBILD is not as bad as that with UIP, the mortality in acute interstitial pneumonitis (AIP) is worse. In the distant past, AIP was sometimes called Hamman-Rich syndrome. This disease damages the lung parenchyma diffusely and is considered a kind of idiopathic adult respiratory distress syndrome. Patients who survive with the help of ventilatory support gradually develop HRCT findings consistent with diffuse fibrosis.

Pearls for Clinicians—Pneumoconiosis, Immunologic and Proliferative Lung Disease

1. When confronted with a chest radiograph showing diffuse infiltrative lung disease, first determine whether the disease is acute or chronic. Prior radiographs are crucial.
2. Try to characterize diffuse infiltrative lung disease seen on a radiograph as a chronic air space pattern or as a linear, nodular, or reticular/reticulonodular pattern (see Table 6-1). If more than one pattern seems to be present, use the dominant pattern.
3. If there is a reticular (net-like) pattern in the lung but you are not sure whether it is caused by bronchial thickening or by infiltrative lung disease, look at the periphery of the lung. If the pattern is most prominent in the lung periphery, an infiltrative disease is more likely the cause.
4. Assess the lung volumes. Unexplained hypoinflation (e.g., no evidence of ascites, obesity, or recent surgery) on multiple chest radiographs may be the sign of infiltrative lung disease that appears before other abnormalities are evident on chest radiographs.
5. High-resolution CT is a very useful tool for diagnosing specific types of infiltrative lung disease, but the clinical history is crucial when CT patterns of different diseases are similar. For instance, the patient's occupational history helps differentiate sarcoid from silicosis, and smoking history differentiates hypersensitivity pneumonitis from RBILD. (Patients with hypersensitivity pneumonitis rarely smoke; patients with RBILD always do.)

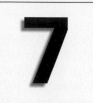

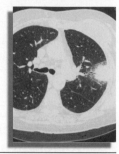

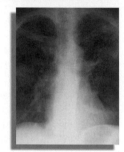

Infectious Lung Disease

For most clinicians, the working definition of pneumonia is the presence of both an abnormal opacity on the chest radiograph and signs and symptoms of respiratory infection (fever, cough, and sputum production). Unfortunately, many other diseases can mimic the radiographic features of infection. Congestive heart failure can cause diffuse interstitial abnormalities or air space disease. The latter more closely imitates pneumonia when it takes on an atypical, asymmetric pattern because of underlying lung disease such as chronic obstructive pulmonary disease (Fig. 7-1). Pulmonary infarction, acute drug toxicity, and pulmonary hemorrhage can all mimic acute pneumonia. The chest radiographs of patients with chronic diseases such as sarcoidosis, lymphoma, and alveolar cell carcinoma may also be indistinguishable from chest radiographs of patients with pneumonia. We often require prior radiographs to differentiate these diseases from acute infection. Even when infection is strongly suspected on clinical grounds, radiographic findings are rarely diagnostic of a specific microorganism (see later discussion).

Despite these limitations, the chest radiograph provides important data for the clinical management of pneumonia. In some cases, the extent of disease seen on the radiograph can have important prognostic significance (e.g., multilobar involvement in pneumococcal pneumonia is associated with increased mortality). The chest radiograph can also identify coexistent abnormalities and complications of pneumonia such as an effusion, empyema, bronchopleural fistula, mass, and hilar or mediastinal adenopathy. Some of the latter findings may be occult on initial radiographs and are visible only following resolution of the acute infection.

Although a specific organism usually cannot be singled out, the radiographic findings *combined* with clinical information can generate a short list of organisms that are the most likely cause of the infection. In order to do this, the clinician needs to categorize the radiographic findings. Is it a lobar pneumonia, a bronchopneumonia, a cavitary pneumonia, or an interstitial pneumonia? Is it focal or diffuse? Chapter 5 describes the appearance of air space disease (for example, lobar pneumonia) and interstitial disease. Although the terms "air space" and "interstitial" disease are pathologically imprecise (see Chapter 6), these terms and the conventional descriptions that follow

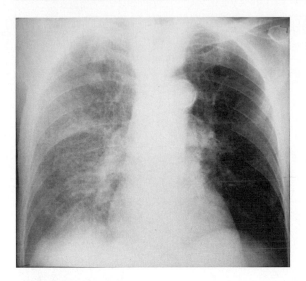

FIGURE 7-1 Posterior-anterior (PA) chest examination: congestive heart failure with asymmetric pulmonary edema (simulating pneumonia). The diffuse reticular pattern is notably asymmetric. The interstitial edema is greater on the right because of the patient's preference to lie on his right side. The cardiac silhouette is only minimally enlarged.

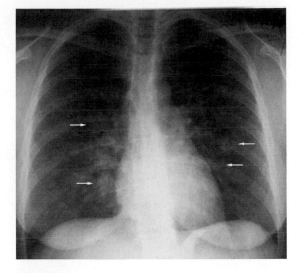

FIGURE 7-2 Posterior-anterior chest radiographs of bilateral bronchopneumonia. Radiograph shows bilateral patchy opacities within the parenchyma accompanied by bronchial wall thickening *(arrows)*. No air bronchograms are visible.

provide a practical way of describing common pneumonias.

Lobar or segmental pneumonia characteristically produces a homogeneous opacity with prominent air bronchograms. This occurs because the inflammatory exudate replaces the air in the alveoli. Because much of the air is replaced with liquid, there is usually not significant volume loss acutely. Accordingly, an opaque lobe that is markedly smaller than normal is much more likely to be due to atelectasis than to lobar pneumonia. The most aggressive infections may cause lobar expansion related to lung necrosis and fluid exudation. If the process progresses to cavitation, lung volume can diminish.

If the infection and inflammation are centered in the bronchiole rather than the alveolus, bronchial wall thickening may be present with few air bronchograms. Small airways are likely to become obstructed because of infection in the bronchioles, resulting in patchy atelectasis. The degree of volume loss, however, is small and difficult to detect. Taken together, these radiographic characteristics, lack of air bronchograms, patchy opacities, and bronchial wall thickening, describe a bronchopneumonia (Fig. 7-2).

Alternatively, inflammatory infiltrates can be confined to the alveolar wall, lobular septa, and perivascular spaces. This produces a linear, mesh-like, or nodular pattern commonly referred to as interstitial disease (see interstitial disease, Chapter 5). Infectious processes may progress from interstitial to air space disease (e.g., *Pneumocystis carinii* pneumonia [PCP]) or show evidence of both patterns at the outset (Fig. 7-3).

Although the radiographic observations are important, it is crucial to consider the host and clinical presentation when generating a list of possible organisms causing the pneumonia. It is important to know whether the patient is ambulatory or hospitalized, an adult or a child. The patient's immune status is pivotal and can be categorized as normal, immunocompromised without acquired immunodeficiency syndrome (AIDS), or immunocompromised with AIDS.

☐ PATTERNS OF PNEUMONIA IN THE NORMAL HOST

Radiographs of pneumonia in normal hosts, patients who are not immunosuppressed, can usually be characterized by one of four patterns: lobar pneumonia, bronchopneumonia, cavitary disease, or interstitial pneumonia. Some patients have radiographs with mixes of more than one pattern.

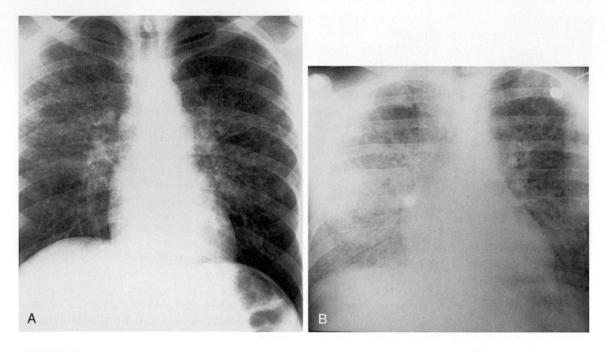

FIGURE 7-3 Posterior-anterior chest examinations: *Pneumocystis carinii* pneumonia (PCP) (interstitial pattern).

A, Perihilar reticular nodular pattern consistent with PCP.

B, Radiograph of an AIDS patient shows progression to air space disease in the right middle and lower lung field. The interstitial component remaining is best defined in the left lung.

Lobar Pneumonia

Lobar pneumonia is characterized by homogeneous opacification with well-defined air bronchograms. Among outpatients, it is most commonly caused by pneumococcus but can be caused by a wide range of organisms including *Legionella* (Fig. 7-4). *Pseudomonas* spp, *Enterobacter* spp, and *Serratia* spp can produce radiographically similar pneumonias but are usually seen in hospitalized patients after they have become colonized with gram-negative rods (Table 7-1).

A few lobar pneumonias increase the volume of the involved lobe, causing the adjacent fissures to bulge. This can be a marker for parenchymal necrosis or gangrene. Classically, this picture is seen with *Klebsiella pneumoniae* pneumonia, but *Staphylococcus aureus*, *Pseudomonas* spp, and other virulent organisms can cause the same appearance (Fig. 7-5). If the necrosis is widespread, the radiographic appearance may change from a homogeneous opacity to a heterogeneous pattern with multiple focal lucencies. In a patient who is acutely ill and clinically deteriorating, patchy radiographic clearing may represent early lung necrosis rather than real improvement. Rarely, confluent air

space disease may appear as a focal spherical shape, termed a round pneumonia (Fig. 7-6). This condition is more common in children than adults and is usually associated with streptococcal pneumonia.

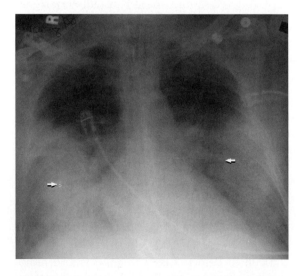

FIGURE 7-4 Posterior-anterior examination: *Legionella* pneumonia. There is bilateral consolidation of the lower lobes with evident air bronchograms *(arrows)*. Rapid extension of consolidation to multiple lobes is characteristic of legionnaires' disease.

TABLE 7-1
Pneumonia in the Normal Host

Radiographic Findings	Most Likely Etiology
Lobar consolidation	*Streptococcus pneumoniae, Legionella,* nosocomial gram-negative rods
Lobar enlargement	*Klebsiella* classically, but any virulent organism
Bronchopneumonia	*Mycoplasma, Streptococcus pneumoniae, Haemophilus influenzae, Branhamella, Chlamydia, Staphylococcus,* SARS*
Cavitation—acute	Anaerobic bacteria, *Staphylococcus,* and virulent *Streptococcus pneumoniae*
Cavitation—chronic	Tuberculosis, histoplasmosis, coccidioidomycosis
Interstitial pneumonia	*Mycoplasma pneumoniae, Chlamydia,* adenoviruses

SARS, severe acute respiratory syndrome.
*Chest radiographs appear similar to bronchopneumonia pattern; however, computed tomography images do not show bronchocentric distribution or evidence of infectious bronchiolitis.

Primary tuberculosis pneumonia can also arise as lobar air space disease, usually involving the lower and middle lobes. This clinical picture is a more common manifestation of tuberculosis in children than in adults. The infection commonly produces hilar adenopathy, which is rare in most pyogenic lobar pneumonias. In fact, pneumonia and hilar adenopathy in a child should alert the physician to the likelihood of primary tuberculosis (Fig. 7-7). The radiographic findings of primary tuberculous infections (as compared with reactivation disease) are listed in Table 7-3. The organisms that can cause air space disease associated with hilar adenopathy also include the agents of plague, tularemia, and fungal pneumonias discussed later. Unfortunately, an underlying neoplasm can also be the cause of hilar adenopathy in an adult with pneumonia and should be considered in patients at risk for bronchogenic carcinoma. Pulmonary anthrax is notably absent from this list of diseases. Rather than attacking the hilar lymph nodes, pulmonary anthrax causes severe mediastinitis with enlarged mediastinal lymph nodes, which dominates the findings on chest radiography and chest computed tomography (CT) (Fig. 7-8).

Granulomatous diseases, that is, fungal and mycobacterial infections, are uncommon causes of lobar pneumonia in the normal adult host. The four fungi that most commonly affect normal hosts are *Coccidioides, Blastomyces, Histoplasma,* and *Cryptococcus.* All of these fungal organisms can cause focal air space disease, but the pneumonias are commonly segmental size pneumonias rather than pneumonias encompassing an entire lobe. These fungal pneumonias are more likely to cause hilar adenopathy than most bacterial pneumonias, but the lack of adenopathy on a chest radiograph does not exclude their diagnosis. As these infections resolve, they often leave behind nodules that can either calcify (histoplasmosis) or remain noncalcified (more commonly with coccidioidomycosis) (Fig. 7-9). In a minority of patients these diseases become chronic, producing cavities and progressive air space disease that mimics tuberculosis. Sometimes these chronic infections produce mass-like lesions that can imitate a bronchogenic neoplasm. When present, satellite lesions, that is, nodules surrounding the mass, are a clue that a lung mass may represent a fungal infection

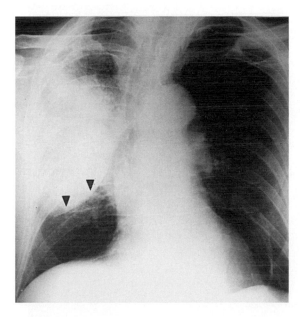

FIGURE 7-5 Posterior-anterior chest: *Klebsiella pneumoniae* pneumonia—bulging fissure sign. *Arrowheads* outline the bulging horizontal (minor) fissure that is inferiorly displaced by the increased volume of the anterior segment of the right upper lobe. Note the homogeneous appearance of this infiltrate.

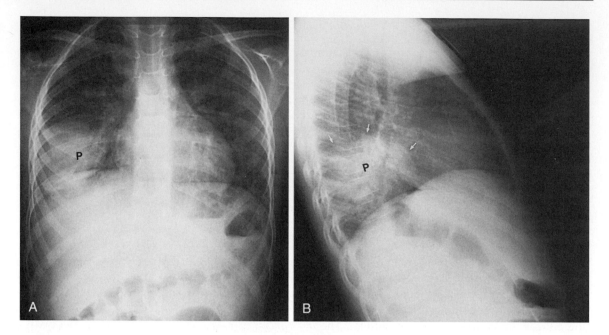

FIGURE 7-6 Posterior-anterior and lateral chest views: round pneumonia.

A, Frontal radiograph shows a well-defined confluent opacity (P) with spherical contours. This appearance can be problematic in adult patients because it can suggest a neoplasm that has a similar radiographic appearance.

B, Left lateral chest view demonstrates the margins of the rounded opacity *(arrows)* in the posterobasilar segment of the right lower lobe. Note that the lower thoracic vertebral bodies are more opaque than normal. This is caused by summation of the opacities of the pneumonia and underlying bone.

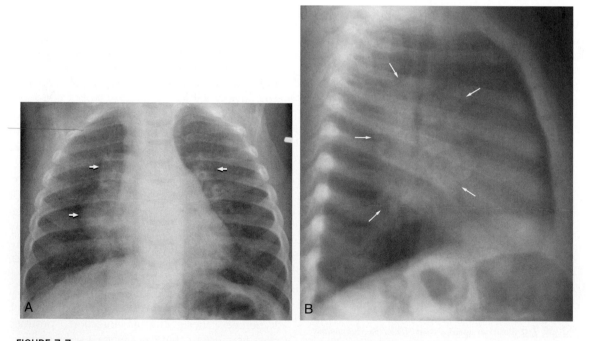

FIGURE 7-7 Posterior-anterior and lateral chest radiographs of a young child with primary tuberculosis.

A, PA projection shows extensive hilar adenopathy, better seen on the right *(arrows)* than the left because of rotation.

B, Lateral view shows adenopathy encircling the hilum, including its inferior margin *(arrows)*, forming a hilar "rosette." No pleural effusion is seen. (Effusions are more common in adults with primary tuberculosis.)

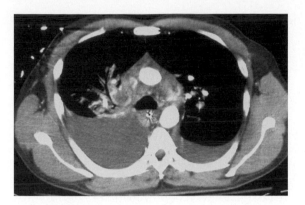

FIGURE 7-8 Computed tomography section from a patient with inhalation anthrax. The mediastinum is markedly edematous, causing the mediastinal fat to appear gray instead of black. Bilateral pleural effusions are also present.

rather than a neoplasm. These satellite lesions are much easier to see on CT scans than on chest radiographs. Typical manifestations of the four common organisms are listed in Table 7-2.

Bronchopneumonia

Bronchopneumonia is caused by inflammation beginning in the small bronchi and bronchioles.

The radiographic densities are patchy and multicentric, representing air space disease that has spread from these foci of bronchitis or bronchiolitis. Untreated, these foci can coalesce into segmental or lobar pneumonia. Not surprisingly, there is considerable overlap between the organisms that cause lobar pneumonias and those that cause bronchopneumonias; for example, pneumococcus appears on both lists. Common community-acquired causes of bronchopneumonia are *Haemophilus influenzae*, *Mycoplasma*, and *Chlamydia pneumoniae*. The latter two are unlikely to present or progress to a lobar pattern. In the hospitalized patient, a nosocomially acquired bronchopneumonia may also be caused by gram-negative rod infection (Fig. 7-10).

Hematogenously spread pyogenic infection can produce multifocal air space disease that resembles bronchopneumonia. The lack of a bronchocentric distribution is often hard to discern on radiographs. Bacterial endocarditis, septic thrombophlebitis, and intravascular catheters can all be sources of septic emboli. *S. aureus* is the most common organism (Fig. 7-11). Radiographic opacities show a predilection for the lower lung fields and may cavitate (see later discussion).

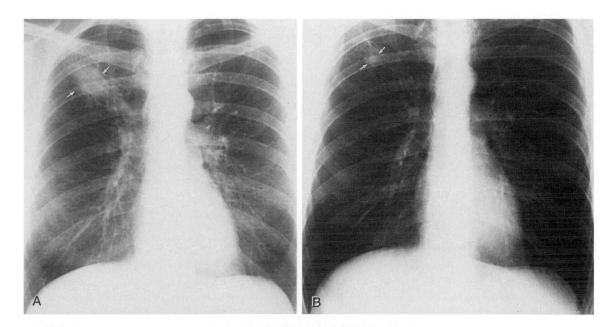

FIGURE 7-9 Posterior-anterior chest examinations: acute and "healed" coccidioidomycosis.

A, PA chest view shows focal air space disease in the right upper lobe *(arrows)*, caused by acute coccidioidomycosis.

B, Two-year follow up shows a right upper lobe nodule *(arrows)*, most opaque at its center because of calcifications.

TABLE 7-2

Typical Manifestations of Fungi in the Normal Host

Organism	Radiographic Manifestation
Histoplasmosis	
Acute	Focal air space or diffuse nodular disease. Resolves to calcified granuloma.
Chronic	Adenopathy Cavitary, can mimic tuberculosis (see Fig. 7-15).
Coccidioidomycosis	
Acute	Focal (can be lobar) or multifocal air space disease. Resolves to noncalcified granuloma. Can excavate if persistent. (Classically thin-walled in upper lobes.) Adenopathy
Chronic progressive	Cavitary, can mimic tuberculosis.
Blastomycosis	
Acute	Focal (can be lobar) or multifocal air space disease. Can be mass-like. Cavitation and adenopathy less common than in histoplasmosis and coccidioidomycosis.
Cryptococcosis	
Acute	Focal air space disease, nodule, or mass. Confined to lung and self-limited in normal hosts. Usually not cavitary in normal host.

Cavitary Disease

Acute infection creates a cavity by forming an abscess. Initially this cavitation may appear as a solid mass or nodule. A central lucency appears only after the necrotic contents have drained into the bronchial tree (Fig. 7-12). These lucencies characteristically have a wall greater than 1 mm thick, differentiating them from emphysematous bullae and blebs. Pneumatoceles, which represent localized intraparenchymal air trapping rather than focal parenchymal necrosis, may mimic a lung abscess. Pneumatoceles can occur during the recovery phases of staphylococcal pneumonia and following pulmonary contusion but are seen most often in patients with chronic adult respiratory distress syndrome. (PCP is a common cause of pneumatoceles but does not occur in normal hosts; see later.)

Anaerobic infections caused by aspiration of dental flora are a frequent cause of discrete abscess, most often in the lower lobes. Pneumonias caused by *S. aureus*, β-hemolytic streptococcus, *Klebsiella* spp, virulent strains of *Streptococcus pneumoniae*, and even *Legionella*

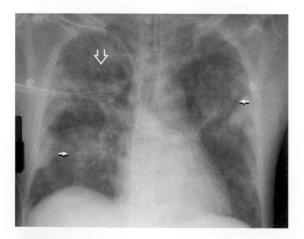

FIGURE 7-10 Anterior-posterior chest: nosocomial gram-negative bronchopneumonia. AP radiograph shows patchy, bilateral opacities *(arrows)* consistent with bronchopneumonia. A few air bronchograms are visible *(open arrow)* in the right upper lobe; the opacities have coalesced into a more lobar pattern.

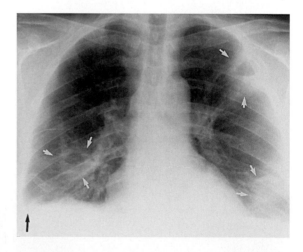

FIGURE 7-11 Posterior-anterior chest examination: septic pulmonary emboli from drug abuse. Multiple ill-defined ("shaggy") soft tissue nodules are present *(arrows)*. Some are cavitary. They have the appearance of hematogenous metastatic lesions, for which they are sometimes mistaken. Metastases are often better defined. Parapneumonic effusion is present *(black arrow)*.

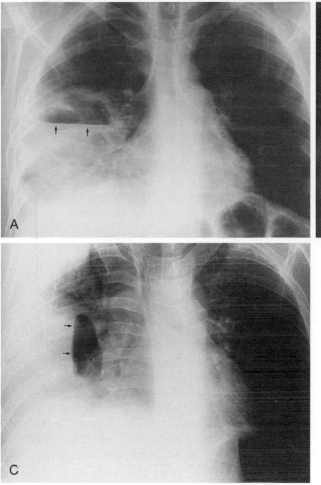

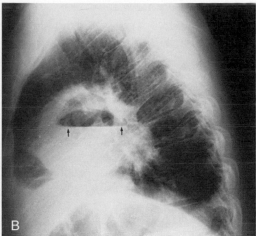

FIGURE 7-12 Multiple chest views: lung abscess.

A, Posterior-anterior upright chest radiograph demonstrates a single large intraparenchymal cavity in the right middle lobe with air-fluid level *(arrows)*.

B and C, Upright lateral and right lateral decubitus films show confinement of the air-fluid level to a roughly spherical cavity *(arrows)*. This shape is more consistent with an abscess than bronchopleural fistula (see Chapter 11).

may result in cavitation in the lung. Mycoplasma and chlamydia almost never produce cavities. (Accordingly, the presence of cavitation argues against empirical therapy with erythromycin or minocycline alone.) When multifocal abscesses are found, the diagnosis of septic pulmonary emboli should be considered.

In addition to pyogenic infections, a parenchymal lung cavity should always raise the possibility of tuberculosis. Classically, this represents reactivation disease and occurs most often in the apical or posterior segments of the upper lobe or superior segment of the lower lobe (Table 7-3). If seen early in the course of reactivation, the sites of infection appear as ill-defined nodules in the same anatomic distribution (Fig. 7-13). Pleural effusions, usually associated with primary tuberculosis, can also occur in reactivation disease. Hilar adenopathy is rare outside the setting of AIDS. Differentiation of active from inactive disease with plain

radiography is unreliable. Even if prior radiographs are available for comparison and appear identical to contemporary studies, the disease is best designated as radiographically stable rather than inactive. CT findings of cavities, consolidation, or centrilobular nodules (small nodules that surround bronchioles) favor active

TABLE 7-3
Findings of (Nondisseminated) Tuberculosis

	Primary*	Reactivation†
Lower lobes	Yes	No
Upper lobes	No	Yes
Cavitation	No	Yes
Adenopathy	Children > adults	No
Pleural effusions	Adults > children	Occasional

*Also late AIDS (low CD4 counts).
†Also early AIDS (preserved CD4 counts).

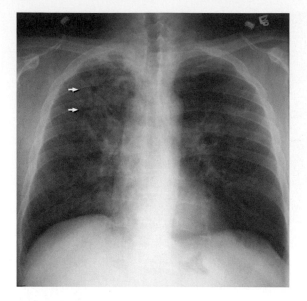

FIGURE 7-13 Posterior-anterior chest in reactivation tuberculosis. PA chest radiograph shows numerous ill-defined nodules in both upper lobes, most apparent on the right *(arrows)*. Findings are consistent with early reactivation (postprimary tuberculosis). These nodules are larger and more ill defined than seen with miliary tuberculosis.

disease (Fig. 7-14). Definitive diagnosis of active disease, however, still relies on sputum culture.

Mycobacterium avium-intracellulare (MAI) complex (MAC) infections can cause upper lobe cavitary disease that is indistinguishable from tuberculosis. Often, but not always, this occurs on a substrate of abnormal lung architecture (e.g., emphysema). MAI can also produce a second radiographic pattern, combining nodular opacities and bronchiectasis. This pattern of MAI classically involves the middle lobe and lingula in 60- and 70-year-old women.

Like MAI infections, histoplasmosis and coccidioidomycosis can also imitate the typical findings of reactivation tuberculosis (Fig. 7-15). These fungal pathogens, however, are more likely than tuberculosis to occur in sites other than the posterior upper lobe segments. Cavities caused by fungal or mycobacterial infections can sometimes be differentiated from those caused by pyogenic bacteria. The cavities caused by fungal pathogens are more likely to be associated with parenchymal scarring, volume loss, and evidence of a healed primary infection, such as hilar node calcification.

Cavitating neoplasms often have a radiographic appearance similar to that of infectious cavities. Primary bronchogenic carcinomas, and metastatic head and neck, colon and gynecologic

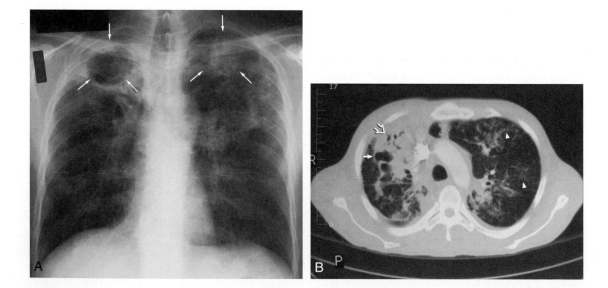

FIGURE 7-14 Posterior-anterior chest examination with computed tomography: reactivation tuberculosis.

A, Frontal radiograph demonstrates typical upper lobe location of reactivation tuberculosis. Cavities are present bilaterally *(arrows)*.

B, CT section from the same patient demonstrates small cavities *(arrows)*, architectural distortion of bronchi *(open arrows)*, and numerous small nodules caused by disease in distal bronchioles *(arrowheads)*. Taken together, these findings are typical of active postprimary tuberculosis.

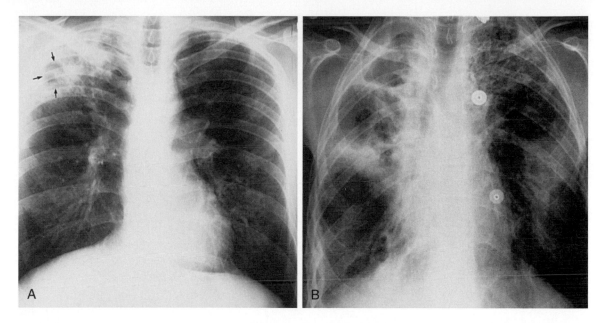

FIGURE 7-15 Posterior-anterior chest views: cavitary histoplasmosis and *Mycobacterium avium-intracellulare*.

A, PA chest radiograph in cavitary histoplasmosis demonstrates findings similar to those shown in Figure 7-14: air space disease and associated cavity are localized to the right upper lobe *(arrows)*. Although acute histoplasmosis pulmonary infection is often associated with hilar lymphadenopathy, none is seen here in this more chronic presentation.

B, Radiograph of a non-AIDS patient with MAI shows extensive cavitary lesions in the right middle and upper lung fields. The coarse reticular pattern seen on the left upper chest probably represents bronchiectasis.

malignancies are potential causes (Fig. 7-16). Criteria for differentiating neoplastic from infectious cavities have been set forth. Cavitary neoplasms, for instance, tend to have cavity walls that are more nodular and thicker (>15 mm) than those seen in infection (<5 mm). Unfortunately, unless old radiographs are available for comparison, there are no plain radiograph or CT findings that are unequivocally diagnostic. If the cavity does not resolve with antibiotic treatment, biopsy is often necessary.

In some cases, both neoplastic and infectious diseases combine to produce lung cavities in the form of a necrotizing pneumonia distal to an obstructing neoplasm. In this situation, thin CT sections (e.g., 1 to 3 mm) can often demonstrate the site of obstruction in one or more of the segmental bronchi.

Immunologic disorders may also cause cavitary pulmonary disease in the normal host, such as rheumatoid nodules and Wegener's granulomatosis (Fig. 7-17). Although these diseases should be included in the differential diagnosis, they are much less common than neoplastic or infectious etiologies. A more complete list of conditions that cause cavitary lesions is included in Table 7-4.

Interstitial Pneumonia

For the purposes of this book, interstitial pneumonia refers to radiographic patterns of linear, reticular, or miliary nodular opacities, described in Chapter 6. In general, interstitial pneumonia is an uncommon radiographic pattern in the normal adult host. Viral infections can cause interstitial pneumonia. Viral infection often starts in the bronchi and bronchioles, causing bronchial wall thickening, and then extends into the interstitium. In other cases, such as in adenovirus infections, inflammation may extend from the bronchioles to the alveoli and cause a bronchopneumonia pattern. Varicella and influenza, two of the most common viral pathogens, do not commonly cause interstitial pneumonia. Chest radiographs in varicella pneumonia, which occurs primarily in adults, usually show innumerable ill-defined (air space) nodules and small (lobular) foci of air space disease (Fig. 7-18). When healed, the infection can leave behind multiple calcified nodules that look similar to healed histoplasmosis (see later discussion). Influenza can cause bronchopneumonia or perihilar air space disease related to hemorrhagic pulmonary edema.

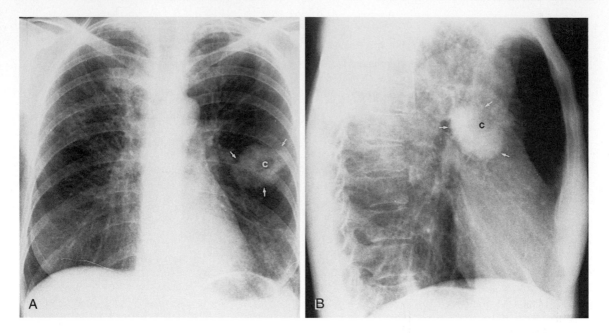

FIGURE 7-16 Posterior-anterior and lateral chest views: cavitating squamous cell carcinoma of the lung.

A and B, A solitary, well-defined, irregularly marginated mass *(arrows)* is identified in the anterior segment of the left upper lobe with a radiolucent cavitary center (C). Note the lack of adjacent air space disease and relative thickness of the wall compared with the images shown in Figures 7-11 and 7-12.

A new viral illness, severe acute respiratory syndrome (SARS), caused by a novel coronavirus has arisen in China and spread to numerous other countries, including Canada. Radiographic manifestations of this disease are pleomorphic but more commonly consist of bilateral ground glass opacities or consolidation rather than a reticular pattern (Fig. 7-19).

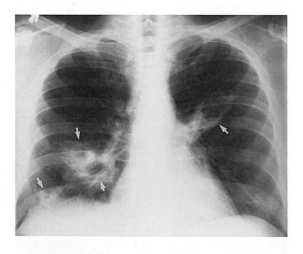

FIGURE 7-17 Posterior-anterior chest radiograph: Wegener's granulomatosis. Multifocal, patchy air space disease associated with multiple, variably sized cavitating lesions is present *(arrows)*. The lower lobe bias seen here is typical.

Mycoplasma is a common cause of interstitial pneumonia in young adults (Fig. 7-20). Approximately one third of patients with mycoplasma pneumonia present with reticulonodular infiltrates. In some cases, the interstitial nature of the opacities can be confirmed by identifying Kerley's B lines. These radiographic findings typically occur in patients with subacute or chronic symptoms. Patients with acute symptoms are more likely to show a bronchopneumonia pattern on a chest radiograph. *C. pneumoniae* strain TWAR, similar to mycoplasma, can cause both interstitial pneumonias and bronchopneumonias.

The miliary nodular pattern is a subgroup of interstitial lung disease. Chest radiographs show multiple small, ill-defined nodules, 2 to 5 mm in diameter. The pattern is diffuse but sometimes spares the peripheral lung fields. Tuberculosis is the most common cause of a miliary pattern; however, other granulomatous infections can be responsible (Fig. 7-21). Disseminated coccidioidomycosis and histoplasmosis are usually confined to immunocompromised hosts. A diffuse pattern that appears similar to miliary disease can occur in a normal host following an acute massive exposure to histoplasmosis spores. This is a reaction to

TABLE 7-4
Causes of Cavitary Lesions

Bacterial infections	Anaerobes, *Staphylococcus*, septic emboli
Granulomatous diseases	Tuberculosis, fungal infections, stage 4 sarcoidosis
Parasitic conditions	*Echinococcus*
Neoplasms	Primary lung tumor, metastatic (e.g., squamous cell carcinoma of the head and neck)
Vascular conditions	Wegener's granulomatosis, rheumatoid nodules
Inhalation	Silicosis or coal workers' pneumoconiosis with complicating tuberculosis, Caplan's syndrome
Pseudocavities	Infected bullae, cystic bronchiectasis, pneumatoceles (trauma, hydrocarbon aspiration, *Pneumocystis carinii* pneumonia)

airborne spores rather than hematogenous spread, and the nodules formed are larger and more ill defined than in miliary disease. Subsequently, these nodules may calcify. Radiographs of patients with noninfectious diseases, including silicosis and coal worker's pneumoconiosis and sarcoidosis, can also look similar to a miliary pattern. These conditions are discussed in Chapter 6.

☐ IMMUNOCOMPROMISED PATIENTS WITH AIDS

The radiographic findings seen in patients with AIDS are best categorized slightly differently than those occurring in nonimmunocompromised hosts. In patients with AIDS, it is practical to characterize parenchymal lung disease as either localized air space disease, diffuse lung disease (interstitial or air space), or multiple nodules (Table 7-5). The presence of hilar, mediastinal, or axillary adenopathy (seen on CT) is also a helpful clue and at times is the sole radiographic manifestation of thoracic disease.

Localized Air Space Disease

As in the normal host, localized air space disease with a segmental or lobar distribution is often bacterial in origin. *S. pneumoniae* and *H. influenzae* are common, followed by *S. aureus* and gram-negative rod pathogens.

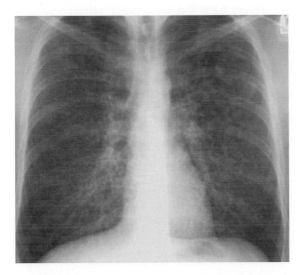

FIGURE 7-18 Posterior-anterior chest view: varicella pneumonia. Although a reticular nodular pattern may be seen early, the radiographic picture usually seen in adults is that of innumerable ill-defined nodules. Parenchymal infiltrates are invariably associated with disseminated skin lesions.

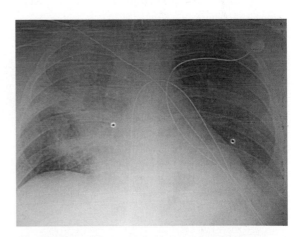

FIGURE 7-19 Portable chest radiograph: severe acute respiratory syndrome. Anterior-posterior chest radiograph shows bilateral air space disease involving the left lower lobe, the periphery of the left lung, and most of the right lung. In SARS patients, consolidation is often predominately in the peripheral lung, but this distribution is more easily appreciated on a computed tomography scan than a chest radiograph. Progression to bilateral disease is often accompanied by ventilatory failure.

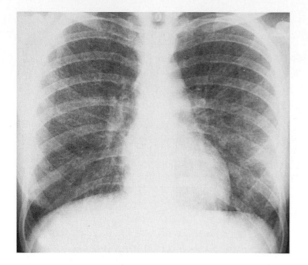

FIGURE 7-20 Posterior-anterior chest radiograph: mycoplasmal pneumonia. Diffuse reticular nodular infiltrates are seen in this adolescent patient with atypical pneumonia. Mycoplasmal pneumonia has this pattern in about one third of the cases.

Concomitant cavity formation or pleural effusion further increases the likelihood that bacterial infection is present. Patients in advanced stages of AIDS are susceptible to unusual bacterial pathogens such as *Nocardia, Rhodococcus equi,* and *Bartonella.*

Mycobacterial infections can also cause focal air space disease. Tuberculosis is relatively

common in patients with AIDS. It can cause cavitary disease in patients early in the course of human immunodeficiency virus (HIV) infection when CD4 T-cell counts are greater than 200/mm³ and after immune restoration by treatment with highly active antiretroviral therapy (HAART). In later stages of AIDS, cavitation is rare and the disease usually has the radiographic appearance of a primary infection. This appearance typically includes air space disease in the middle and lower lobes, thoracic adenopathy, and occasionally pleural effusions (see Table 7-3).

Diffuse Lung Disease

PCP is an important cause of diffuse lung disease in AIDS. (*Pneumocystis carinii* has recently been renamed *Pneumocystis jiroveci,* but the acronym PCP is still commonly used to refer to pneumonia caused by the organism.) Early in the history of the AIDS epidemic, PCP was by far the most common cause of diffuse infiltrative lung disease. PCP, however, usually does not occur until CD4 counts are very low, less than 200/mm³. This level of immune compromise currently occurs much less commonly where HAART is available. In addition, prophylactic therapy for PCP is now widely prescribed for patients with CD4 counts below 200/mm³. On chest radiographs, PCP classically

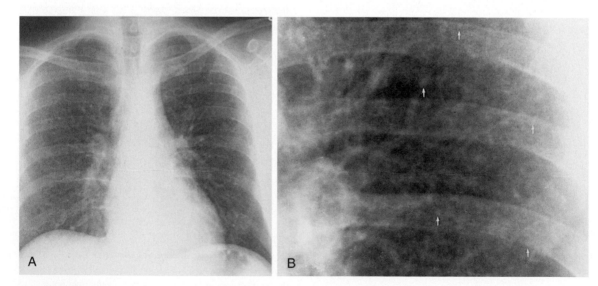

FIGURE 7-21 Posterior-anterior chest view with detail: miliary coccidioidomycosis.

A, Multiple ill-defined 2- to 5-mm nodules are diffusely scattered throughout the pulmonary parenchyma by hematogenous dissemination.

B, Close-up of small miliary (millet seed size) nodules *(arrows).* Miliary disease is more common in tuberculosis than in coccidioidomycosis. See discussion of high-resolution computed tomography of miliary tuberculosis, Chapter 6.

TABLE 7-5
Causes of Pneumonia in Immunocompromised Host with AIDS—Chest Radiograph Patterns

Localized air space disease	Community-acquired bacterial pneumonias, tuberculosis, atypical bacteria such as *Nocardia, Rhodococcus*, fungal infections (e.g., *Cryptococcus*)
Diffuse air space disease	PCP, (Kaposi's sarcoma),* overwhelming bacterial or fungal pneumonia
Diffuse interstitial pneumonia	PCP, cytomegalovirus, MAC, (lymphoma, Kaposi's sarcoma, lymphocytic interstitial pneumonia, CHF from AIDS-related cardiomyopathy)
Multiple nodules	Septic emboli,† atypical bacterial infections,† *Cryptococcus, Mycobacterium*† (Kaposi's sarcoma, AIDS-related lymphoma)
Lymphadenopathy alone	MAC, tuberculosis, (AIDS-related lymphoma)

*Noninfectious diseases are in parentheses.
†May be cavitary.
AIDS, acquired immunodeficiency syndrome; CHF, congestive heart failure; MAC, *Mycobacterium avium* complex; PCP, *Pneumocystis carinii* pneumonia.

causes bilateral, often symmetric opacities that have a granular or reticular pattern. Without treatment, these opacities can progress to diffuse consolidation (see Fig. 7-3).

Upper lobe predominance and focal disease may occur and have become more common findings in patients with *Pneumocystis* than early in the AIDS epidemic. Thin-walled cysts, pneumatoceles, may also form and can be a striking finding (Fig. 7-22 and Table 7-6). On high-resolution CT (HRCT), PCP often causes ground glass opacities (see Chapter 6) that are distributed in a perihilar or mosaic-like pattern (Fig. 7-23). The CT scan may also reveal pneumatoceles, which cannot be appreciated on chest radiographs. These cysts can later rupture and lead to pneumothorax, especially in patients who require mechanical ventilation.

Infections other than PCP can also cause disease in AIDS patients, including disseminated bacterial infections. Recurrent bacterial infections may also cause thickening and dilatation of bronchioles and bronchi, sometimes called "pyogenic airway disease." These thickened

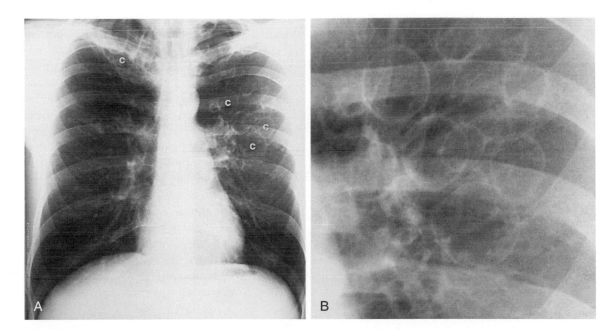

FIGURE 7-22 Posterior-anterior chest radiograph and close-up: *Pneumocystis carinii* pneumonia interstitial disease with parenchymal cyst formation.

A, Multiple thin-walled parenchymal cysts (c), the sequelae of PCP, are identified bilaterally in the upper lung fields, much more numerous on the left. Incidence of these sequelae approaches 30% in some series.

B, This close-up view demonstrates a cluster of the thin-rimmed cysts in the left middle lung field.

TABLE 7-6

Findings in *Pneumocystis carinii* Pneumonia in AIDS Patients

Common
Diffuse air space disease
Bilateral interstitial disease (symmetric or asymmetric)

Occasional
Apical lung disease (e.g., with inhaled pentamidine)
Pneumatoceles (10% of patients or more)

Uncommon
Acute lobar and/or cavitary disease

Very rare
Adenopathy
Pleural effusion

airways appear as a reticular pattern on chest radiographs, particularly in the lung bases, and are sometimes mistaken for PCP. Disseminated fungal infections, particularly coccidioidomycosis and histoplasmosis, cause diffuse infiltrative disease with a miliary nodular pattern, sometimes accompanied by hilar adenopathy. Cytomegalic inclusion virus infections are seen in late stages of AIDS when immunocompromise is severe and can appear identical to PCP.

Noninfectious conditions may also arise as diffuse infiltrative lung disease in patients with AIDS. Lymphocytic interstitial pneumonia, infiltration of the interstitium with lymphocytes and plasma cells, can cause a nodular or reticulonodular pattern on a chest radiograph and is more common in children with AIDS. Although the radiographic appearance is nonspecific, stability over time may suggest the diagnosis. Lymphocytic interstitial pneumonia may also occur in non-AIDS patients with immunologic diseases such as Sjögren's disease. Both AIDS-related lymphoma and Kaposi's sarcoma may present as diffuse infiltrative disease but more commonly appear as nodular disease.

Nodules and Masses

The nodular pattern described here is not the same as the nodular pattern in a morphologic, interstitial, or diffuse infiltrative lung disease. The nodules caused by these diseases are larger and less numerous. AIDS-related lymphoma, Kaposi's sarcoma, mycobacterial disease, and fungal infections can all cause nodules or masses in patients with AIDS. AIDS-related lymphoma occurs in patients with severe immunocompromise and is related to Epstein-Barr virus infection in most cases. It is an aggressive B-cell lymphoma that is commonly extranodal but involves the chest in a minority of cases. Thoracic lymphadenopathy can occur but is not present as consistently as in thoracic lymphoma among normal hosts, and extranodal disease often dominates the radiologic findings (Fig. 7-24). Kaposi's sarcoma is the most common neoplasm that occurs in AIDS patients and is strongly associated with human herpes virus 8 infection. It rarely involves the lungs without first involving the skin or oropharynx. Nodules caused by Kaposi's sarcoma tend to be indistinct, sometimes flame shaped, and follow a bronchovascular distribution (Fig. 7-25). In later stages of the disease, conglomerate masses and effusions may be present. The most common fungal infectious agent among AIDS patients is *Cryptococcus*. The disease usually presents as meningitis but can also affect the lungs, where it can cause nodules, masses, or less well-defined air space opacities similar to those caused by bacterial infections.

Adenopathy

Many of the diseases already described can cause intrathoracic adenopathy in AIDS, including AIDS-related lymphoma, Kaposi's sarcoma, mycobacterium tuberculosis, and fungal infections.

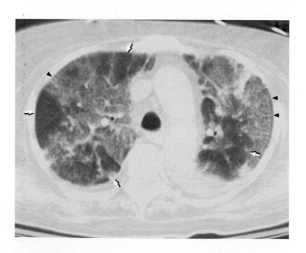

FIGURE 7-23 Computed tomography section: *Pneumocystis pneumonia.* CT section viewed in lung parenchymal window shows areas of ground glass opacity *(arrowheads)*, some of them containing thickened interlobular lines (1 to 2 cm long). There are well-marginated foci of nearly normal appearing lung as well *(white arrows).* This combination of well-defined ground glass and normal-appearing lung is termed a mosaic pattern.

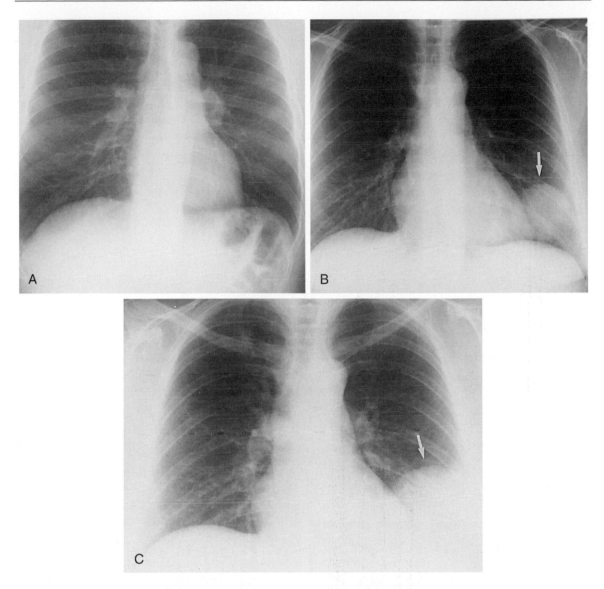

FIGURE 7-24 Posterior-anterior chest view: AIDS-related lymphoma. A large left lower lobe nodule *(arrows)* developed in the 6-week interval between studies shown in parts **A** and **B**. The nodule doubled in size in the following 2 weeks (**C**). AIDS-related lymphomas may grow rapidly, mimicking infection. (Courtesy of Dr. David Levin, UCSD.)

MAC may also cause extensive intrathoracic adenopathy and occurs in AIDS patients with very low CD4 counts (<50/mm³) (Fig. 7-26). The infection is widely disseminated and may be present in the blood and bone marrow without apparent chest radiographic abnormalities. When the lung parenchyma is involved, diffuse nodules or patchy air space disease may be present. Patients with undiagnosed MAC infections may develop lymphadenitis when begun on therapy with HAART. This paradoxical response to partial immune restoration may result in worsening lymphadenopathy or parenchymal lung disease.

PCP is notably absent from this list of diseases. The presence of adenopathy on the chest radiograph of a patient with AIDS indicates that either the suspected infection is not PCP or there is disease caused by another organism in addition to PCP.

☐ IMMUNOCOMPROMISED PATIENTS WITHOUT AIDS

There are many causes of immunocompromise in non-AIDS patients, and these conditions

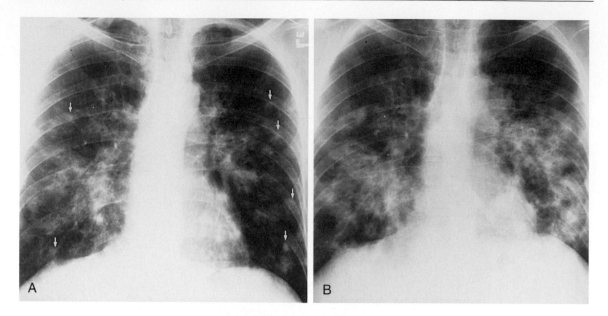

<u>FIGURE 7-25</u> Serial posterior-anterior chest radiographs: Kaposi's sarcoma.

A, Bilateral, relatively indistinct, shaggy nodules are identified in the middle and lower lung fields *(arrows)* on a background of diffuse interstitial disease. (High-resolution computed tomography would show these nodules to be clustered along the bronchovascular bundles.)

B, With progression, these areas appear as patchy air space disease and could be difficult to distinguish from pulmonary infections.

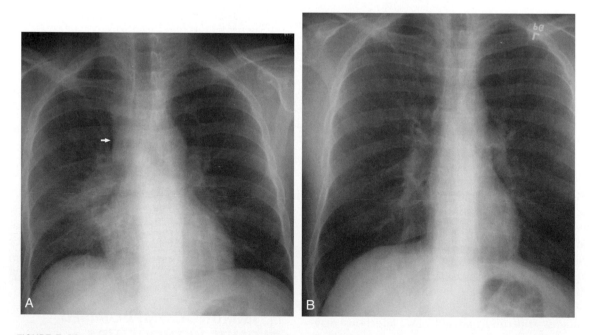

<u>FIGURE 7-26</u> Serial chest radiographs in a patient with AIDS and systemic *Mycobacterium avium-intracellulare* infection.

A, Posterior-anterior chest radiograph shows marked bilateral hilar and right paratracheal *(arrow)* lymph node enlargement.

B, Radiograph taken several months earlier when patient's CD4 counts were much higher shows no evidence of mediastinal or hilar adenopathy.

TABLE 7 7
Causes of Pneumonia in Immunocompromised Host without AIDS*

Focal air space disease	Gram-negative rods,[†] *Staphylococcus, Aspergillus*[†] (hemorrhage, leukemic infiltrate, infarction), *Nocardia*[†]
Diffuse pneumonia	PCP, cytomegalovirus, (drug reactions) Overwhelming bacterial and fungal infections
Solitary or multiple nodules	*Nocardia, Legionella micdadei*, fungi, (pulmonary infarcts, post-transplantation lymphoproliferative disease)

*Noninfectious diseases are in parentheses.
[†]May be cavitary.
PCP, *Pneumocystis carinii* pneumonia.

result in different types of immune defects. Granulocytopenia, depressed cell-mediated immunity, and hypogammaglobulinemia can occur by themselves or in various combinations. These different types of immunosuppression predispose to different types of pulmonary infection. The radiographic manifestations are therefore varied. Using radiographic categories similar to those proposed for immunocompromised hosts with AIDS, we can make a few generalizations (Table 7-7).

The duration of disease helps focus the differential diagnosis. Diseases resulting from bacterial infections usually develop over a few days, and infections with fungi and mycobacterial disease develop over a minimum of several days and often over a few weeks. In patients who have undergone organ transplantation, the duration of immunosuppression further refines the differential diagnosis. Bacterial infections occur within the first month after transplantation, whereas cytomegalovirus, PCP, and fungal infections usually occur more than a month after the initiation of immunosuppression.

Focal Air Space and Cavitary Disease

Regardless of the underlying immunologic abnormality, acute focal air space disease often represents bacterial infection. Nosocomial infection with gram-negative rods is common and may result in cavitation. In patients with prolonged leukopenia and in patients 1 to 4 months after solid organ transplantation, focal air space disease may also be caused by invasive fungal disease or *Nocardia*.

Aspergillus is probably the most common fungal lung infection in neutropenic hosts. Invasive infection with this pathogen usually begins as multiple ill-defined nodules that may later coalesce. Further evaluation with chest CT characteristically shows a dense central opacity with a surrounding halo of ground glass opacity (Fig. 7-27). These findings are said to represent infarcted tissue and surrounding inflammation caused by vascular invasion by the organism. Infections with *Mucor* species can produce an identical pattern. As the patient's immune system returns toward normal, these masses may cavitate. A portion of the necrotic center of the cavity may remain attached to the cavity wall. This necrotic mass is outlined by a rim of air that is known as the air crescent sign (Fig. 7-28).

The focal lung necrosis and crescent-shaped air collections caused by invasive *Aspergillus* should not be confused with aspergilloma formation. Aspergillomas do not occur in immunosuppressed hosts but instead are found in patients with normal immune systems and underlying distortion of the lung architecture. Cavities related to tuberculosis, sarcoidosis, and histoplasmosis

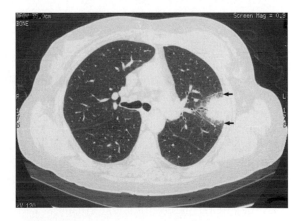

FIGURE 7-27 Computed tomography: invasive *Aspergillus* in a patient with leukemia. CT section viewed in a lung parenchyma window shows a left upper lobe mass with a peripheral rim of ground glass opacity *(arrows)*. In this clinical setting, the findings strongly suggest fungal infection with *Aspergillus* or less commonly mucormycosis.

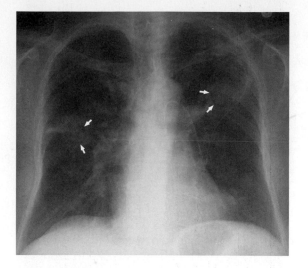

FIGURE 7-28 Frontal chest radiograph: invasive aspergillosis. Posterior-anterior chest of a patient recovering from severe neutropenia. There are at least two lung masses that now contain necrotic material that has retracted away from the surrounding tissue, forming an air crescent *(arrows)*. Note that the air in the cavity on the left has not risen to the most cephalad portion of the cavity because the necrotic tissue is still attached superiorly.

become home for this saprophytic fungal growth (Fig. 7-29). The fungus ball appears as a soft tissue mass within the cavity that changes in location with changes in the patient's position (e.g., on decubitus films). Unlike invasive aspergillosis, these fungal growths do not make patients systemically ill. Occasionally they cause serious hemoptysis. Life-threatening pulmonary hemorrhage can be treated with surgical resection, bronchial artery embolization, and intracavitary antifungal agents.

There are two other manifestations of aspergillosis (Table 7-8). Allergic bronchopulmonary aspergillosis occurs in patients with asthma when *Aspergillus* colonizes the central airways. The resulting hyperimmune response causes central bronchiectasis (see Chapter 3). Semi-invasive aspergillosis occurs in patient with mild immunocompromise and can be thought of as an intermediate state between aspergilloma and invasive aspergillosis. Like an aspergilloma, semi-invasive aspergillosis often occurs in a lung with underlying architectural abnormalities. Like invasive aspergillosis, the fungus invades tissue, but it remains a local infection and does not spread hematogenously.

Noninfectious processes may also cause air space disease in immunocompromised hosts. The diagnosis of pulmonary infarction is often

overlooked in the rush to identify an infectious agent. Further evaluation with CT pulmonary angiography should be considered in at-risk patients, such as those who have recently had a renal transplant. Asymmetric pulmonary edema and pulmonary hemorrhage (e.g., in the patient with untreated acute leukemia) may produce focal findings but are more likely to cause diffuse air space disease.

Multiple Nodules

Like patients with AIDS, patients with immunocompromise of other origins can also develop multiple pulmonary nodules as a manifestation of infectious and noninfectious disease. *Nocardia* and fungal pathogens, particularly *Aspergillus* and *Cryptococcus*, are common causes of multiple lung nodules. Occasionally, bacterial agents, notably *Legionella micdadei*, also cause nodular infiltrates. Mycobacterial disease is much less common than among AIDS patients, and Kaposi's sarcoma does not occur. Transplant patients may develop post-transplantation lymphoproliferative disease, which can produce mediastinal lymphadenopathy and lung nodules. Fortunately, the prevalence of this disease has waned with the use of newer immunosuppressive regimens.

Diffuse Disease (Interstitial or Air Space)

The differential diagnosis for diffuse lung disease is similar in the immunocompromised host with and without AIDS. Diffuse disease may be caused by cytomegalovirus (the most common pneumonia in transplant recipients), PCP, or a variety of noninfectious etiologies. Kaposi's sarcoma is notably absent from the differential diagnosis in patients without AIDS. Instead, reactions to drugs need to be considered as potential causes of diffuse lung disease, particularly in patients undergoing chemotherapy. Drug reactions may have several different radiographic patterns ranging from interstitial edema with Kerley's B lines and patchy opacities to diffuse consolidation similar to that in adult respiratory distress syndrome (see Chapter 8). The latter pattern represents diffuse alveolar damage and is most commonly related to cytotoxic agents such as bleomycin, used in cancer chemotherapy (see Fig. 8-14). HRCT may detect diffuse infiltrative disease before plain radiographic findings are evident, but the appearance

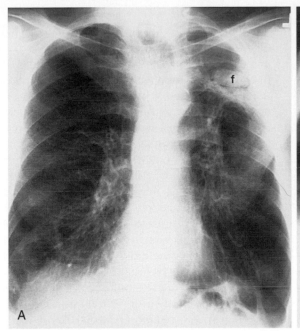
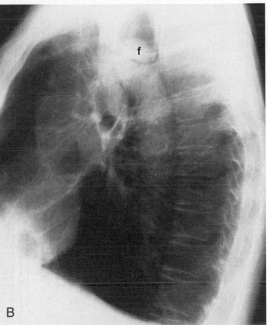
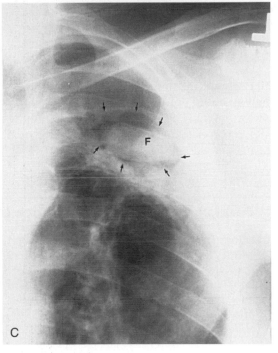

FIGURE 7-29 Posterior-anterior chest view with detail:
noninvasive aspergillosis (aspergilloma).

A, A large left upper lobe fungus ball (f) is present in a
background of parenchymal fibrosis, compatible with sequelae of
tuberculosis. Note the appearance of the solid ovoid mass
(aspergilloma) within the large, thin-walled cavity.

B, Lateral study showing fungus ball (f) in apical posterior
segment of the left upper lobe.

C, Close-up of the view shown in part A demonstrates a
well-defined fungus ball mass (F) inside the cavity *(arrows)*.

TABLE 7-8
Types of *Aspergillus* Infection

Syndrome	Underlying Problem	Radiographic Signs
Invasive aspergillosis	Neutropenia, immunosuppressives	Multiple large nodules, air crescent sign (halo sign on computed tomography)
Semi-invasive aspergillosis	Chronic obstructive pulmonary disease, radiation fibrosis, tuberculosis (postprimary)	Slowly progressive upper lobe opacities
Aspergilloma	Cavitary lung disease	Mass within preexisting lung cavity
Allergic bronchopulmonary aspergillosis	Asthma	Central bronchiectasis, finger in glove pattern, transient consolidation

of disease on HRCT is not sufficient to make a specific diagnosis. A high index of suspicion for drug toxicity is needed since a biopsy may be necessary to confirm the diagnosis.

☐ COMPLICATIONS OF PNEUMONIA

During the acute stages of pneumonia, patients who are improving clinically need not have frequent follow-up chest radiographs. If fevers are persistent or the patient's clinical status changes markedly, a chest radiograph should be ordered. For instance, if there is newly developed dullness to percussion and localized decrease in breath sounds, pleural effusions may have developed. In this case, the goal is to confirm the presence of a parapneumonic effusion and to determine whether the effusion represents an empyema or is likely to become one. Parapneumonic effusions are discussed with pleural diseases in Chapter 11.

Delayed resolution of the parenchymal infiltrate after treatment for pneumonia is often a major clinical concern. It raises the possibility that the infiltrate is not infectious (e.g., represents a bronchoalveolar carcinoma) or that

an underlying neoplasm is causing bronchial obstruction.

Clinical decisions are based on the natural history of pneumonias. For instance, consolidation from bacteremic pneumococcal pneumonia usually resolves within 8 weeks. Volume loss, stranding densities, and pleural thickening can persist longer and may be present in one third of patients. Other pneumonias may resolve more slowly. Chest radiographs in patients with legionnaires' pneumonia may take several months to clear. Advanced age, underlying chronic obstructive pulmonary disease, alcoholism, and other comorbid conditions may prolong convalescence and resolution of the radiographic findings.

All of these factors—age, organism, and underlying diseases—should be weighed when evaluating the patient. If, based upon the overall clinical presentation, further work-up is needed, a practical next step is CT of the chest. Scanning should be done using both intravenous contrast and thin sections (e.g., 3 mm) to evaluate for evidence of an underlying lung mass and to look for endobronchial obstruction. If neither a discrete mass nor an endobronchial lesion is seen, some patients require biopsies of the lung to exclude noninfectious causes of chronic air space disease (see Chapter 6).

Pearls for Clinicians—Infectious Lung Disease

1. Know the immune status of your patient when looking at the radiograph of a pneumonia.
2. Look carefully for lung cavities or enlarged hilar lymph nodes; the presence of either on the chest radiograph limits your differential diagnosis.
3. If you see parenchymal disease in the apical-posterior segments of the upper lobes or the superior segment of the lower lobe, think of tuberculosis even if a definite cavity is not visible on the chest radiograph. Put a mask on the patient and avoid being

hounded by the infection control team later.
4. When confronted by diffuse lung disease on a chest radiograph, keep an open mind to the possibility that you are may, in fact, be looking at heart failure or a drug reaction.
5. Among immunocompromised patients large nodules and masses suggest infection with a fungus (*Cryptococcus* in AIDS, *Aspergillus* in non-AIDS) or *Nocardia*. Think about empirical therapy or a transthoracic needle biopsy early on.

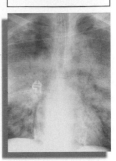

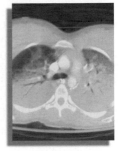

8

Traumatic and Toxic Lung Disease

Physical trauma to the lung parenchyma can be accidental or iatrogenic (e.g., postoperative). In most settings, primary care practitioners are not acutely called upon to care for victims of major accidental trauma. However, they are confronted with delayed sequelae of accidental lung injury or with postoperative complications.

☐ ACCIDENTAL LUNG TRAUMA

Contusions, Pneumatoceles, and Hematomas

Acute blunt chest trauma can cause pulmonary contusions, areas of alveolar edema and hemorrhage that are seen on chest radiographs as localized or asymmetric diffuse air space disease. The radiographic findings are most pronounced at the periphery under the site of impact (Fig. 8-1). Contusions occur within several hours following blunt trauma and, if they do not become infected, typically resolve in 4 to 5 days. Pulmonary hematomas and lung cysts (pneumatoceles) may also form after blunt chest trauma (Fig. 8-2). These injuries are formed when a hole is torn in the lung and fills with

blood or air, respectively. Hematomas present as pulmonary nodules, either "solid" or cavitating. Unlike contusions, hematomas may persist for weeks or months. As a result of this prolonged resolution, a patient may or may not relate a history of recent trauma. Some patients with hematomas (or contusions) also lack evidence of acute or healing rib fractures. In young adults, the chest wall is flexible enough that the lung tissue can be compressed without fracture of the overlying ribs.

Fat Emboli

Accidental trauma can also affect the lung indirectly by producing fat emboli. Fat emboli originate from long bones when they are fractured and can occur after trauma or after surgical manipulation. Clinical findings include respiratory distress, petechiae, and central nervous system abnormalities. These findings are manifest 1 to 3 days after the accident. Although the chest radiograph is frequently normal, bilateral air space disease occasionally occurs. These radiographic opacities are usually distributed peripherally, sometimes with a basilar bias. Unlike contusions, this air space disease is

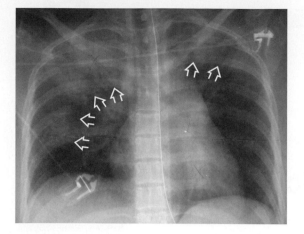

FIGURE 8-1 Anterior-posterior portable chest radiograph of pulmonary contusion. Frontal radiograph shows asymmetric parenchymal opacities that are most severe in the right upper and midlung zones *(arrows)*. The opacities are most evident peripherally, consistent with a pulmonary contusion.

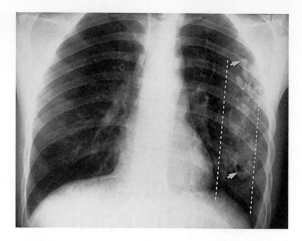

FIGURE 8-2 Posterior-anterior chest view: post-traumatic hematomas. This examination was obtained a week after blunt trauma to the left chest. Shearing injury resulted in tears in the lung parenchyma that filled with blood, now seen as solid and cavitating nodules *(arrows)*. Note the linear area of impact to the chest wall *(dashed lines)* associated with these hematomas. Unlike contusions, hematomas take weeks to months to resolve.

relatively symmetric (Fig. 8-3). Fat emboli also differ from contusions in that the latter are seen immediately after the injury and begin to improve within 24 to 48 hours, which is the time when fat emboli first begin to appear. Disease from fat emboli tends to clear within 7 to 10 days after the injury.

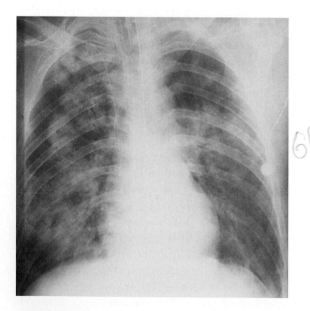

FIGURE 8-3 Posterior-anterior chest radiograph: post-traumatic fat emboli. Radiograph obtained 72 hours after a femur fracture demonstrates diffuse bilateral symmetric alveolar opacities (a basilar predilection is reported to be more common).

Alveolar Rupture and Pneumomediastinum

A sudden rise in intrathoracic pressure can cause alveolar rupture. Sufficient increases in intrathoracic pressure to rupture alveoli can be generated by a bout of coughing, vomiting, or straining or by mechanical ventilation. Once the alveolar rupture has occurred, air dissects along the bronchi to enter the mediastinum and may extend from there into the subcutaneous tissues. Air may also dissect peripherally into the pleural space, where it causes a pneumothorax. Although in the past pneumomediastinum, pneumothorax, or subcutaneous air occurred in up to 15% of patients receiving mechanical ventilation, the incidence of baro-trauma (injury to the lung caused by the mechanical ventilator) has probably decreased with the current use of smaller tidal volumes.

On chest radiographs, subcutaneous air is often seen outlining the fibers of the pectoral muscles (see Chapter 11). When severe, these air shadows in the subcutaneous tissues make it very difficult to assess the lung parenchyma with chest radiographs. Pneumomediastinum can be recognized by displacement of the mediastinal pleura laterally, which creates a dark line adjacent to the heart and mediastinal structures. Low-density (dark) streaks of air are often seen extending upward into the neck.

Similar dark lines may encircle the right pulmonary artery on lateral view, causing a "ring around the artery." The visualization of the central portion of the diaphragm (the continuous diaphragm sign), especially in supine patients, is also a helpful clue to the presence of pneumomediastinum (Fig. 8-4). The continuous diaphragm sign occurs when air tracks between the diaphragm and pericardium. Subtle radiographic differences distinguish pneumomediastinum from pneumopericardium. In pneumopericardium, air surrounds the heart but does not extend upward past the origin of the great vessels. Pneumopericardium and pneumomediastinum may coexist, and for the most part differentiating them is not clinically important. Neither condition is likely to be physiologically significant in adults. (A tension pneumopericardium occasionally causes tamponade in infants.)

Most of the time a pneumomediastinum causes few symptoms and resolves spontaneously without therapy. On occasion, pneumomediastinum may be a sign of esophageal rupture. Rupture can occur because of esophageal instrumentation and after severe vomiting (Boerhaave's syndrome). Because perforations in Boerhaave's syndrome usually occur in the distal esophagus, the injury is often accompanied by a left pleural effusion or hydropneumothorax. If it is not promptly diagnosed and treated, the outcome can be catastrophic. Pneumomediastinum is also important in the setting of mechanical ventilation, where it is a sign of barotrauma. The same barotrauma that produces the pneumomediastinum can later produce pneumothoraces. Therefore, if a pneumomediastinum is detected in a mechanically ventilated patient, one needs to be vigilant and it is a good idea to have a chest tube set nearby.

☐ THE POSTOPERATIVE CHEST

Surgical resection of lung parenchyma is not uncommon. Although limited resection of lung tissue (e.g., segmentectomy) can be used to preserve lung parenchyma, lobectomies and pneumonectomies are still commonly performed for the treatment of lung carcinoma and occasionally for trauma or infection. Following left upper lobe lobectomy, the major fissure on that side is not visible because it is no longer outlined by aerated lung on both sides. After a right upper lobe resection, a "neofissure" is visible because the middle lobe expands to form a pleural border along the length of the lower lobe. A "juxtaphrenic peak," a sharp upward point along the contour of the diaphragm where the lower lobe is anchored, is a sign that the upper lobe on that side has been removed or collapsed. After most lobectomies (of any lobe), the remaining lobes gradually expand to fill the hemithorax so that the postoperative hemithorax is only slightly smaller than normal (Fig. 8-5). If the mediastinum is markedly displaced toward the side of a lobectomy, there is probably atelectasis of the remaining lung tissue.

After pneumonectomy, the hemithorax gradually fills with fluid (Fig. 8-6). Within 4 to 7 days, about one half to two thirds of the chest cavity is opacified. Over the next several weeks to months, the cavity usually opacifies completely. During this time, the hemidiaphragm elevates and the mediastinum shifts gradually toward the side of the resected lung. The position of the mediastinum becomes permanent after about 8 to 9 months. Any movement of the mediastinum in the opposite direction (away from the side of surgery) is abnormal and suggests formation of an empyema or malignant effusion. Infection can also cause breakdown of the surgical stump and result in

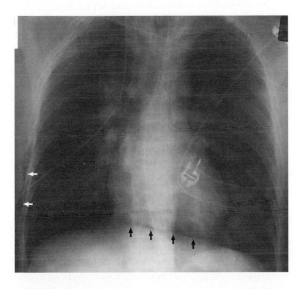

FIGURE 8-4 Anterior-posterior chest: pneumomediastinum. A lucent (dark) line is seen passing under the cardiac silhouette *(black arrows)*, outlining the superior margin of the diaphragm. This "continuous diaphragm sign" is caused by pneumomediastinum. A small amount of subcutaneous emphysema is also seen along the right lateral chest *(white arrows)*.

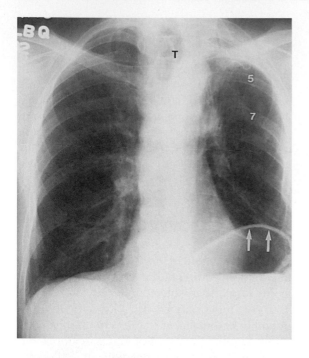

FIGURE 8-5 Posterior-anterior chest view: after left upper lobectomy. There is left hemithorax volume loss and the left hilum is abnormally elevated. Although radiographs obtained shortly after the surgery may show mediastinal shift, studies obtained later, as in this case, do not. There may be elevation of the left hemidiaphragm if the remaining lung cannot hyperinflate enough to fill the hemithorax *(arrows)*. Note the postsurgical absence of the sixth posterior rib. T, trachea.

a bronchopleural fistula. This is seen radiographically as a sudden drop in the amount of fluid in the hemithorax (Fig. 8-7).

Abdominal and nonpulmonary thoracic surgery can also affect the lung parenchyma (Fig. 8-8). The most common parenchymal complication of these surgical procedures is atelectasis. Most often this involves part or all of the left lower lobe, particularly after cardiac surgery. It is easily detected on routine chest radiographs by recognizing loss of the silhouette of the descending aorta and medial aspect of the left hemidiaphragm. It is helpful to look for the presence of a central air bronchogram in the atelectatic lobe. If these are present, the atelectasis is probably diffuse, peripheral, and unlikely to be caused by a central obstruction. If air bronchograms are absent, a central mucus plug may be present and the atelectasis is more likely to respond to specific treatment (such as suctioning or bronchoscopy). Occasionally, a central mucous plug can cause acute respiratory decompensation before volume loss or

increased opacity in the affected lung is evident on chest radiograph. The clinical presentation may mimic that of a pulmonary embolism or early adult respiratory distress syndrome (ARDS), leading to further evaluation with a computed tomography (CT) angiogram or a radionuclide lung scan. These examinations can detect mucous plugging of the central bronchi by direct visualization of the occluded airway on CT or by demonstration of decreased ventilation (radionuclide lung scan) (Fig. 8-9).

☐ RADIATION INJURIES

Radiation injuries to the lung are usually the result of radiation therapy treatments directed to an area within the lung (bronchogenic neoplasm), mediastinum (lymphoma, testicular carcinoma), or other part of the thorax (breast). The severity of radiation injuries increases with the radiation dose administered, the lung volume irradiated, and the rate of administration. Radiation pneumonitis rarely occurs with fractionated doses less than 2000 rad, whereas a dose of 6000 rad almost always causes severe pneumonitis. In patients receiving therapeutic radiation, the pulmonary complications are usually asymptomatic and radiographic abnormalities occur more frequently than significant respiratory symptoms. Radiographic abnormalities appear about 8 weeks after therapy or sooner at doses greater than 4000 rad.

There are two stages in the radiologic-pathologic findings after radiation therapy: (1) the acute phase of radiation pneumonitis and (2) the late stage of pulmonary fibrosis. Acute radiation pneumonitis presents as areas of air space disease (with air bronchograms), often with associated volume loss. These opacities can be differentiated from infection because their borders follow the radiation ports instead of the usual anatomic boundaries of lobes or segments (Fig. 8-10). Sometimes this geometric distribution can be more easily seen with cross-sectional images on a CT scan of the chest. Rarely, a patient who has had high-dose localized radiation has diffuse radiographic changes not confined to the radiation port. The diffuse lung damage may represent a widespread immunologically mediated response to a localized radiation injury.

Acute radiation pneumonitis can either resolve completely or progress to the late

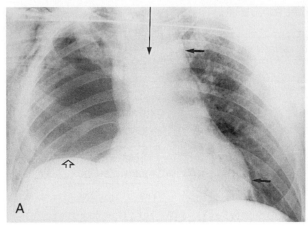

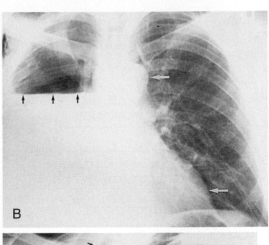

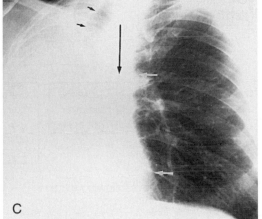

FIGURE 8-6 Serial chest films: right pneumonectomy.

A, Initial postoperative chest radiograph in the recovery room shows loss of lung markings on the right. There is no mediastinal shift *(arrows)*. The right hemidiaphragm is elevated *(open arrow)*. Subcutaneous emphysema is seen overlying the right chest.

B, Follow-up upright posterior-anterior radiograph taken 1½ weeks after surgery demonstrates that approximately two thirds of the hemithorax is already filled with fluid *(small arrows)*. No significant mediastinal shift is noted *(large arrows)*.

C, Follow-up at 2 months. The right hemithorax is fluid filled and mediastinal shift is indicated by the position of the trachea *(small black arrows)* and left mediastinal border *(white arrows)*. The midline is indicated by the *long black arrow*.

FIGURE 8-7 Serial posterior-anterior chest examinations: postoperative bronchopleural fistula.

A, Chest radiograph taken after left pneumonectomy demonstrates the expected left hydrothorax with prominent elevation of the left hemidiaphragm *(open arrows)* indicated by high stomach bubble (SB). *White arrows* indicate normal mediastinal shift.

B, Radiograph obtained 1 week after that shown in part A demonstrates marked loss in volume of the left effusion with multiloculated fluid *(white and black arrowheads)*. This indicates a bronchopleural fistula. Also note that there is now an abnormal mediastinal shift to the right *(white arrow and arrowhead)*.

ALGORITHM FOR POSTOPERATIVE RESPIRATORY DISTRESS

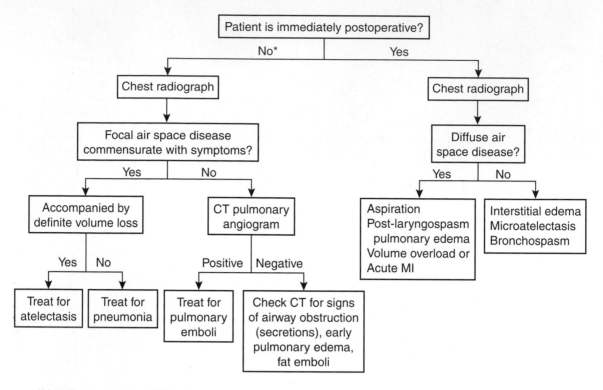

*Usually several days following surgery

FIGURE 8-8 Algorithm: postoperative respiratory distress. CT, computed tomography; MI, myocardial infarction.

fibrotic stage. The resulting damage usually stabilizes within a year. It can cause enough volume loss to radiographically mimic tuberculous postinflammatory changes (Fig. 8-11). Fibrotic tissue and tumor are both opaque on chest radiographs and may have similar densities on chest CT. Therefore, it may be difficult to detect local recurrence of a tumor in an area of radiation fibrosis. Early detection of tumor, however, is not crucial following radiation for

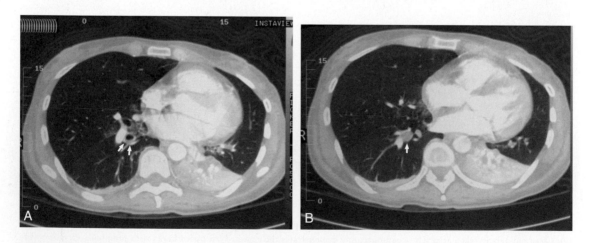

FIGURE 8-9 Computed tomography (CT) sections through the lower lobes: endobronchial plugging.
    A, CT image from a CT pulmonary angiogram performed on a patient with postoperative respiratory distress. The left lower lobe is atelectatic. Secretions partially fill the right lower lobe bronchus (arrow).
    B, CT image slightly caudal to A. The right lower lobe bronchus is completely filled with secretions (arrow).

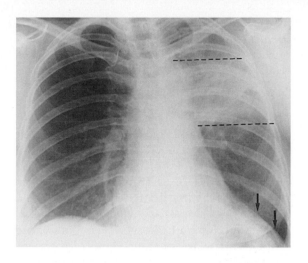

FIGURE 8-10 Posterior-anterior chest view: acute radiation pneumonitis. Focal air space disease is present with associated air bronchograms. The radiation port can be geometrically outlined by the parenchymal reaction seen *(dashed lines)*. There is associated volume loss, as is often the case (secondary to surfactant loss and mucous plugging), indicated here by elevation of the hemidiaphragm *(arrows)*.

bronchogenic carcinoma because of the limited therapeutic options for patients with recurrent disease.

The issue of tumor recurrence after radiation therapy is more often of clinical importance in the treatment of mediastinal lymphoma. Masses caused by Hodgkin's disease often contain a

large amount of fibrous tissue, and some tissue remains even after the lymphoma cells are eradicated. This persistent mass makes the decision whether to stop or continue treatment more difficult. Currently, positron emission tomography (PET) imaging of fluorodeoxyglucose (FDG) combined with CT is the best way to determine whether viable lymphoma is still present in the chest. PET imaging of FDG differentiates neoplastic tissue from fibrous tissue by identifying increased glucose metabolism in the tumor (see Chapter 9). Following treatment of lymphoma, the combination of a persistent or enlarging mass and increased uptake of FDG is likely to represent residual or recurrent tumor.

☐ TOXIC LUNG DAMAGE

Aspiration

Pulmonary aspiration may cause disease in one of three ways: (1) airway obstruction by large particulate matter, (2) infection from aspirated bacteria, or (3) direct damage to the lung parenchyma from gastric contents. Large particulate matter may produce resorptive atelectasis, and infections from aspirated bacteria may lead to lung abscesses. Both processes are discussed in other chapters.

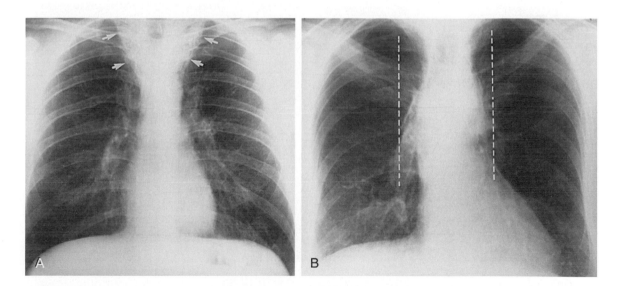

FIGURE 8-11 Posterior-anterior chest radiograph: chronic radiation fibrosis.

A, Intense interstitial fibrosis that is relatively focal is seen *(arrows)*. Architectural distortion that takes place in chronic radiation fibrosis may not demarcate the radiation ports as closely as do changes in acute pneumonitis.

B, A second patient with chronic radiation change following radiation for Hodgkin's disease. Note the dense hilar fibrosis, which makes detection of local recurrence in the area difficult. *Dashed lines* define approximate radiation port.

Aspiration of gastric contents containing a high concentration of hydrochloric acid causes increased-permeability pulmonary edema. This is manifest radiographically as air space disease, which is usually bilateral and sometimes extensive. Radiographic changes occur rapidly, often within a few hours. Violent coughing and deep inspirations caused by the irritation of the acid may spread the gastric contents and cause diffuse lung damage; lesser degrees of aspiration may lead to more focal air space disease. Localization of the radiographic changes is governed by the patient's position at the time of aspiration: lower lobes are more commonly involved if the patient is upright, and the superior segment and posterior upper lobes are involved if the patient is supine. On portable chest radiographs the latter appears as perihilar air space disease. Because the posterior distribution of disease is not appreciated without a lateral view, the pattern can be mistaken for cardiogenic pulmonary edema.

If the opacities are caused by direct damage from gastric acid, not complicated by infection or airway obstruction, the radiograph tends to clear within a few days (Fig. 8-12). Repeated, small quantity aspirations can lead to focal fibrosis that appears as coarse reticular shadows and volume loss, usually in the lower lobes. Reviewing previous radiographs can be useful in documenting the long-term consequences of recurrent aspiration.

Toxic Inhalation Injury

Aspiration of other substances, including fresh and salt water, and hydrocarbons can appear similar to gastric acid aspiration on chest radiography. The development of diffuse disease may be delayed 24 to 48 hours following the aspiration of hydrocarbons. Toxic gases are a less common cause of diffuse parenchymal injury. Chlorine and phosgene gas both cause diffuse alveolar damage and increased-permeability pulmonary edema. The onset of symptoms and radiographic changes may occur within several hours after exposure. Silo filler's disease, caused by nitrous dioxide produced from silage, can also produce diffuse lung damage. It differs from other exposures in that it may ultimately lead to the delayed development of bronchiolitis obliterans (see Chapter 4).

Drug-Induced Pulmonary Disease

Drugs can affect the lung parenchyma, mediastinum (e.g., phenytoin [Dilantin]-induced adenopathy), and pleura. Pleural disease is

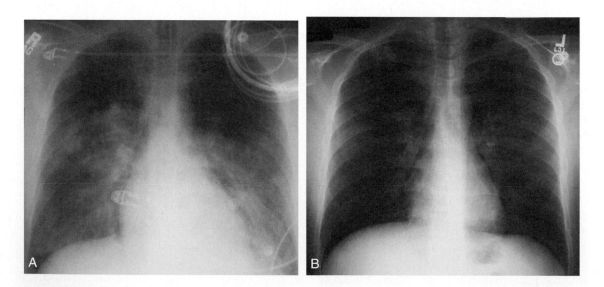

FIGURE 8-12 Serial chest radiographs: aspiration pneumonia.

A, Posterior-anterior (PA) upright chest radiograph obtained several hours after a patient was endotracheally intubated during severe upper gastrointestinal bleeding. Gross aspiration was observed clinically. There are bilateral midlung and basilar opacities.

B, Follow-up PA chest view approximately 3 days after the radiograph in A shows nearly complete resolution of the parenchymal disease. Rapid resolution can be seen in gastric aspiration that is not complicated by airway obstruction from solid material or by superinfection.

TABLE 8-1
Pulmonary Disease Induced by Drugs

Radiographic Presentation	Drug
Diffuse air space disease (adult respiratory distress syndrome)	Heroin, morphine, methadone, aspirin
Subacute/chronic reticular pattern (fibrosis)	Busulfan, bleomycin, methotrexate, cyclophosphamide, nitrofurantoin (chronic), amiodarone
Patchy opacities (often peripheral), interstitial edema	Nitrofurantoin (acute), methotrexate, sulfonamides, isoniazid, amiodarone
Pleural disease from drug-induced lupus erythematosus	Procainamide, hydralazine

often a result of drug-induced lupus and is discussed further in Chapter 11. Within the lung parenchyma, drugs can cause one of three general categories of disease: diffuse alveolar damage, subacute or chronic fibrosis, and hypersensitivity reactions (Table 8-1). Diffuse alveolar damage results in ARDS when severe and is seen on chest radiographs as diffuse air space disease. Subacute or chronic diffuse infiltrative disease that results in fibrosis usually produces a reticular pattern on chest radiographs. Hypersensitivity reactions appear as pleural effusions and interstitial edema or as patchy alveolar opacities. These patchy opacities are often peripheral and on biopsy may reveal bronchiolitis obliterans with organizing pneumonia (BOOP) or eosinophilic pneumonia. (Remember that idiopathic BOOP and eosinophilic pneumonias both cause peripheral opacities; see Chapter 6.)

Aspirin and heroin are classic examples of drugs capable of causing ARDS, but cytotoxic agents are also common causes of this type of drug reaction. Lung damage caused by these agents cannot be distinguished radiographically from damage from other causes of ARDS (Fig. 8-13). Cytotoxic agents such as bleomycin, busulfan, and cyclophosphamide can also cause diffuse infiltrative disease resulting in fibrosis. Bleomycin toxicity, for example, can cause either diffuse alveolar damage or diffuse fibrotic lung disease (Fig. 8-14), both of which can rapidly progress with the administration of supplemental oxygen. This is probably due to increased generation of oxygen radicals that accelerate the lung toxicity.

Other agents, such as methotrexate and nitrofurantoin, can also produce two distinctly different syndromes—one a chronic or subacute infiltrative disease leading to fibrosis, the other a more acute hypersensitivity reaction (Fig. 8-15).

The hypersensitivity reactions can cause patchy air space disease or effusions and interstitial edema in patients undergoing chemotherapy, making it difficult to differentiate the radiographic changes of drug toxicity from radiographic findings caused by atypical pulmonary infections (e.g., *Pneumocystis carinii* pneumonia). In these cases, high-resolution CT (HRCT) findings can help with the differential diagnosis but usually cannot preclude lung biopsy.

Amiodarone toxicity is common and also bridges several drug reaction categories. It can cause a diffuse infiltrative disease resulting in fibrosis or bilateral air space disease that resembles BOOP or eosinophilic pneumonia. Unlike the findings in other forms of air space disease, the iodine content of the drug causes the diseased lung tissue to absorb x-ray photons.

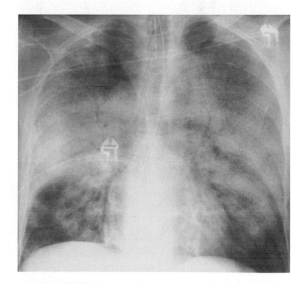

FIGURE 8-13 Posterior-anterior chest radiograph: adult respiratory distress syndrome secondary to acetylsalicylic acid overdose. This frontal chest examination demonstrates bilateral diffuse acute air space disease with associated air bronchograms.

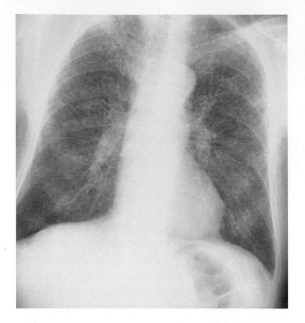

FIGURE 8-14 Posterior-anterior chest radiograph: bleomycin toxicity. Bleomycin toxicity is manifest as chronic diffuse infiltrative lung disease causing a reticulonodular pattern. Lung volumes are preserved, suggesting that there may be an element of underlying obstructive lung disease.

The difference in x-ray absorption is not great enough to be seen with plain radiographs but can be apparent on CT if areas of consolidation are present (reticular opacities are usually not confluent enough to assess their density on CT).

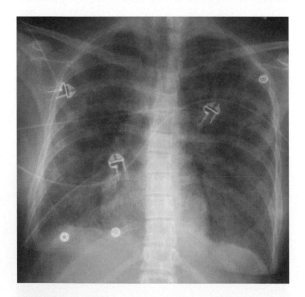

FIGURE 8-15 Posterior-anterior chest radiograph: nitrofurantoin hypersensitivity. Portable chest radiograph shows linear interstitial pattern and small bilateral pleural effusions. No evidence of heart disease was found. The patient improved rapidly after cessation of nitrofurantoin.

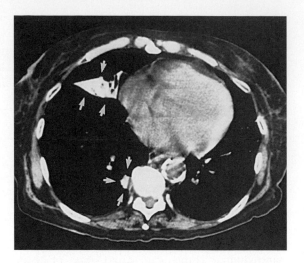

FIGURE 8-16 Contrast-enhanced conventional computed tomography: amiodarone lung toxicity. Although plain radiographic findings are nonspecific (see text), deposition of iodine within the lung parenchyma can be identified by CT. The iodine deposition is seen as areas of increased attenuation *(arrows)* and is especially evident displayed on the mediastinal window setting.

The finding can aid in the diagnosis of amiodarone lung toxicity (Fig. 8-16).

Adult Respiratory Distress Syndrome

ARDS is high-permeability pulmonary edema, leakage of fluid from the alveolar capillary bed that is not caused by increased hydrostatic pressure (e.g., heart failure). It is a common product of many different assaults on the lung parenchyma and, in that respect, is no more a specific disease than is pedal edema or upper gastrointestinal bleeding. Disseminated lung infection can produce ARDS. More often, ARDS is caused by systemic or nonpulmonary infections that release hematogenous mediators that damage the lung parenchyma. Similar mechanisms are probably responsible for ARDS following burns, multisystem trauma, and pancreatitis. In other cases, toxins reach the lung through the airways (e.g., in near drowning or exposure to toxic gases) (Table 8-2).

Acute ARDS usually appears as diffuse air space disease. Nearly all such patients require mechanical ventilation. The day-to-day changes in mechanical ventilation technique, particularly in the use of positive end-expiratory pressure (PEEP), can cause marked fluctuation in the apparent opacity and extent of the parenchymal disease. Increasing the PEEP can improve

TABLE 8-2
Causes of Adult Respiratory Distress Syndrome

Mechanism	Disease
Release of systemic mediators	Septic shock, multiple transfusions, trauma, pancreatitis
Respiratory infection	Nosocomial pneumonia
Inhaled toxins	Aspiration, near drowning, toxic gas inhalation

both oxygenation and the radiographic appearance of the disease, but it does not improve the underlying lung pathology. CT scanning in ARDS shows that the most dependent portions of the lung appear to be the most involved, the most densely consolidated. This is because the fluid-filled lung is more susceptible to atelectasis in its dependent portions (Fig. 8-17). PEEP improves the radiograph by opening up some of the lung that is partially atelectatic but not yet completely airless.

If the patient survives the acute stage of ARDS, after 3 to 7 days more chronic pathologic changes occur. These changes gradually convert the radiographic appearance from that of confluent air space disease to a coarse reticular pattern (Fig. 8-18). At this stage, patients may show evidence of barotrauma. Clinical trials

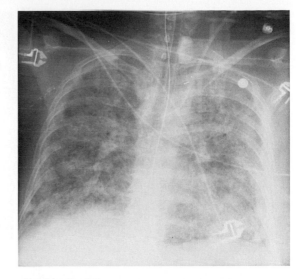

FIGURE 8-18 Anterior-posterior supine chest: chronic adult respiratory distress syndrome. This radiograph shows a mixture of a coarse, diffuse reticular pattern (consistent with interstitial fibrosis) and persistent areas of air space disease with air bronchograms. The lung volume is diminished.

have shown that a considerable amount of lung injury in ARDS is actually attributable to barotrauma rather than the underlying disease. More recent ventilation techniques that decrease the lung volumes delivered to patients in mechanical ventilation have decreased the prevalence of barotrauma.

If barotrauma occurs, the earliest radiographic finding may be interstitial emphysema caused by air leaking from ruptured alveoli and dissecting along the bronchi. The air can superimpose a bubbly or stippled appearance on preexisting areas of pneumonia or ARDS. This change can be mistaken for radiographic improvement. If barotrauma progresses further, pneumatoceles, pneumomediastinum, and pneumothoraces can occur. The pneumothoraces produced may be loculated and difficult to detect on radiographs. The areas of increased lucency that are created by these pneumothoraces may also be mistaken for improvement in the parenchymal disease (Fig. 8-19).

Unfortunately, nosocomial pneumonia often occurs during the chronic period of ARDS. The diagnosis of this infection is problematic and has led to trials of specialized culture techniques (e.g., quantitative cultures of bronchoalveolar lavage fluid and protected bronchial brushings) to distinguish nosocomial pneumonia from worsening ARDS. Findings on portable chest radiographs

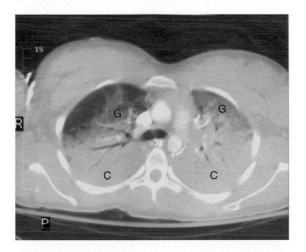

FIGURE 8-17 Computed tomography in adult respiratory distress syndrome. CT section through the upper lobes shows consolidation (C) in the most posterior portion of the lungs. Just ventral to (above) the consolidation are areas of ground glass opacity (G), and anterior to these are relatively normal-appearing lung. In reality, the lung is diffusely damaged and edematous. The dependent lung is most opaque because it is compressed by the lung tissue anterior to it.

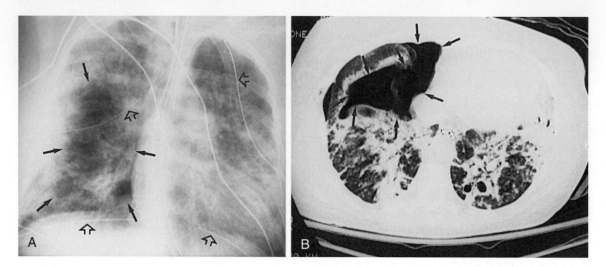

FIGURE 8-19 Anterior-posterior (AP) supine chest radiograph and computed tomography: patient with adult respiratory distress syndrome (ARDS) with loculated pneumothorax.

A, The AP supine chest view demonstrates the diffuse, coarse, reticular nodular opacities of chronic ARDS. A focal area of increased lucency is seen in the right midlung field and extends into the inferomedial aspect of this hemithorax *(arrows)*. Bilateral chest tubes are seen *(open arrows)*.

B, A single axial CT slice displayed with lung windows shows a loculated pneumothorax *(arrows)* that is sequestered anteriorly in the right hemithorax.

are usually nonspecific because of the many other factors that may affect the appearance of ARDS on a day-to-day basis (Table 8-3).

Much has been written about differentiating ARDS from cardiogenic pulmonary edema radiographically. A few differentiating points are listed in Table 8-4. In practice, radiographic findings by themselves are not sufficient to differentiate ARDS from cardiogenic edema. The clinician must rely upon multiple pieces of data including records of fluid input and output, physical examination, and sometimes reading from a pulmonary artery catheter to assess adequately the patient's intravascular volume.

TABLE 8-3
Changes in Appearance of Adult Respiratory Distress Syndrome

Appears Worse	Appears Better
Decreased exposure of radiograph	Increased exposure of radiograph
Decreased positive end-expiratory pressure	Increased positive end-expiratory pressure
Pleural effusion (late)	Interstitial emphysema
Pneumonia	Pneumothorax
ARDS worsening	ARDS improving

TABLE 8-4
Radiographic Findings in ARDS versus CHF

	ARDS	CHF
Air space disease	Peripheral	Basilar or perihilar (initial)
Heart size	Normal (usually)	Increased (usually)
Kerley's B lines	No	Yes (occurs early)
Pleural effusions	No (occurs late)	Yes (occurs early)

ARDS, adult respiratory distress syndrome; CHF, congestive heart failure.

Pearls for Clinicians—Traumatic and Toxic Lung Disease

1. Pulmonary contusions cause peripheral air space disease that crosses anatomic boundaries and develops over the first 24 hours after injury. Deterioration more than 48 hours after injury suggests superimposed pneumonia, pulmonary thromboemboli, or fat emboli. The last, fat emboli, is a clinical and not a radiologic diagnosis.

2. Aspiration pneumonitis is an important cause of acute perihilar air space disease and may mimic the appearance of acute volume overload. Both frequently follow cardiopulmonary resuscitation.

3. Radiographic changes from radiation pneumonitis usually stabilize at 1 year. New opacities that develop after a year suggest new or recurrent disease.

4. Pneumomediastinum is most often a benign finding. However, if it is accompanied by left basilar parenchymal disease and pleural effusion, think about the possibility of distal esophageal perforation.

5. Drug-induced lung disease can cause three of the four radiographic patterns of infiltrative lung disease: reticular/reticulonodular, linear, and chronic air space disease (see Chapter 6). Always consider this etiology in the differential diagnosis of diffuse lung disease.

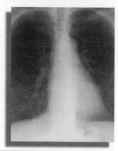

Pulmonary Neoplasms

☐ SOLITARY NODULE GENERAL PRINCIPLES

The earliest radiographic indication of a primary pulmonary neoplasm is a solitary pulmonary nodule. Classically, a solitary pulmonary nodule is defined as a well-circumscribed parenchymal mass 3 cm or less in diameter. Well circumscribed, however, is a subjective term, and many malignant nodules have indistinct margins on chest radiographs, particularly when obscured by overlying structures such as blood vessels. Because malignant lung nodules are often ill defined and incompletely opaque, most are not detected until their diameter exceeds 1 cm. Once a nodule is discovered by routine chest radiography, distinct or ill-defined, the most important questions become: Is it new? Is it really in the lung? and Can it be shown to be benign?

The first question can best be answered with examination of prior radiographs (or, second best, reading of prior radiograph reports). The most valuable "diagnostic study" may be a telephone call to another institution to locate the patient's prior radiographs. A parenchymal lung lesion that has doubled in size in 3 weeks or first appeared within the last 3 weeks is unlikely to be a neoplasm and is most likely caused by infection, infarction, or trauma. Only a few very aggressive metastatic tumors, germ cell neoplasms, lymphomas, sarcomas, and melanomas can mimic this appearance. More important, if an intrathoracic lesion can be shown to be absolutely stable for 2 years or more, it is benign and does not require further work-up. However, this is more difficult to prove than it might seem if the nodule is small. When nodules are small, a minor increase in diameter can represent a doubling in nodule volume (volume = πR^3). For instance, a nodule 1 cm in diameter that increases to 1.25 cm in diameter has doubled in volume. This is the critical factor to remember when examining serial radiographs. Some carcinomas, such as bronchoalveolar cell carcinoma, are very slowly growing tumors. Thus, small changes in nodule size are potentially of great importance.

If no prior radiographs are available or if their arrival from elsewhere is pending, one should try to determine whether the lesion definitely lies within the lung parenchyma. This may seem obvious, but skipping this step can raise unnecessary alarm and waste time and money.

140

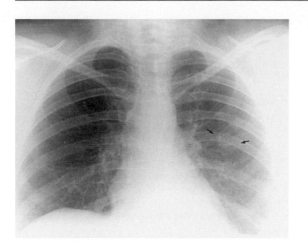

FIGURE 9-1 Posterior-anterior chest radiograph: healed rib fracture simulating lung nodule. This frontal chest radiograph demonstrates an area of increased opacity overlying the left midlung parenchyma that is caused by a healing fracture of the posterior seventh rib *(arrows)*. A similar fracture is also present at the sixth rib.

A variety of overlying structures can masquerade as intraparenchymal lung nodules, including nipple shadows, healed rib fractures (Fig. 9-1; see Fig. 2-18), osteophytes, bone islands, and skin lesions. Often these lesions can be excluded by "low-tech" methods, such as nipple markers. If it is suspected that the lesion lies within a rib, shallow oblique or inspiratory-expiratory views may be helpful to confirm its osseous origin by showing that the nodule continues to project within rib despite changes in the patient's position.

If the suspected nodule cannot be proved to be sufficiently old or to lie outside the lung parenchyma, computed tomography (CT) of the chest should be the next step. Most thoracic CT scanning is currently performed using spiral technique, in which continuous imaging is performed as the patient is slowly moved through the scanning beam by a moving table. With this technique, images are not obtained one slice at a time. Instead, information is gathered from a cylinder-shaped volume of space that contains the patient (see Chapter 1). Each three-dimensional cylinder-shaped volume is called one (data) acquisition. After the scan is performed and the data are stored, a large number of "slices" can be carved from this cylinder. If a single-slice CT scanner is used, the slices must be the same width as the original scan beam but the slices can be positioned along the cylinder such that they overlap. This makes it less

likely to overlook nodules that are smaller than the width of the scan beam. If the nodule is very small, an additional scan is usually done using a very thin beam confined to the area containing the nodule. This is particularly important in order to detect calcium (see later). The newest CT scanners offer multidetector scanning in which multiple x-ray detectors rotate around the patient at the same time. This allows the CT to scan large areas of the body quickly despite using a very thin x-ray beam (less than 5 mm). Thin-section multidetector CT scanning avoids the need for performing an extra acquisition to characterize a small lung nodule but at the cost of a moderate increase in radiation dose.

☐ SOLITARY NODULE DIFFERENTIAL DIAGNOSIS

Common Diagnoses

Once the nodule has been confirmed as intraparenchymal, the entire differential diagnosis is long. The number of common causes, however, is short (Table 9-1). The relative frequency of the two most common causes, granulomas and bronchogenic carcinoma, depends on the age and smoking history of the patient and other clinical parameters of the population. Together, granulomas and bronchogenic carcinoma account for more than 80% of solitary nodules. Many granulomas have classical radiographic appearances with a clearly calcified central nidus (Fig. 9-2). Unfortunately, some granulomas may remain uncalcified or slowly enlarge. This may occur more commonly with coccidiomycosis than with other fungi or mycobacteria (Fig. 9-3).

Although not rare, solitary metastases, bronchial carcinoids, hamartomas, rounded atelectasis, organizing pneumonia, and pulmonary infarcts present as solitary nodules less commonly than granulomas or bronchogenic neoplasms. Solitary metastasis is always an important consideration in patients with known extrathoracic malignancies. Overall, colon carcinoma is the most common malignancy to present as a solitary metastasis. Often it is important to determine whether a new solitary nodule is more likely to represent a metastasis or a primary lung carcinoma. The likelihood that the nodule is caused by a metastasis depends on both the site of the primary neoplasm and its stage.

TABLE 9-1

Common Causes of Solitary Pulmonary Nodules

Diagnosis	Radiologic Clues to Diagnosis
Most common	
Primary lung carcinoma	Spiculated border >1.5 to 2.0 cm diameter
Granuloma	Dense central calcifications occupy greater than 20% of nodule
Histoplasmosis	
Coccidiomycosis	
Mycobacterium	
Others	
Less common	
Solitary metastases	More common in middle to lower lung
Bronchial carcinoid	Endobronchial location, marked enhancement after intravenous contrast
Hamartoma	Intralesional fat on computed tomography
Rounded atelectasis	*Must* be adjacent to pleural thickening
Organizing pneumonia	May have concave borders

In general, if the patient's prior malignancy was a squamous cell carcinoma of the head and neck, a new primary bronchogenic carcinoma is more likely to be the cause of a solitary lung nodule than is a metastasis. In patients with prior colon or renal carcinoma, a solitary metastasis and a new bronchogenic carcinoma are about equally common. In most cases, patients with soft tissue sarcomas or melanomas are more likely to have a solitary metastasis than a primary lung neoplasm. In any of these instances, chest CT should be performed when a single nodule is discovered on chest radiography. Discovery of additional (multiple) lesions within the lung increases the likelihood that the nodule seen on plain radiographs represents a metastasis (see "Multiple Nodules").

Bronchial carcinoids are not benign but rather are low-grade malignancies. They are not common, and only a minority arise as

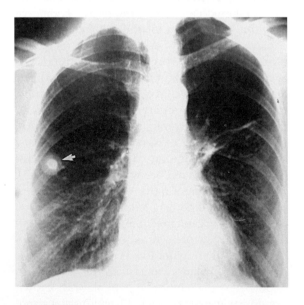

FIGURE 9-2 Posterior-anterior chest radiograph: calcified granuloma. The examination shows a large solitary nodule with a central, densely calcified nidus *(arrow)*, which is diagnostic of healed granulomatous disease. Occasionally, granulomas with a noncalcified "rind" of tissue as seen in this figure grow slowly because of continued inflammatory reaction. These are usually caused by histoplasmosis and are sometimes called histoplasmomas.

FIGURE 9-3 Posterior-anterior chest radiograph: noncalcified granuloma. This routine chest radiograph of a middle-aged man demonstrates a solitary, noncalcified intraparenchymal nodule *(arrow)*. In this instance, old films were available and showed that no change had occurred in 2 years, but the patient opted for surgical removal. The diagnosis was coccidioidomycosis granuloma.

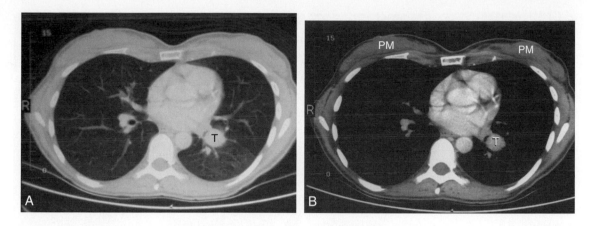

FIGURE 9-4 Computed tomography with intravenous contrast: bronchial carcinoid.

A, Section displayed in lung windows shows a tumor (T) obstructing the left lower lobe bronchi. The mass has a large extraluminal component.

B, The same section displayed in mediastinal windows shows that the mass (T) is higher in attenuation than skeletal muscles (pectoralis major, PM). Carcinoid tumors are vascular and often show enhancement following administration of intravenous contrast material. In some cases, their postenhancement attenuation may mimic pulmonary vasculature.

solitary nodules. Most arise centrally, with an intraluminal component at main or segmental bronchial bifurcations (Fig. 9-4). Accordingly, they are more likely to arise as recurrent lobar obstruction (in a younger patient) than to be the cause of a solitary parenchymal nodule. These tumors can be very vascular and enhance brightly after intravenous contrast material is given. Accordingly, some clinicians may be reluctant to perform transbronchial biopsies when the diagnosis of carcinoid is suspected.

Pulmonary hamartomas are the most common benign noninflammatory cause of single pulmonary nodules. Rather than developmental lesions, hamartomas probably represent slow-growing neoplasms. They most commonly occur in patients 45 to 50 years of age and constitute up to 5% of resected nodules. The classical "popcorn" calcifications that are often talked about are the exception rather than the rule (Fig. 9-5). More hamartomas (slightly less than half of the cases) can be recognized by the presence of intralesional fat. A well-defined nodule that contains tissue with fat density on CT (−80 to −120 Hounsfield units) or fat and calcium is almost certainly a hamartoma. There is a potential pitfall, however. The fat density must be measured using thin sections through the center of the nodule. If measurements are made too close to the edge of the nodule, the CT scanner may combine the attenuation of the lung (about −700 HU) with that of the nodule.

This is called volume averaging and can produce spurious low-density measurements of the nodule that are in the range of fat. It is critical to avoid this problem when assessing a solitary pulmonary nodule.

Rounded atelectasis is an important diagnosis to consider when a peripheral lung nodule or mass is seen adjacent to an area of pleural thickening. This form of atelectasis occurs when a section of the lung parenchyma becomes engulfed by the pleura, probably during resolution of a pleural effusion. Characteristically, it occurs in the setting of asbestos-related pleural disease but it can occur adjacent to pleural thickening of other causes (see discussion Chapter 5). Rounded atelectasis can often be diagnosed from CT findings (Fig. 9-6). If it is necessary to confirm the diagnosis, the mass can be biopsied easily with a transthoracic needle because of its proximity to the pleural surface.

Uncommon Diagnoses

Acute pneumonia is a rare cause of a discrete pulmonary nodule or mass in immunocompetent adults (see Fig. 7-6). A true "round pneumonia" is most commonly a pediatric condition, often secondary to pneumococcus. In immunocompromised patients, however, acute infection with atypical organisms (*Aspergillus, Nocardia*) is a potential cause of a solitary nodule.

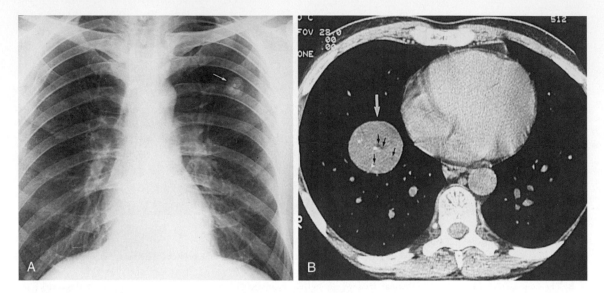

FIGURE 9-5 Posterior-anterior chest radiograph and computed tomography: hamartoma.

A, The 3-cm, smoothly lobulated, well-defined peripheral mass in the left upper lobe *(arrow)* demonstrates classic ("popcorn") calcifications. Unfortunately, these calcifications are present in a minority of hamartomas.

B, CT in another patient shows areas of low attenuation (fat; *small arrows*) and small calcifications in smoothly marginated hamartoma *(large arrow)*. The presence of fat is diagnostic of a hamartoma.

Pulmonary vasculitis (e.g., Wegener's granulomatosis) or pulmonary infarction caused by emboli may cause a solitary nodule but more often produces multiple opacities.

Developmental anomalies are a rare cause of pulmonary nodules or masses in adults. Most developmental anomalies arise from varying combinations of abnormal bronchi and alveoli and abnormal pulmonary vasculature.

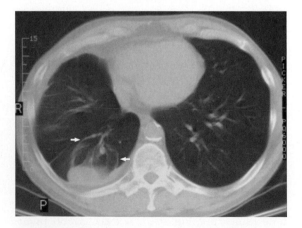

FIGURE 9-6 Computed tomography section of rounded atelectasis. The CT section shows a rounded mass that makes acute angles with the chest wall in an area of pleural thickening. Note that vessels enter the mass, curving toward its center *(arrows)*.

Bronchogenic cysts and bronchial atresia, for example, are composed nearly entirely of abnormal bronchi, and arteriovenous malformations (discussed in Chapter 10) are formed entirely of blood vessels.

Bronchogenic cysts may first detected in adults. They usually appear as a unilocular cyst near the carina and are more commonly mediastinal than intraparenchymal (Fig. 9-7). The cyst may be filled with fluid or with air. Bronchial atresia causes secretions to be trapped in a blind-ending bronchus and always appears as an intraparenchymal mass. Because of the diminished ventilation to the surrounding lung, the number of blood vessels is also decreased and the lung adjacent to the mass appears hyperlucent (Fig. 9-8).

Bronchopulmonary sequestrations are anomalies containing both abnormal bronchoalveolar tissue and an abnormal vascular supply. These congenital masses lack normal connections with the tracheobronchial tree and receive blood supply from the aorta. Sequestration may present as a discrete mass but more commonly appears to be an area of persistent pneumonia in a lower lobe, usually the left. Extralobar sequestrations (located outside the lung's visceral pleura) usually present in neonates and are removed surgically in infancy. Intralobar sequestrations consist of nonfunctional

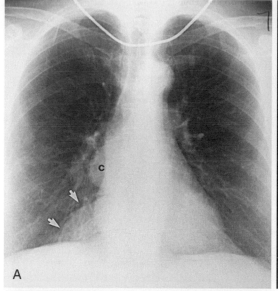

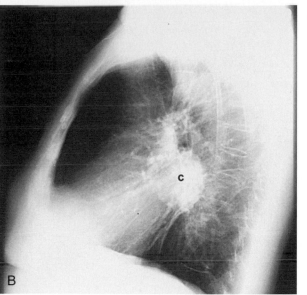

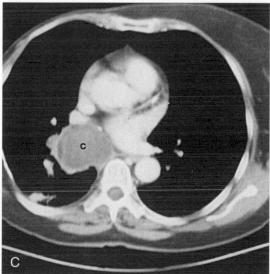

FIGURE 9-7 Posterior-anterior and lateral chest radiographs and contrast-enhanced computed tomography: bronchogenic mediastinal cyst.

A, Frontal radiograph demonstrates the right infrahilar mass (c), convex laterally, with smooth, well-defined margins and homogeneous opacity. Note the proximity of the mass to the carina. A right pericardial fat pad is seen inferior to the mass *(arrows)*.

B, Lateral radiograph demonstrates the mass (c) as subcarinal and midmediastinal in position.

C, Contrast-enhanced CT at the level of the mass (c) demonstrates right middle mediastinal position with characteristic thin wall and homogeneous cystic center (approximately 5 HU). Bronchogenic cysts can be higher in density if they contain proteinaceous fluid.

bronchopulmonary tissue located within the visceral pleura of a lobe. This type of sequestration may be first discovered in childhood or adulthood when it becomes infected (Fig. 9-9). Spiral CT with intravenous contrast can often make the diagnosis by showing the anomalous arterial blood supply arising from the aorta.

☐ CHARACTERIZING THE NODULE

The next step is to determine whether the nodule is benign or malignant. A high degree of certainty must accompany this determination

to exclude the diagnosis of lung cancer. The 2-year survival rate of patients with unresectable bronchogenic carcinoma is less than 20%. Accordingly, when a radiologist states that there is 95% likelihood that a nodule is benign, there is still a 1 in 20 chance that the lesion is in fact a carcinoma that will ultimately lead to the patient's death.

Although observations of growth rate can give reasonable assurance of benignity, lesion size and contour are only marginally helpful. Nodules larger than 2.0 cm, particularly those with spiculated borders, are assumed to be malignant until proved otherwise. Lesions smaller than 2.0 cm with smooth margins are

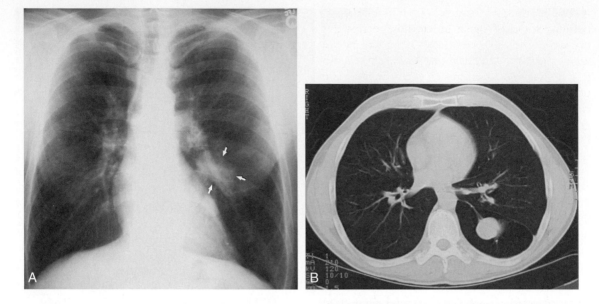

__FIGURE 9-8__ Posterior-anterior radiograph and computed tomography of bronchial atresia.

A, Frontal radiograph shows lobulated well-defined mass *(arrows)* below the left hilum.

B, CT confirms the smooth borders of the mass and shows the surrounding lung parenchyma to be hyperlucent.

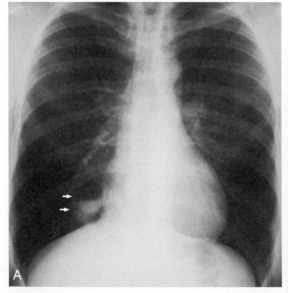

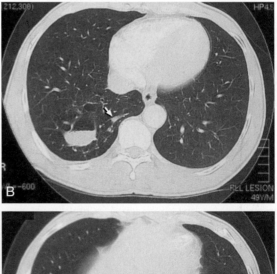

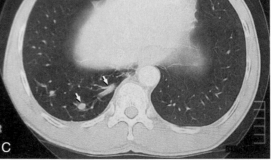

__FIGURE 9-9__ Posterior-anterior chest radiograph and computed tomography: sequestration.

A, Sequestration is present at the right medial base *(arrows),* where it appears as a mass containing an air-fluid level. Most sequestrations are found on the left.

B and C, CT sections confirm the presence of an air-fluid level and show an abnormal vessel *(arrow)* that supplies blood to the sequestration from the descending aorta. (Courtesy of Chris Bauman, MD.)

indeterminate and may be either malignant or benign. Some of these indeterminate nodules, however, can be classified as benign by the identification of calcifications. On a chest radiograph a very small nodule (≤5 mm) that is more opaque than the adjacent rib is almost certainly calcified. Unfortunately, detecting nodule calcium on radiographs by comparing the opacity of the nodule with the opacity of the ribs is not reliable for larger nodules or masses.

Fortunately, CT is much more effective than chest radiography in detecting calcifications. The CT sections, however, must be no thicker than half the diameter of the nodule to avoid missing the calcifications because of volume averaging (see "Partial Volume Artifacts" in Chapter 2). Benign calcifications are symmetrically distributed (central nidus, laminated) and make up more than 10% to 20% (often more than 50%) of the nodule's cross-sectional area or volume. Nodules smaller than 2 cm in diameter with benign calcifications and smooth contours are very likely benign (see Fig. 2-13). Because "very likely benign" falls short of "certainly benign," even nodules that meet these criteria should be monitored prospectively for growth over a 2-year period.

☐ DYNAMIC CONTRAST COMPUTED TOMOGRAPHY AND POSITRON EMISSION TOMOGRAPHY

In many cases, lung nodules do not contain adequate calcium to be classified as benign and diagnostic evaluation has to be taken to the next level. Two techniques are available to determine whether these nodules are likely to be benign or malignant, namely, dynamic contrast CT and nuclear medicine imaging with fluorine 18 fluorodeoxyglucose (FDG). Dynamic contrast CT makes use of CT scanning performed before and after an intravenous contrast agent is given to identify granulomas. After the administration of the intravenous contrast agent, the density of granulomas increases little, usually less than 15 HU. Although nodules enhancing more than 15 HU are probably not granulomas, they are not necessarily malignant. In addition to carcinomas, hamartomas and organizing pneumonia can enhance more than 15 HU. Another disadvantage of dynamic

CT is that nodules containing a few specks of calcium or air can produce false-negative or false-positive results unless precisely the same part of the nodule is measured both before and after the contrast agent is given. Because of these limitations and the rapid proliferation of positron emission tomography (PET) scanners, dynamic enhancement is not frequently used in the United States.

The most common radiology study now done to evaluate indeterminate nodules is nuclear medicine imaging with FDG. This radionuclide is preferentially taken up and trapped within metabolically active cells, such as those in malignant tumors. Imaging can be done with a PET scanner or a gamma camera (a type of instrument used for conventional nuclear medicine studies) that has been specially modified. Both the PET scanner and the modified gamma camera detect the energy products of positron emission from FDG. The PET scanner is more efficient at detecting these photons, and its spatial resolution is slightly better than that of the modified gamma cameras. FDG-PET can evaluate nodules as small as 7 to 8 mm in diameter, and modified gamma cameras are accurate in the evaluation of nodules 1 cm or larger (Fig. 9-10).

The sensitivity of FDG-PET in detecting malignancy is approximately 95% for nodules 1 cm or larger. Specificity is somewhat lower because other metabolically active cells, such as those found in infections, can also take up FDG. Positive nodules should be biopsied or excised with the understanding that this decision results in the biopsy of some active infections in addition to malignancies. If scanning with FDG is negative and the clinical suspicion of malignancy is not high (because of radiographic appearance and other patient-related risk factors), nodules may be monitored and observed for growth. Bronchoalveolar cell carcinoma and carcinoid tumors, however, may yield false-negative PET scans. If these tumors are suspected or if there is a high likelihood of malignancy, biopsy should be considered despite a negative PET scan. Patients for whom the suspicion of carcinoma is high should proceed directly to biopsy. Noninvasive imaging adds little to the evaluation in these situations and may lead to confusion and false security. For instance, if a lung nodule has been documented to double in size over the past year, a biopsy or excision should be performed regardless of the

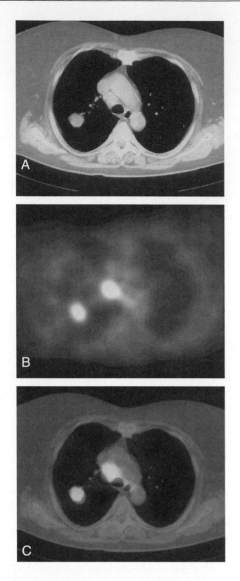

FIGURE 9-10 Computed tomography, positron emission tomography, and coregistered CT and PET of non–small cell lung carcinoma.

A, CT shows a right upper lobe lung nodule and a slightly enlarged right paratracheal lymph node.

B, Axial PET scan through the upper chest reveals two foci of increased fluorodeoxyglucose (FDG) uptake.

C, Coregistered PET and CT confirms that the areas of increased FDG uptake are the lung nodule and the paratracheal lymph node. Findings are consistent with bronchogenic lung carcinoma with ipsilateral mediastinal spread.

results of a PET scan. Similarly, a spiculated 3-cm mass in a heavy smoker that does not resolve after antibiotics and several weeks of observation has such a high risk of being a malignant that biopsy should be performed regardless of PET results. PET, therefore, should not be performed in the diagnostic evaluation of these nodules. (This differs from the role of PET in staging lung carcinoma, which is discussed later.)

☐ BIOPSY

Options for biopsy include transthoracic needle biopsies (TTNBs), bronchoscopic biopsies, and thoracoscopy. TTNBs have a sensitivity and specificity of 90% or greater in diagnosing bronchogenic cancer. This is much higher than that of bronchoscopy, particularly for lesions less than 2 cm in diameter. TTNB, however, does carry an increased risk of pneumothorax compared with bronchoscopy. (Between 5% and 10% of patients require chest tubes.) The likelihood of a successful bronchoscopic biopsy is much higher if CT shows that a segmental or larger airway terminates within the mass, and bronchoscopy is often reserved for patients with these findings. Thoracoscopy offers the advantage of an excisional biopsy, with the option of proceeding to tumor staging and a more definitive procedure, depending on the pathologic findings. One school of thought holds that likely malignancies should be excised without prior biopsy in patients with a low operative risk. Nonexcisional biopsies (i.e., by transthoracic needle or bronchoscope) would be reserved for patients at high risk for surgery, patients with suspected metastatic disease, and patients in whom an infectious etiology is likely on clinical grounds (i.e., in an immunocompromised host). An algorithm for work-up of a solitary parenchymal lung is presented in Figure 9-11.

☐ LUNG CANCER SCREENING

The preceding part of this chapter describes the evaluation of a lung nodule found on chest radiographs; however, many nodules are now first seen on a CT scan. The vast majority of these small lung nodules are incidental findings on CT scans performed for other reasons. Most of these nodules are not evident on chest radiographs, even if one goes back and looks at the radiograph again after reviewing the CT scan. CT scanning's ability to find nodules that are occult on radiographs and the dismal outlook for survival from late-stage lung cancer have generated interest in CT scan screening for early-stage lung carcinoma.

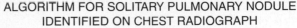

ALGORITHM FOR SOLITARY PULMONARY NODULE
IDENTIFIED ON CHEST RADIOGRAPH

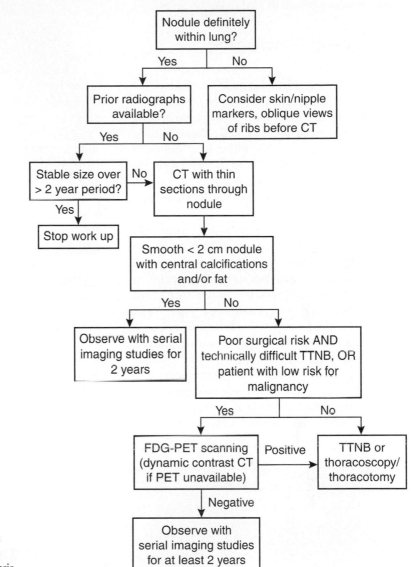

FIGURE 9-11 Algorithm: solitary pulmonary nodule identified on chest radiograph. CT, computed tomography; FDG, fluorodeoxyglucose; PET, positron emission tomography; TTNB, transthoracic needle biopsy.

Results of several large trials have shown conclusively that CT screening can detect more early-stage lung cancers than are detected in unscreened populations. These cancers can often be cured by surgical resection. Despite this good news, enough controversy remains to generate impassioned editorials. Part of the controversy has been caused by the sheer number of small nodules detected with chest CT. Although the prevalence of cancer in patients undergoing their first screening CT is about 2% to 3%, up to 70% of patients screened

may have at least one small nodule. Most of these nodules are less than 1 cm in diameter and therefore are difficult to biopsy percutaneously and too small to evaluate accurately with PET scanning. At this time, the best we can do is to follow these small nodules serially with CT scans to look for growth (see algorithm). The prevalence of malignancy in these nodules smaller than 1 cm is probably less than 10% in patients being screened for lung cancer. This high rate of false-positive studies, often requiring follow-up serial CT scans over a

2-year period, has led some experts to doubt the value of screening chest CT, especially in patients who are not at high risk.

Evaluation of Bronchogenic Carcinoma

When evaluating bronchogenic carcinoma for treatment, it is practical to classify tumors as either small cell (making up 20% to 25% of lung carcinomas) or non–small cell. This division basically represents the difference between chemotherapy (small cell) and consideration for surgical resection (non–small cell). Non–small cell carcinoma can be divided further into squamous cell, adenocarcinoma (of which bronchoalveolar is probably a subtype), large cell, and mixed. There are some differences in the classical presentation of the types of non–small cell carcinoma. Squamous carcinoma tends to be central and recur locally and is the most common subtype to cavitate (see Fig. 7-16). Adenocarcinoma is more likely to present as a solitary peripheral pulmonary nodule and is currently the most common form of lung carcinoma (Fig. 9-12). Large cell carcinoma is less common and characteristically appears as a mass greater than 3 cm in size. Bronchoalveolar cell carcinoma may present with one of three

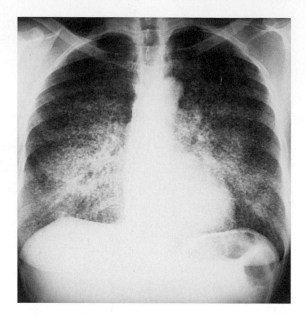

FIGURE 9-13 Posterior-anterior chest radiograph: bronchoalveolar carcinoma. Bilateral uncountable small nodules. These coalesce on the right side to form an area of confluent air space disease that could be mistaken for a pneumonia.

general patterns. It may appear as a single nodule, as diffuse nodules, or as an area of consolidation. The last pattern can be initially mistaken for a pneumonia (Fig. 9-13; see Fig. 6-2). In most instances, however, there is considerable

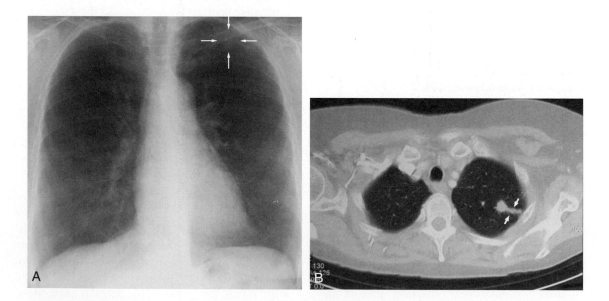

FIGURE 9-12 Posterior-anterior chest radiograph and computed tomography of a peripheral adenocarcinoma.

A, Frontal chest radiograph shows a small nodule *(arrows)* partially hidden by anterior and posterior ribs and the clavicle.

B, CT section through the upper lobes reveals a 1-cm peripheral nodule with irregular border and a linear opacity extending to the pleura *(arrows)*, a pleural "tail." These findings are more commonly seen with adenocarcinoma than with other bronchogenic neoplasms.

overlap between the radiographic manifestations of the subtypes of non–small cell lung carcinoma. Regardless of the subtype and the various modes of presentation, the key in evaluating a patient with lung cancer is to determine the stage of the disease. It is the tumor stage that determines whether the tumor can be resected, and only surgical resection is curative (Fig. 9-14).

If the patient has enough reserve lung function to tolerate surgery, the pivotal issue in staging is whether the tumor is anatomically resectable. The International System for Staging Lung Cancer was modified in 1997 and is widely published in its entirety. Malignancies are graded on the basis of the primary tumor size (T), nodal spread (N), and the presence of distal metastases (M). According to this system, patients do not undergo surgery for resection if the tumor has (1) invaded the heart, great vessels, trachea, vertebral body, or esophagus, caused a malignant effusion, or formed a satellite

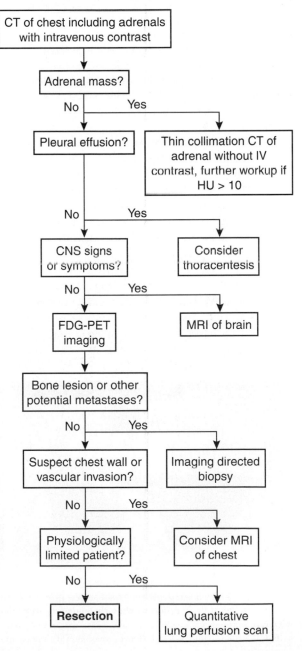

STAGING BRONCHOGENIC CARCINOMA

FIGURE 9-14 Algorithm: staging bronchogenic carcinoma. CNS, central nervous system; CT, computed tomography; FDG, fluorodeoxyglucose; HU, Hounsfield units; IV, intravenous; MRI, magnetic resonance imaging; PET, positron emission tomography.

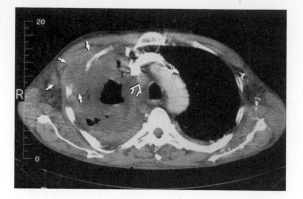

FIGURE 9-15 Computed tomography: chest wall invasion by non–small cell lung cancer. The tumor can be seen growing through the chest wall *(arrows)*. Although chest wall invasion alone does not designate the tumor as inoperable, resection is usually not performed if there is also evidence of ipsilateral mediastinal node involvement. In this case, positron emission tomography (not shown) was positive in the right paratracheal node *(open arrow)*.

nodule in the same lobe as the primary tumor (T4 lesion); (2) metastasized to contralateral mediastinal or hilar nodes or any scalene node (N3 disease); or (3) metastasized to distant sites including any lobe of the lung other than that containing the primary tumor (M1). Note that T3 lesions, e.g., tumors presenting with chest wall invasion, pericardial invasion, and main bronchus involvement within 2 cm of the carina, are technically still operable (Fig. 9-15). The same is true for patients with ipsilateral mediastinal node involvement (N2 disease). However, the overall survival of these patients

is low and the morbidity of resection high. Surgery is usually limited to selected patients.

The radiograph on which the tumor is detected is the first step in the staging procedure. Chest radiographic findings that affect staging include tumor size, evidence of atelectasis, mediastinal or hilar adenopathy, pleural effusion, and bone invasion. After the chest radiograph, chest CT is routinely performed in staging lung carcinoma. It is very useful in evaluating large central tumors that may be T3 or T4 by virtue of invading pulmonary arteries, pulmonary veins, pericardium, and main bronchi (Fig. 9-16). In addition, CT is more sensitive than chest radiography for the detection of mediastinal and hilar adenopathy. The right paratracheal nodes are a common pathway for the lymphatic drainage of both lungs and are frequently involved if there is mediastinal spread (Fig. 9-17). Subcarinal adenopathy and aorticopulmonary window adenopathy are also common. If the tumor is left sided, it is important to look for enlarged para-aortic and aorticopulmonary nodes with CT. These lymph nodes are not accessible with standard cervical mediastinoscopy. In order to sample them a mini-thoracotomy, a percutaneous needle biopsy or thoracoscopy is usually needed.

Until recently, the radiologic evaluation of mediastinal and hilar nodes prior to resection of lung carcinoma was accomplished with CT scanning alone. Nodes that had a diameter greater than 1 cm were classified as positive and required further evaluation with biopsy. Unfortunately, using these CT criteria to

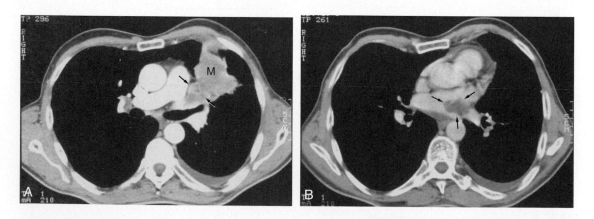

FIGURE 9-16 Computed tomography section of a patient with tumor invasion of the pulmonary vein.

A, CT section at the level of the right main pulmonary artery shows a left upper lobe mass (M) that extends into the left superior pulmonary vein *(arrows)*.

B, CT section slightly below A shows extension of the tumor into the left atrium *(arrows)*.

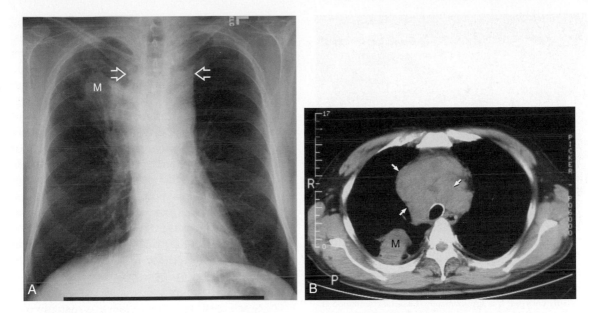

FIGURE 9-17 Posterior-anterior chest radiograph and computed tomography section of a patient with adenocarcinoma and bilateral mediastinal metastases.

A, Frontal radiograph demonstrates a right upper lobe mass (M). The mediastinal contour is abnormally widened, particularly above the aortic arch *(open arrows)*.

B, CT without intravenous contrast shows the primary tumor (M) and enlarged bilateral high paratracheal lymph nodes *(arrows)*. The left-sided nodal involvement represents N3 lymph node disease and renders this tumor inoperable.

differentiate metastatic adenopathy from benign inflammatory adenopathy is only about 60% to 70% specific and sensitive. FDG-PET scanning has now become commonly used for lung carcinoma staging and has a specificity 85% and a sensitivity of about 90%. Combining PET and CT images together on the same image is becoming increasingly popular. This technique of combining CT and PET images, sometimes called image fusion or image coregistration, may allow more precise localization of nodes containing metastases and improve the accuracy of staging.

Nevertheless, even when combined with CT, PET is not perfect. Patients undergoing lung cancer staging commonly harbor inflammatory mediastinal lymph nodes, such that the negative predictive value of FDG-PET is 95% but the positive predictive value is only 75%. Because the positive predictive value is only moderate, PET-positive nodes should be biopsied whenever their involvement determines whether the tumor is resectable. The price of a false positive in this situation (i.e., denying the opportunity of cure to a patient with resectable tumor) is too high to accept.

The likelihood of systemic metastases of non–small cell carcinoma varies with cell type.

Adenocarcinomas may metastasize systemically even when the primary tumor is small, whereas squamous carcinomas usually do not spread to distant organs until the tumor is advanced locally. Both CT and PET play a role in the detection of distant metastases. When a CT scan of the chest is used to stage a bronchogenic neoplasm, portions of the upper abdomen are routinely included in the scan. The liver and adrenal gland are the key sites that are examined, and the frequency of metastases is generally greater in the adrenal gland. The liver is usually not optimally imaged in this fashion, and if there is clinical concern for liver metastases (e.g., liver enzyme abnormalities) or a hepatic abnormality is suggested on the CT study of the chest, the CT scan should be repeated using a protocol specific for liver pathology.

The identification of adrenal metastases is confounded by the frequency of nonfunctioning adrenal adenomas, which are present in 1% of the population. Even in patients with lung cancer, about half of adrenal masses are adenomas rather than metastases. Adenomas are often low in attenuation (e.g., <10 HU before the administration of intravenous contrast) because they contain lipids (Fig. 9-18). This distinction

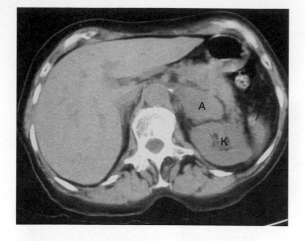

FIGURE 9-18 Computed tomography: adrenal metastases from bronchogenic carcinoma. CT without intravenous contrast, section through the upper abdomen. The left adrenal (A) is markedly enlarged. It is approximately the same attenuation as the kidney (K), higher than the attenuation of most benign adrenal adenomas.

between an adenoma and a metastatic lesion can often be made on a routine CT scan done to evaluate the lung; however, sometimes the patient must return for repeated CT scanning with thinner sections through the adrenals in order to measure accurately the density of the mass (see "Partial Volume Artifacts" in Chapter 2). If thin section scanning through the adrenal without intravenous contrast does not yield a definite answer, CT scanning can be done immediately after the administration of an intravenous contrast agent and repeated again about 15 minutes later. This can usually differentiate metastases from an adenoma because intravenous contrast material washes out of adenomas faster than it washes out of metastases, causing the density of adenomas to fall more quickly over time.

When PET scanning is performed as part of the evaluation of the mediastinal and hilar lymph nodes, the rest of the body is usually imaged as well. These whole-body PET images can detect unsuspected metastases, such as bone metastases, in about 10% of patients. PET scanning with FDG is not as sensitive for detection of metastases to the brain as it is for detection of metastases to other parts of the body because the normally functioning brain takes up large amounts of FDG. For a metastasis to be visible as a "hot spot" on PET scanning, it must take up and trap still more FDG than the surrounding brain tissue. Similar problems occur when

searching for cardiac metastases. PET scanning is also capable of detecting adrenal metastases, but its role in differentiating metastases from adenomas is not yet fully defined.

It is sometimes helpful to evaluate further patients who have borderline pulmonary physiology and anatomically resectable disease with a quantitative lung perfusion scan. The amount of lung perfusion to the area planned for resection is combined with pulmonary function testing to predict the postoperative pulmonary function. Patients with a postoperative pulmonary function (forced expiratory volume in 1 second or diffusing capacity) of less than 40% of the predicted normal value often undergo preoperative exercise testing, and patients with predicted function less than 30% may not be treated with surgery.

Small cell lung carcinoma is usually not treated surgically, and therefore imaging is not done to determine anatomic or physiologic resectability. This tumor rarely arises as a peripheral nodule and usually manifests with marked mediastinal or hilar abnormalities without an identifiable primary lesion (Fig. 9-19; Table 9-2). Two thirds of patients with small cell carcinoma have disseminated disease when they are first diagnosed. Staging for small cell carcinoma is geared to separate patients with limited disease (confined to one hemithorax) from those with extensive involvement. This is important for prognostic purposes and in order to consider combining local radiation therapy with chemotherapy in patients with limited disease. Abdominal CT is routinely performed to detect liver metastases, and the central nervous system is imaged with CT or magnetic resonance imaging. In approximately 10% of patients brain metastasis is apparent on head CT at the time of staging.

Multiple Nodules

Multiple pulmonary nodules may appear on chest radiographs as round homogeneous opacities within the lung parenchyma with well-defined borders and smooth edges. They are often round and usually do not have air bronchograms. These characteristics may distinguish multiple nodules from multifocal air space disease. Some lung opacities, however, are poorly seen on radiographs and can be determined to be nodules or masses only on CT scanning. Although there is considerable

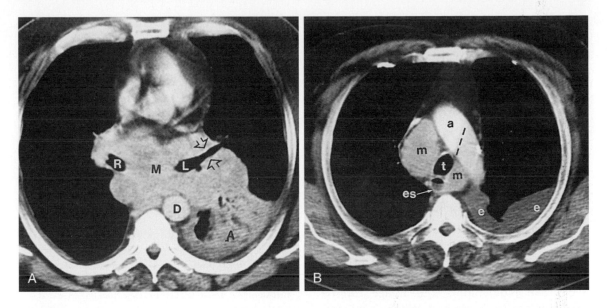

FIGURE 9-19 Posterior-anterior chest radiograph and contrast-enhanced computed tomography: small cell carcinoma with mediastinal adenopathy.

A, Contrast-enhanced CT axial image utilizing mediastinal windows, obtained 3 cm below the carina, demonstrates a mass (M) made up of a conglomerate of mediastinal nodes extending to encase the lingular bronchus *(arrows)* as well as right (R) and left (L) main stem bronchi. There is associated atelectasis of the left lower lobe (A). D, descending aorta.

B, Nodal masses (m) in the superior aspect of the middle mediastinum in the same patient. The anterior paratracheal mass compresses the superior vena cava. This caused superior vena cava syndrome in this patient. a, aorta; e, effusion; es, esophagus; t, trachea.

overlap with either radiographic pattern (Table 9-3), multiple nodules are more likely to be caused by metastatic disease and multifocal air space disease is more often caused by an inflammatory process.

The patient's clinical history and prior radiographs are both very helpful in determining the most likely diagnoses. Ill-defined opacities that condense into multiple nodules over time are more consistent with evolving granuloma or infarctions. Knowledge of the presence of primary malignancy elsewhere in the body is

TABLE 9-2
Radiologic Clues to Specific Lung Malignancies

Clue	Suggested Diagnosis
Central mass with distal atelectasis of lobe(s)	Squamous cell
Small peripheral mass, may have pleural "tail"	Adenocarcinoma
Large peripheral mass	Large cell
Inapparent mass, extensive mediastinal adenopathy	Small cell or aggressive adenocarcinoma
Air bronchograms on radiographs*	Bronchoalveolar cell or lymphoma

*Adenocarcinomas often contain air bronchograms on CT images.

TABLE 9-3
Multiple Nodules

Neoplasm
Metastatic malignancy
Bronchoalveolar carcinoma*
Lymphoma*
Multiple hamartomas

Noninfectious inflammatory
Sarcoidosis*
Rheumatoid nodules

Infections
Granulomas
Septic emboli*
Parasites
Opportunistic infections* (*Aspergillus, Cryptococcus, Nocardia*)

Vascular
Infarcts*
Hematomas
Multiple arteriovenous malformations
Wegener's granulomatosis

*Also cause multifocal air space disease.

of obvious importance. Most neoplasms (central nervous system primary tumors being a notable exception) can metastasize to the lungs. Eighty percent of patients with pulmonary metastases have a known primary lesion. At most, only 20% of patients have pulmonary metastases at the time of the initial diagnosis of cancer. Choriocarcinoma, testicular and renal cell carcinoma, and, to a lesser extent, thyroid carcinoma are the most likely neoplasms to have already metastasized to the lungs at the time the primary tumor is discovered. Primary lung cancer is an uncommon cause of multiple lung nodules.

Metastatic disease may arise as a countable or uncountable number of nodules. The latter are classically seen in cases of thyroid carcinoma. The radiographic appearance can be very similar to the pattern of miliary infections, sarcoid, and some pneumoconioses. Usually high-resolution CT (HRCT) can differentiate metastases from the latter two, but differentiating miliary infections from "miliary" metastases relies on clinical history and sometimes on biopsy.

Some other radiographic characteristics of metastatic lung nodules may suggest a specific diagnosis. "Cannonball" lesions are classically seen in metastatic sarcomas and colon carcinoma but may originate from other primary tumors as well (Fig. 9-20). Cavitary lesions are most likely secondary to head and neck squamous cell carcinoma, and ossified metastases can be seen with osteogenic sarcoma (Figs. 9-21 and 9-22). There is significant overlap between the radiographic presentations of different neoplasms.

Lymphoma may also cause multiple parenchymal nodules. The intrathoracic manifestations of lymphoma vary considerably, depending on the clinical setting. In patients with acquired immunodeficiency syndrome (AIDS), lymphoma arises as multiple parenchymal nodules that are usually well defined. In this way, lymphoma differs from Kaposi's sarcoma, which usually causes more ill-defined pulmonary nodules and may be accompanied by a pleural effusion.

Lymphoma is an uncommon cause of multiple nodules in patients without AIDS, and when it does occur it is usually a manifestation of systemic involvement. Primary intrathoracic lymphomas (lymphomas that originate in the lung) are rare and tend to be of the non-Hodgkin's type. Large nodules and masses

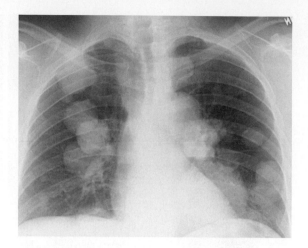

FIGURE 9-20 Posterior-anterior chest radiograph: cannonball metastases—carcinoma of the esophagus. These hematogenous metastatic lesions range from one to several centimeters in diameter and are not "too numerous to count." Their size variation indicates different episodes of pulmonary parenchymal seeding. Large metastatic lesions are typically seen with soft tissue sarcomas, gastrointestinal metastases (especially colon carcinoma), testicular tumors, and uterine carcinoma. Lower lung field predominance of nodules is expected in metastatic disease but is not prominent in this radiograph.

caused by both primary and systemic parenchymal lymphoma characteristically contain air bronchograms that are visible on CT imaging (Fig. 9-23). Parenchymal disease caused by systemic Hodgkin's and non-Hodgkin's lymphoma

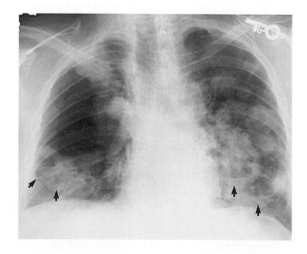

FIGURE 9-21 Posterior-anterior view of the chest: multiple cavitary lesions. Same patient as shown in Figure 9-20, only 8 months later. Some of the nodules have progressed to central necrosis and cavitation *(arrows)*. Note the thickness of the walls, which suggests cavitary metastases rather than cavitary infectious disease.

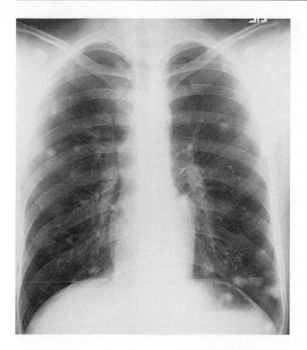

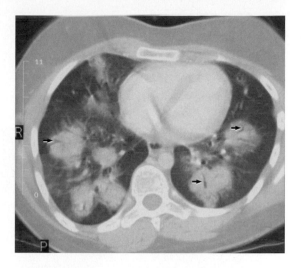

FIGURE 9-23 Computed tomography: lymphomatous involvement of the lung parenchyma. Multiple large nodules are present bilaterally, some containing air bronchograms *(arrows)*.

FIGURE 9-22 Posterior-anterior chest radiograph: calcified metastasis. This frontal radiograph demonstrates multiple nodules with smooth, well-defined borders. The opacity of the nodules relative to the rest of the chest tissue is greater than that usually seen with parenchymal nodules of this size. These are calcifying metastases from primary osteosarcoma of the left femur. (Healed histoplasmosis and varicella can also produce large numbers of calcified nodules, but they are usually smaller in size.)

is almost always accompanied by hilar or mediastinal adenopathy, or both, if seen before treatment. Primary lymphoma of the lung and recurrent Hodgkin's disease, however, may appear to affect the parenchyma alone.

Special Manifestations of Pulmonary Metastases

Diffuse involvement of the lymphatic system (lymphangitic carcinoma) may occur with many malignancies. The majority of primary neoplasms are adenocarcinomas (e.g., stomach, lung, and breast). Most often, lymphangitic carcinoma is the result of hematogenous rather than lymphatic metastases, and therefore lymphadenopathy is commonly absent on the chest radiograph. Patients with this condition

present with dyspnea and nonproductive cough and radiographs characteristically show a linear or reticulonodular pattern that is most extensive at the lung bases (Fig 9-24). When the linear pattern is present, Kerley's B lines are prominent, and therefore this diagnosis should be considered in patients with an atypical heart failure pattern on their chest radiographs. Occasionally, a patient may be symptomatic before any abnormal findings are evident on the chest radiographs. HRCT of the lungs is able to detect the disease at earlier stages and can strongly suggest the correct diagnosis. HRCT images usually show nodular thickening on interlobular septa, peribronchial tissues, and pleural fissures (see Chapter 6).

Endobronchial metastases are an uncommon presentation of metastatic malignancy. They should be considered in patients with known melanoma and primary lesions of the colon, breast, and kidney who show signs of obstructive atelectasis on chest radiographs. These radiographic changes may be indistinguishable from those that appear with centrally occurring primary bronchogenic lesions. Bronchoscopic biopsy is usually successful in obtaining a definitive answer.

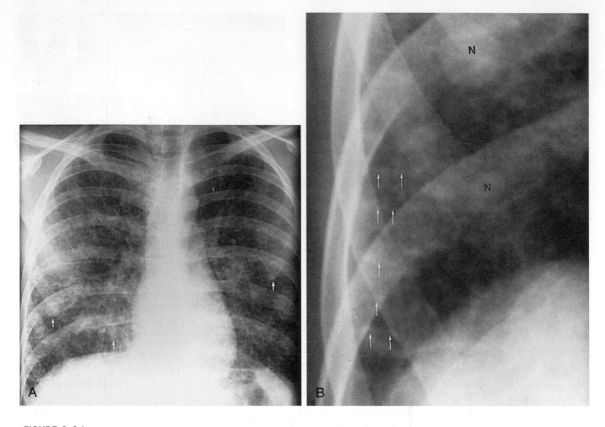

FIGURE 9-24 Posterior-anterior chest radiograph: hematogenous metastases with lymphangitic spread.

A, Frontal chest radiograph demonstrates the nodules from hematogenous metastases *(arrows)* and the presence of lymphangitic spread. Note the prominent Kerley's B lines.

B, Close-up of lymphangitic spread: Kerley's B lines are well defined *(arrows)*. Linear opacities extend to the lateral pleural surface, indicative of involvement of the interlobular septa. N, nodule.

Pearls for Clinicians—Pulmonary Nodules and Neoplasms

1. "Smart is good but old films are better"—Robert Green, MD.
2. When searching for lung carcinoma on chest radiographs, do not focus on tiny nodules (<5 mm), which are usually granulomas or vessels seen on end. Missed cancers are more commonly nodules and masses 1.5 to 3 cm in size, which are partially obscured by ribs and normal structures in the hila and mediastinum.
3. Small nodules (less than 1 cm in diameter) are very common incidental findings on chest CT. Even among smokers, about 90% of these nodules are stable over 2 years of CT follow-up and are probably benign. Small nodules are more likely to be malignant in patients with a known malignancy.

4. PET imaging is very useful in staging known lung carcinoma but can be overused in the evaluation of lung nodules. Generally, PET scanning is not useful for evaluation of nodules that are likely to be malignant on the basis of clinical and CT evaluation. These nodules should be biopsied or excised (see Figs. 9-11 and 9-14).
5. Consider PET evaluation of a lung nodule when the risk of malignancy is low or the risks of both surgery and biopsy are high. If the PET is negative, these nodules should *still* be followed with CT for interval growth (see Fig. 9-11).

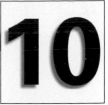

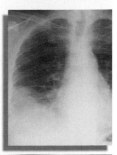

Pulmonary Vascular Lung Disease

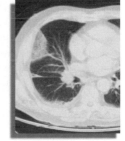

☐ EMBOLI AND FOCAL DISEASE

Pulmonary Emboli

Acute Emboli

Pulmonary emboli are the most common vascular cause of lung disease. No matter what algorithm is chosen for subsequent work-up a chest radiograph is the best first step in the evaluation of pulmonary emboli. The radiograph is essential to ensure that the patient's symptoms are not related to some other disease process (e.g., a pneumothorax or adult respiratory distress syndrome). Contrary to a popular myth, among patients with pulmonary emboli, chest radiographs are usually not normal. One large multi-institutional study showed that only 12% of patients with documented pulmonary emboli had normal radiographs. Unfortunately, the radiographic abnormalities that are caused by pulmonary emboli are nonspecific, most commonly atelectasis or small effusions. Still, these findings can be helpful when combined with history. For instance, small effusions in young adults with acute pleuritic pain are more compatible with pulmonary emboli than viral pleurodynia. Young patients with effusions but

without evident pneumonia should receive further evaluation for pulmonary emboli.

Although the chest radiograph is usually abnormal, the more specific or "classical" plain radiographic signs are rarely present. Westermark's sign, a zone of relative radiolucency related to hypoperfusion, is generally recognized on radiographs only if the reader has been given a "running start" (e.g., a history of pleuritic chest pain) (Fig. 10-1). A peripheral wedge-shaped consolidation with the apex directed toward the hilum is called Hampton's hump and is a sign of pulmonary infarction (Fig. 10-2). A single hump is nonspecific and easily attributed to a pneumonia. Multiple areas of peripheral consolidation are more worrisome but rarely appreciated on chest radiographs.

In the vast majority of cases, the key in detecting pulmonary emboli is considering the diagnosis on clinical grounds rather than recognizing specific radiographic findings. What is the best way to evaluate a patient with suspected pulmonary emboli? Although there are still many points of controversy, over the past 5 to 10 years the computed tomography (CT) pulmonary angiogram has become the cornerstone of the evaluation for pulmonary emboli (Fig. 10-3).

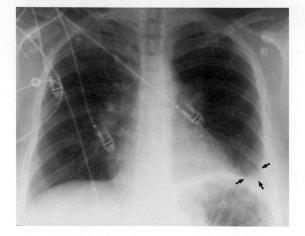

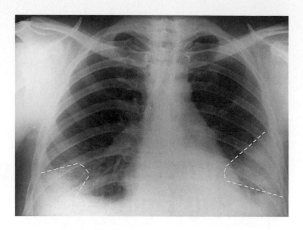

FIGURE 10-1 Chest radiograph: Westermark sign. Anterior-posterior radiograph of a patient with a large pulmonary embolism to the left lung shows the left hemithorax to be diffusely lucent with few vessels seen within the parenchyma. A small opacity is also seen at the costophrenic angle *(arrows)*, possibly representing an infarct.

FIGURE 10-2 Posterior-anterior radiograph of the chest: Hampton's hump. This frontal radiograph shows triangular pleura-based opacities *(dashed lines)*. The apices of the triangles point medially. Eighty-five percent of pulmonary emboli are bilateral and most frequently occur in the lower lobes because of the increased blood flow to these areas.

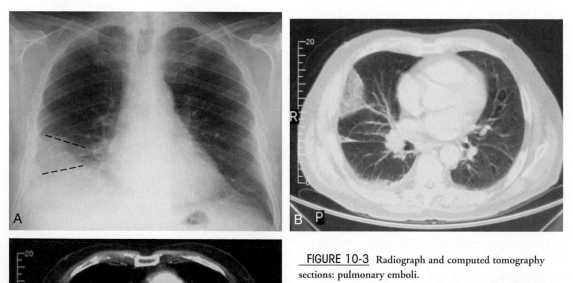

FIGURE 10-3 Radiograph and computed tomography sections: pulmonary emboli.

A, Pleura-based opacity *(dashed lines)*, similar to those shown in Figure 10-2, is present in the right middle lobe. The right hemidiaphragm is also elevated.

B, Contrast-enhanced CT section through the right middle lobe, lung window. There is a triangular subpleural opacity in the middle lobe matching the radiographic findings in A.

C, Contrast-enhanced mediastinal window at the same level as B. Large, low-density clots *(arrows)* are seen in the right descending and right middle lobe arteries. Although both the middle and lower lobes were affected by pulmonary embolism, an infarct occurred only in the middle lobe.

CT pulmonary angiograms depend on three things: rapid scanning using a spiral CT scanner, thin collimation, and intravenous (IV) contrast. Rapid scanning is important because the best images are obtained during a single breath-hold. Although adequate images can sometimes be obtained during slow, shallow breathing, images during a breath-hold are more likely to be free of motion artifacts. The volume averaging that occurs during respiratory motion can cause apparent defects in the pulmonary arteries that are mistaken for emboli. Thin slices improve the spatial resolution of the CT angiogram and also lessen volume-averaging

artifacts. With single-detector spiral CT scanners the slice thickness usually cannot be decreased to less than 3 mm, before the scanning time (and breath-hold) becomes intolerably long for the patient (Fig. 10-4). With the invention of multidetector CT (MDCT), thin slices and scan speed are no longer mutually exclusive. Using 16-row MDCT, slice thickness of 1 mm or less can usually be used while scanning through all of the segmental pulmonary arteries during a single breath-hold (Fig. 10-5).

Exceptionally thin slices and dazzling speed are still not much help unless there is adequate contrast material in the vessels. Under optimal conditions, contrast material is administered through an antecubital fossa vein at

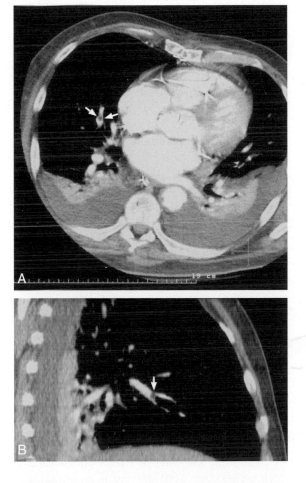

FIGURE 10-4 Single-detector computed tomography scans of pulmonary embolism.

A, Axial CT image from a single-detector scanner shows a small pulmonary embolism *(arrows)* in a segmental branch of the right pulmonary artery.

B, Reformatted image in the sagittal plane depicts only a small portion of the artery but does confirm the presence of an embolism *(arrow)* surrounded by contrast material.

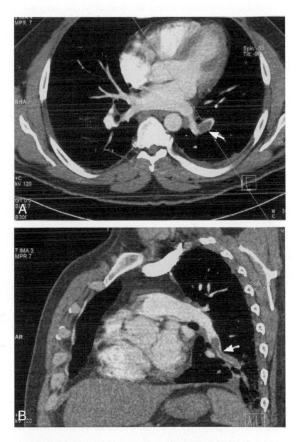

FIGURE 10-5 Multidetector computed tomography: pulmonary emboli.

A, Axial image shows left lower lobe pulmonary embolus *(arrow).*

B, Reformatted (reconstructed) sagittal image shows extension of emboli into the basal segments of the left lower lobe *(arrow).* Because of the thin sections used by the multidetector CT scanner, the reformatted image shows better resolution of detail (spatial resolution) than the image in Figure 10-4.

3 to 5 mL/sec and scanning is begun after an "empirical" delay of 15 to 25 seconds. Unfortunately, in many clinical settings conditions are not optimal. The patient may have a prolonged circulation time because of a cardiomyopathy, or the only IV site may be a small vein in the back of the patient's hand. Under these circumstances a small amount of contrast material, a test bolus, can be injected just before the diagnostic scan to determine the optimal delay between starting the contrast injection and starting the scan. Software has been developed that uses sequential imaging of a target vessel to detect the arrival of the contrast bolus in the pulmonary vessels and then automatically triggers the spiral CT acquisition.

CT pulmonary angiograms, particularly those performed with multidetector scanners, produce large numbers of images. In order to follow accurately the course of the pulmonary arteries to the segmental level, these images must be reviewed on a workstation rather than on film. Workstations allow the reader to scroll rapidly up and down through the images while following a particular artery and also allow the reader to reconstruct (reformat) the data in various planes. These reconstructions are performed after slicing the "cylinder" of data acquired with a spiral CT. Thin initial sections pack the data in the cylinder more densely than thick sections and therefore make possible more detailed reconstructions in sagittal, coronal, and oblique planes (see Chapter 1). Because MDCT makes it possible to obtain very thin axial sections over a long section of the body, it can be used to image pulmonary vessels accurately in multiple planes.

Workstations also make possible more complex computer processing of the image data such as creation of three-dimensional images, but these techniques are usually not necessary to make the correct diagnosis (Fig. 10-6). More important than complex postprocessing, high-quality interpretation still requires a solid knowledge of pulmonary anatomy. Hilar lymph nodes, pulmonary veins that are unopacified with contrast material, and secretion-filled bronchi can all be mistaken for emboli by inexperienced readers.

How good are CT pulmonary angiograms? Reports vary depending on slice thickness, but with a single-detector scanner the sensitivity and specificity for segmental emboli are probably between 85% and 90%. Sensitivity and

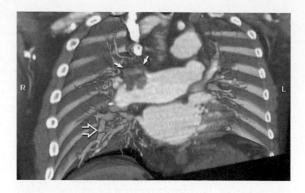

FIGURE 10-6 Computed tomography of pulmonary emboli displayed with volume rendering. CT image after postprocessing using a technique called volume rendering, which creates an image with a three-dimensional appearance. A large embolism in the right main pulmonary artery extends into the right upper lobe *(arrows)*. Thrombus also fills the right descending pulmonary artery *(open arrow)*. (Courtesy of David Levin, MD, San Diego, California.)

specificity for multidetector scanners exceed 90%. Sensitivity and specificity for small, subsegmental, emboli are lower, and there is still considerable uncertainty regarding the best management of isolated small emboli (those not accompanied by larger clots). Fortunately, isolated subsegmental emboli are relatively uncommon in symptomatic patients.

In light of these advances, a good-quality CT pulmonary angiogram usually obviates the need for catheter-directed pulmonary angiography (Fig. 10-7). Knowledge of the patient's pretest likelihood of having had an embolism is less critical when using MDCT than when interpreting ventilation-perfusion scans, but it is still important. Patients with a very high suspicion of having had an embolism may require further work-up despite a negative CT angiogram, especially if a single-detector CT scanner is used. Sometimes a repeated CT angiogram with thinner sections through a portion of the pulmonary vasculature that was partially obscured by the patient's motion or other artifacts suffices.

Although the rate of major complications from pulmonary angiography is less than 1%, the study is time consuming and now is usually reserved for patients with technically limited CT angiography (Fig.10-8). Pulmonary angiography has the advantage of a long track record of efficacy; patients with negative pulmonary angiograms have been shown to be at very low risk for recurrent pulmonary emboli. Like CT

DIAGNOSTIC ALGORITHM FOR SUSPECTED PULMONARY EMBOLISM

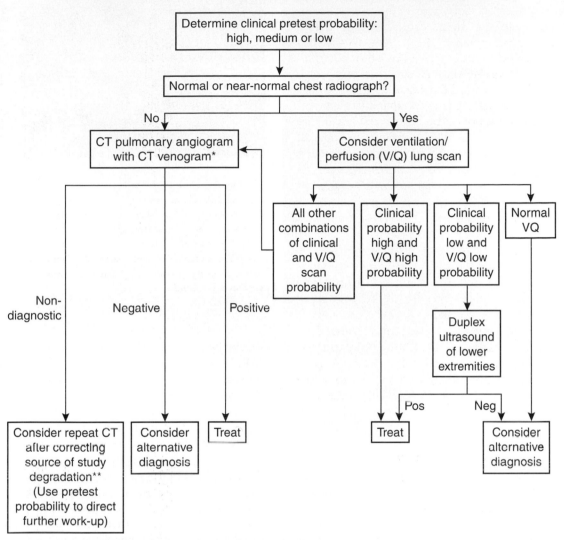

*Duplex ultrasound may be substituted for CT venography.
**Check bolus timing, use thinner sections in area of poorly visualized vessels, etc.

FIGURE 10-7 Algorithm: pulmonary embolism. CT, computed tomography.

angiography, however, catheter-directed angiography is much less accurate in identifying sub-segmental emboli than it is in detecting larger clots.

Is there still a role for the ventilation-perfusion radionuclide lung scan (V/Q scan)? Probably yes. Patients with allergies to contrast material or decreased renal function and patients who have difficulty in holding their breath (if a single-detector CT is used for angiography) may be best served by a ventilation-perfusion scan. In these situations, it is usually best to combine the results of the ventilation-perfusion scan with other diagnostic information such as duplex scanning of the lower extremity veins and the levels of D-dimer isomers in the patient's peripheral blood. Combining all of this clinical information with knowledge of the patient's pretest probability of an embolism significantly increases the accuracy of the final diagnosis.

Review of the chest radiograph is an important step before proceeding to a ventilation-perfusion scan in these patients. First, review of the radiograph is needed to exclude other causes of hypoxia such as adult respiratory distress syndrome or pneumothorax (Fig. 10-9). Equally

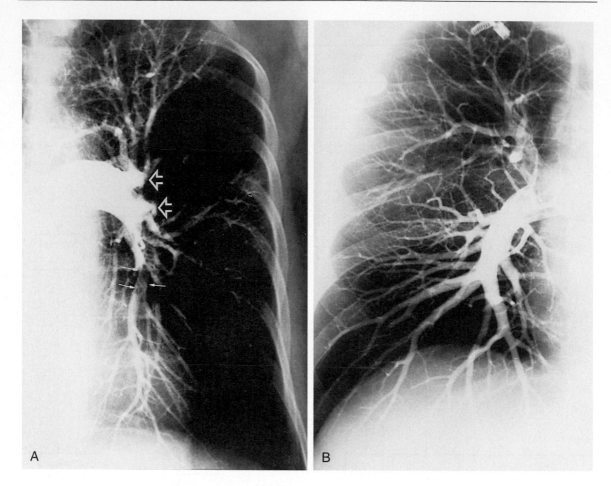

FIGURE 10-8 Pulmonary angiogram: acute pulmonary embolus (and normal angiogram for comparison).

A, Selective left pulmonary angiogram, anterior-posterior projection, demonstrates amputation of the pulmonary arteries *(open arrows)* and intraluminal filling defects *(arrows)* outlined by a thin rim of contrast material. The abrupt cutoff of a pulmonary artery and an intraluminal filling defect are definitive findings of pulmonary embolus. Chest radiograph was unremarkable.

B, Normal right selective pulmonary angiogram, same projection, for comparison. The homogeneous intraluminal contrast opacity is demonstrated throughout the central and more peripheral pulmonary arterial vessels with a normal branching pattern.

important, ventilation-perfusion scanning is most likely to be diagnostic in patients with nearly normal chest radiographs. At some institutions patients with normal or near-normal chest radiographs may undergo V/Q scanning as the initial diagnostic procedure in evaluation for pulmonary emboli.

In ventilation-perfusion scanning, areas of abnormal lung perfusion (Q) cause defects (cold areas) in the lung images made after IV injection of radiolabeled particles (made of macroaggregated albumin). Ventilation (V) abnormalities are seen as areas of decreased inflow of radioactive xenon gas (cold areas) or xenon trapping (persistent hot areas). If the ventilation abnormality

and the perfusion defect are the same size and shape, a matched defect is present. Pulmonary emboli manifest themselves as areas where perfusion is absent but ventilation is preserved, known as areas of mismatch.

A normal perfusion lung scan has no areas of perfusion defect. Lung scans that indicate a low probability for pulmonary embolism show small (less than 25% of a lung segment in size) matched perfusion defects or show perfusion defects much smaller than corresponding radiographic abnormalities. Lung scans that are classified as high probability for pulmonary embolism must show evidence of two or more large (≥75% of a lung segment) perfusion defects or their

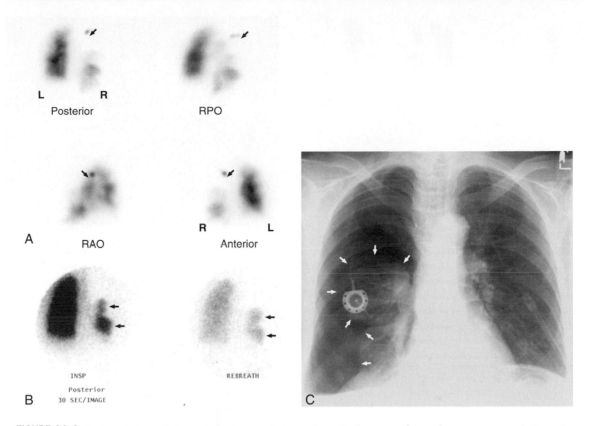

FIGURE 10-9 Radionuclide ventilation-perfusion scan and chest radiograph of a pneumothorax. Contrary to protocol, the nuclear medicine study was obtained before a chest radiograph was performed.

A, Perfusion scan shows minimal perfusion in the right lung. The radionuclide was injected through the patient's chemotherapy port and a small focus of residual activity remains in the port *(arrow)*.

B, Ventilation scan (obtained in the posterior projection) shows ventilation to only a small portion of the right lung, seen in the inferior aspect of the chest *(arrows)*.

C, Chest radiograph revealed a large right-sided pneumothorax *(arrows)*.

equivalent in moderate defects (25% to 75% of a segment) without accompanying ventilation or radiographic abnormalities (V/Q mismatch) (Fig. 10-10). If radiographic abnormalities are present, the scan can still indicate high probability if the perfusion defects are much larger than abnormalities that are evident on the plain radiograph.

Intermediate scans are all those falling between the low- and high-probability definitions. For example, a scan with a single segmental perfusion defect in a lower lobe unmatched by a plain radiograph or ventilation abnormality is indicative of intermediate probability of an embolism. With these definitions in hand, only the following few rules need be remembered:

1. If the perfusion scan is normal, the patient (almost) never has pulmonary embolism.

2. If the clinician's before-test estimate of the likelihood of a pulmonary embolism was low and the scan is low probability, the chance that a pulmonary embolism is present is less than 5%.

3. If the clinician's before-test estimate of the likelihood of a pulmonary embolism was high and the scan is high probability, the chance that a pulmonary embolism is present approximates 95%.

4. All patients who do not fit into above categories 1 to 3 need further evaluation.

The preceding discussion does not address the source of pulmonary emboli. The thrombi that become emboli most commonly originate in the lower extremities, occasionally the pelvis, and rarely the upper extremities. Some form of evaluation of the lower extremities is included

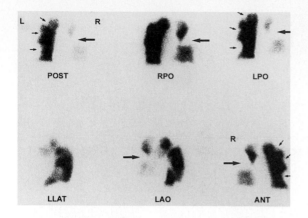

FIGURE 10-10 Ventilation-perfusion scan: high probability. Perfusion scan demonstrates multiple moderate-sized (25% to 75% of the segment; *small arrows*) and large (>75% of the segment; *large arrows*) perfusion defects bilaterally. The chest radiograph of the same patient (see Fig. 10-2) shows large bibasilar infarcts. A lung scan indicates a high probability for pulmonary emboli if it shows two large perfusion defects or their equivalent (e.g., two moderate and one large defect) that are not matched by ventilation defects.

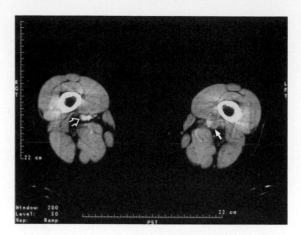

FIGURE 10-11 Computed tomography of lower extremity venous thrombosis. CT images of both thighs show low-attenuation clot in the left superficial femoral vein, part of the deep venous system *(arrow)*. The right superficial femoral vein is normal *(open arrow)*.

in most algorithms for evaluating acute pulmonary emboli, but the sequence of diagnostic studies varies widely. Lower extremity duplex ultrasonography is very accurate in detecting thrombi in veins running from the inguinal ligament to the popliteal fossae, the source of most emboli. This study should be considered in patients with a nondiagnostic CT pulmonary angiogram or ventilation-perfusion scan who have any signs or symptoms suggesting deep venous thrombosis.

CT venography can also evaluate the lower extremity veins and in addition can evaluate the iliac vessels, inferior vena cava, and pelvic vessels that cannot be well examined using Doppler ultrasonography. Delayed CT scanning of the pelvis and lower extremities is a convenient method for obtaining a CT venogram. This technique makes use of the contrast material already injected for evaluation of the chest, by waiting 2 to 3 minutes to allow the material to enter the lower extremity veins (Fig. 10-11). This additional information about the venous system is obtained at the cost of increased radiation exposure, a more significant concern in children and young adults than in older patients.

Chronic Emboli

If pulmonary emboli are documented, a follow-up CT angiogram or V/Q lung scan should be considered during the patient's convalescence (within several months after diagnosis). Although many patients' studies return to normal, other patients may develop permanent abnormalities. A convalescent CT pulmonary angiogram or a radionuclide perfusion scan is potentially useful if the patient returns with recurrent symptoms.

Detection of chronic pulmonary emboli is also important because some of these patients go on to develop pulmonary hypertension and right-sided heart failure. Other patients present with symptoms related to chronic pulmonary hypertension without a documented episode of acute emboli. If chronic emboli can be documented, the patient may be a candidate for pulmonary endarterectomy. In selected cases this surgical intervention can dramatically improve the patient's functional capacity and overall condition. On CT pulmonary angiograms, chronic embolic characteristically can be seen as adherent to the artery wall rather than causing a filling defect in the artery lumen. CT angiograms and catheter angiography may also show abrupt tapering of segmental pulmonary arteries with diffuse narrowing of the distal lumen (Fig. 10-12).

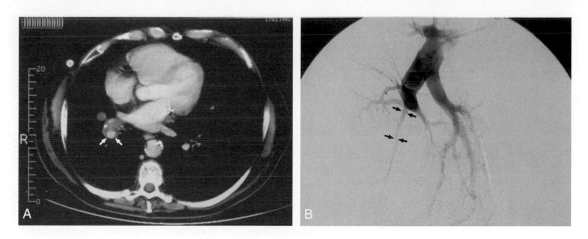

FIGURE 10-12 Computed tomography and pulmonary angiogram of chronic emboli.

A, CT shows peripheral chronic embolism adherent to the pulmonary artery wall with recanalization *(arrows)* of the central portion of the thrombus.

B, Pulmonary angiogram from a different patient with chronic emboli shows abrupt tapering of the descending pulmonary artery and diffuse narrowing of a distal segmental branch *(arrows)*. Unlike the appearance of acute emboli, no intraluminal filling defects are seen.

Other Focal Vascular Disease

Septic pulmonary emboli, caused by intravascular spread of small pieces of infected thrombi, are commonly seen in the setting of right-sided endocarditis from IV drug use and occasionally from septic thrombophlebitis. Infectious symptoms dominate the clinical presentation because the emboli are small and usually do not cause sufficient obstruction of the pulmonary vasculature to cause pulmonary infarction or pulmonary hypertension. Chest radiographs show multiple ill-defined nodules that may or may not have apparent cavitations. CT imaging almost always detects cavitation in at least one nodule (Fig. 10-13).

Other pulmonary vascular diseases cause focal lung disease much less commonly. Tumor emboli occur in advanced stages of several malignancies but are usually very small and difficult to detect on imaging studies. Pulmonary vasculitis more typically causes diffuse disease but can cause focal opacities as well. Wegener's granulomatosis can appear radiographically similar to pulmonary infarction. Although less common than pulmonary infarction from emboli, it is far from being a textbook curiosity. The diagnosis should be considered in the differential diagnosis of multiple nodules, especially when the opacities cavitate or change in size or location rapidly (see Fig. 7-17).

☐ DEVELOPMENTAL VASCULAR ABNORMALITIES

Developmental anomalies may also cause focal pulmonary vascular diseases. In general, these anomalies arise from varying combinations of abnormal bronchi and alveoli and abnormal

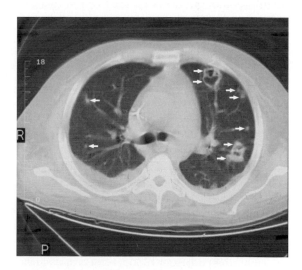

FIGURE 10-13 Computed tomography: septic emboli. CT images shows multiple nodules of varying sizes *(arrows)*. Most of these nodules are located peripherally and the largest two are cavitary.

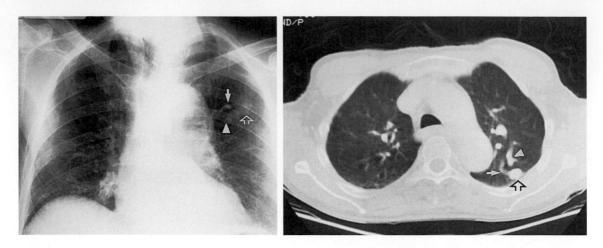

FIGURE 10-14 Posterior-anterior chest radiograph and contrast-enhanced computed tomography: arteriovenous malformation of the lung.

A, The chest radiograph shows a peripheral multilobulated opacity in the left middle lung field *(open arrow)*. The feeding and draining vessels are visible *(arrowhead and arrow)*.

B, Contrast-enhanced CT at the level of the arteriovenous malformation, lung window. The arteriovenous malformation *(open arrow)* and its feeding and draining vessels *(arrowhead and arrow)* are well defined.

pulmonary vasculature. Pulmonary arteriovenous malformations (AVMs) are at one end of the spectrum of congenital abnormalities: lesions with abnormal vasculature but no associated lung parenchymal abnormalities. Most often they arise in the third decade of life with symptoms that include dyspnea, cyanosis, and hemoptysis. Approximately half of the cases of pulmonary AVMs occur in patients with hereditary hemorrhagic telangiectasia (Osler-Weber-Rendu syndrome). These patients often have multiple pulmonary AVMs at multiple sites throughout the body as well as in the pulmonary vasculature. Plain chest radiographs of patients with AVMs usually show a focal opacity with enlarged feeding and draining vessels (Fig. 10-14). Spiral CT is the best method to confirm the presence an AVM. CT scans of lung nodules caused by common diseases (granulomas, metastases, and lung carcinomas) often show a single vessel of normal caliber that appears to connect with the nodule. On the other hand, CT images of AVMs show blood vessels that are larger than adjacent blood vessels at a similar distance from the hilum (e.g., the vessels do not taper normally but remain large as they extend into the lung periphery). Usually there are vessels leading both to and away from the nodule or mass. If the appearance is characteristic, using IV

contrast is not essential. Pulmonary angiography is now rarely done for diagnosis alone but is performed as part of a therapeutic procedure during which the AVM is permanently occluded with wire coils or detachable balloons. AVMs with a feeding vessel greater than 3 mm in diameter should be occluded, even if asymptomatic, to prevent strokes or brain abscess caused by small thrombi or bacteria that bypass the normal lung vasculature (Fig. 10-15).

Scimitar or venolobar syndrome is another congenital anomaly that may be seen in adults. Like AVMs, it primarily affects the lung vasculature, but it also affects the parenchyma, causing the entire lung to be small. The full syndrome includes hypoplasia of the right lung and right pulmonary artery, anomalous venous drainage from the right lower lobe to the inferior vena cava, and anomalous arterial supply from the abdominal aorta to the right lower lobe. The key radiographic finding is the appearance of the anomalous vein (shaped like a scimitar), which courses from the hilum to the diaphragm (Fig. 10-16). Although this anomaly causes some increased pulmonary blood flow because of left-to-right shunting, adults are often asymptomatic. Frequently the finding is of more interest to the radiologist than to the clinician.

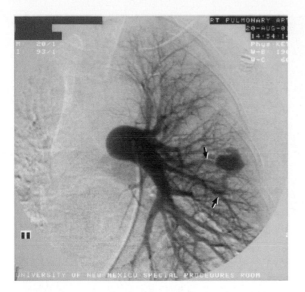

FIGURE 10-15 Angiogram of pulmonary arteriovenous malformation from a different patient than in Figure 10-14 showing both the feeding and draining vessels *(arrows).* The feeding vessel measured just over 3 mm.

Developmental vascular abnormalities other than AVMs or venolobar syndrome are very rare and include an abnormal origin of the left pulmonary artery (from the right pulmonary artery), agenesis of the right pulmonary artery,

and pulmonary varices (Fig. 10-17). Patients with the latter two congenital abnormalities are often asymptomatic and may be diagnosed in adulthood. Pulmonary varices may be congenital or acquired. Acquired varices consist of dilatation of a pulmonary vein near its entrance into the left atrium and are usually associated with mitral valve disease.

☐ DIFFUSE DISEASE

Pulmonary vasculitis most commonly presents as diffuse parenchymal opacities from pulmonary hemorrhage. This can occur in patients with lupus erythematosus, or it can be associated with renal disease, such as in Goodpasture's syndrome. Wegener's granulomatosis can also arise with diffuse lung hemorrhage rather than discrete lung masses (Fig. 10-18). In the appropriate clinical setting, acute pulmonary hemorrhage should be included in the differential diagnosis of coalescent air space disease. For instance, it should be considered routinely in patients with leukemia who exhibit pneumonia-like chest radiographic densities. These patients are almost always thrombocytopenic and often have a concurrent pulmonary infection that triggers the hemorrhage. If pulmonary

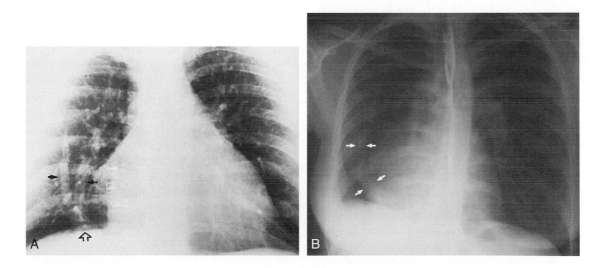

FIGURE 10-16 Posterior-anterior (PA) chest radiographs of scimitar syndrome.

A, The radiograph demonstrates the typical anomalous vein *(arrows)*, extending from midlung to the medial border of the right hemidiaphragm *(open arrow)* and draining into the inferior vena cava. In this case, the right lung size is normal.

B, PA radiograph of a different patient with the complete constellation findings of scimitar syndrome. The right lung is small, causing the heart to shift to the right (dextroposition of the heart). An anomalous pulmonary vein is also present in the inferior aspect of the right lung but is less well seen than in part A.

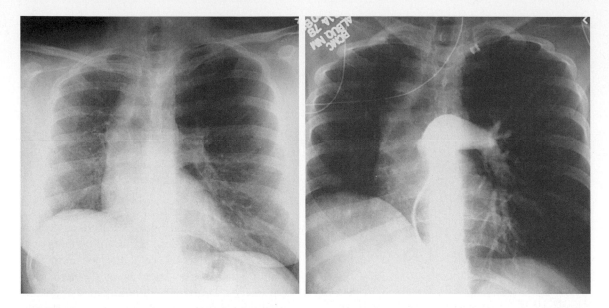

FIGURE 10-17 Posterior-anterior chest and pulmonary angiogram: agenesis of right pulmonary artery.
A, The right lung is hypoplastic, but the normal left lung appears more lucent.
B, Pulmonary angiogram shows absence of contrast-filled vessels in the right lung.

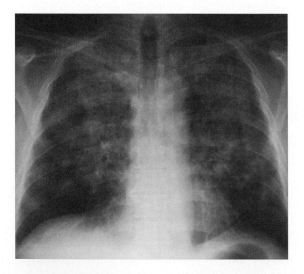

FIGURE 10-18 Posterior-anterior chest radiograph: Wegener's granulomatosis. Radiograph shows bilateral diffuse air space disease that spares the periphery of the lung, the characteristic distribution of acute pulmonary hemorrhage. Acute volume overload can produce a similar pattern, but no ancillary findings of intravascular volume overload are seen on the radiograph.

hemorrhage is caused by recurrent or chronic illness, such as in mitral stenosis, hemosiderin may be deposited in the interstitium. This produces a reticular pattern of interstitial disease, which may underlie the air space disease caused by acute hemorrhage.

Patients with chronic liver disease may acquire diffuse small pulmonary vascular malformations. Hepatopulmonary syndrome is present when these malformations are associated with persistent hypoxia. These patients form a subgroup of those with chronic liver disease and hypoxia. (Hypoxia in liver disease is usually multifactorial.) Patients with the hepatopulmonary syndrome develop right-to-left shunting from dilatation of the intrapulmonary vasculature. This shunting can be documented noninvasively by radionuclide perfusion scans of the lung. These scans shows escape of radionuclide from the lung vasculature into extrathoracic organs, that is, the brain and kidneys (Fig. 10-19). Pulmonary angiography can also be diagnostic, but the arteriovenous connections are generally very numerous and very small and are not amenable to treatment by embolization.

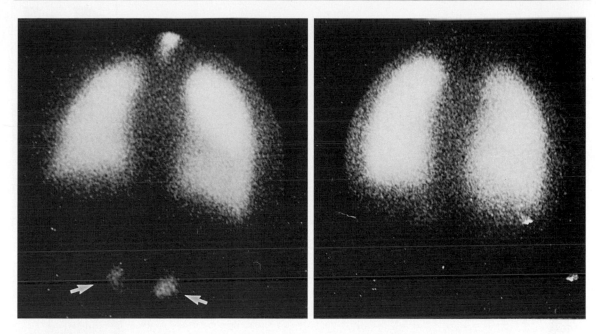

FIGURE 10-19 Right-to-left shunt on lung perfusion scan. Shunting is characterized by the appearance of radionuclide in the capillary bed of both kidneys *(arrows)*. (From Mettler FA, Guiberteau MJ. Essentials of Nuclear Medicine Imaging, 2nd ed. San Diego: Grune & Stratton, 1986.)

Pearls for Clinicians—Intraparenchymal Vascular Disease

1. The accuracy of CT pulmonary angiography for acute pulmonary emboli increases as thinner slices are used, and the sensitivity and specificity for multidetector CT scanners exceed 90%. Institutions with 16-detector CT scanners almost never perform invasive pulmonary angiography to make a diagnosis of acute pulmonary emboli.

2. Nuclear medicine ventilation-perfusion scans may be useful to exclude pulmonary emboli in young patients with normal or nearly normal chest radiographs.

3. Chronic pulmonary emboli, particularly in peripheral vessels, can be more difficult to detect than acute emboli. Make sure these studies are reviewed by an experienced reader provided with an accurate history.

4. Occasionally, pulmonary nodules from many causes appear to be connected to a single vessel on chest CT but pulmonary AVMs should be connected to two vessels, a feeding artery and a draining vein.

5. Although it is uncommon, consider the possibility of pulmonary vasculitis in the diagnostic differential for diffuse bilateral symmetric air space disease and in the differential for multiple pulmonary masses or large nodules.

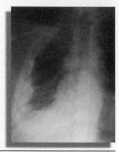

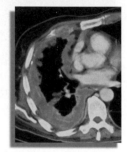

11

Pleura and Diaphragm

☐ PNEUMOTHORAX

Pneumothoraces may occur spontaneously or be secondary to trauma (penetrating injury, blunt injury, or barotrauma). Spontaneous pneumothoraces are termed primary if the patient has no prior lung disease. These usually occur in young patients (often males) and are probably secondary to rupture of apical blebs. Secondary pneumothoraces are those that occur in patients with underlying abnormal lung parenchyma, most often emphysema or infiltrative lung disease that has associated cystic changes. Usually chest radiographic findings can distinguish a primary from a secondary pneumothorax. This is clinically important. Patients with secondary pneumothoraces have more severe symptoms, frequently need chest tubes, and require longer treatment.

In the upright patient, identification of a pneumothorax is based on the detection of a thin visceral pleural line, outlined by air on each side (Fig. 11-1). Lung tissue within this line does not appear to be of increased density unless the degree of collapse is great. This is in contradistinction to a skin fold, which is occasionally confused with a pneumothorax. Because of the folding of overlying soft tissues, the apparent opacity of the lung tissue gradually increases laterally until it reaches an edge where the opacity abruptly decreases. This edge represents the lateral margin of the folded tissues (Fig. 11-2). Often pulmonary vasculature is visible distal to the skin fold line.

In some patients, indirect signs of pneumothorax are useful. A small air-fluid level in the costophrenic angle (manifested by a horizontal air-fluid interface) may be a clue to a subtle pneumothorax (Fig. 11-3). This sign is reliable only on an upright radiograph and cannot be seen in supine patients (see later discussion). The absence of peripheral vasculature is an indirect sign of pneumothorax that seems to be favored by house officers, but it can be misleading. Normal lung vasculature cannot be seen within 1 or 2 cm of the chest wall, and it may be further attenuated by apical blebs or bullae, leading to a false diagnosis of pneumothorax. In trauma victims and in patients receiving mechanical ventilation, the presence of a pneumomediastinum increases the likelihood that a pneumothorax may be present and should lead to a careful search for a pleural line. Pneumomediastinum, however, may also

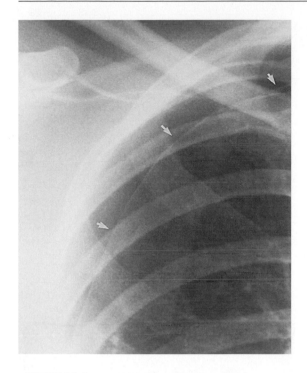

FIGURE 11-1 Posterior-anterior chest radiograph: pneumothorax. Close-up demonstrates the white (visceral) pleural line *(arrows)* and also the lack of pulmonary vascular markings lateral to the pleural line. Also see Figure 11-3.

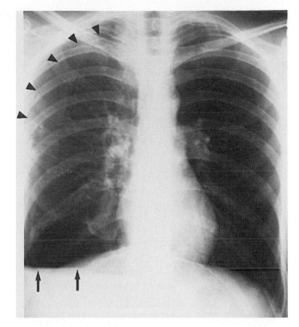

FIGURE 11-3 Posterior-anterior upright chest view: small pneumothorax with air-fluid level in costophrenic angle. Full radiograph of the patient shown in Figure 11-1 demonstrates an air-fluid level *(arrows)* that is well defined at the right costophrenic angle. In some instances, the size of the air-fluid level is very small and the only indication of free air within the pleural space. The white (visceral) pleural line *(arrowheads)* is better seen in the close-up (Fig. 11-1).

occur as an isolated finding (see Chapter 8) (Fig. 11-4). Subcutaneous emphysema is rarely an isolated finding and is almost always associated with either pneumomediastinum or a pneumothorax (Fig. 11-5).

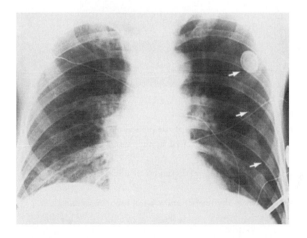

FIGURE 11-2 Posterior-anterior chest radiograph: skin folds simulating pneumothorax. The apparent pleural line *(arrows)* is well defined and was not seen to extend beyond the thoracic margin in this case. The salient finding is a gradual increase in lung opacity from medial to lateral, becoming most opaque at the inner edge of the "line," where it abruptly decreases. See text.

If the diagnosis of pneumothorax is uncertain, the next step should be an expiratory or lateral decubitus view. A pneumothorax should *appear* larger on the expiratory view because the underlying lung decreases in size but the amount of air trapped in the pleural space does not change. On decubitus films, a pneumothorax moves to the uppermost portion of the chest. Whenever a decubitus view is ordered to detect a pneumothorax, the radiologist and radiology technologist must be told the purpose of the study. Otherwise, they assume that the decubitus film is being taken to look for fluid and may center the image on the dependent ("down" side) rather than the nondependent ("up" side) portion of the decubitus chest.

The detection of pneumothorax in a supine, rather than an upright, patient may be more problematic. Often the supine individual is intubated and mechanically ventilated, making detection of pneumothorax more critical. Rather than occurring apically, pleural air collections in the supine patient characteristically occur

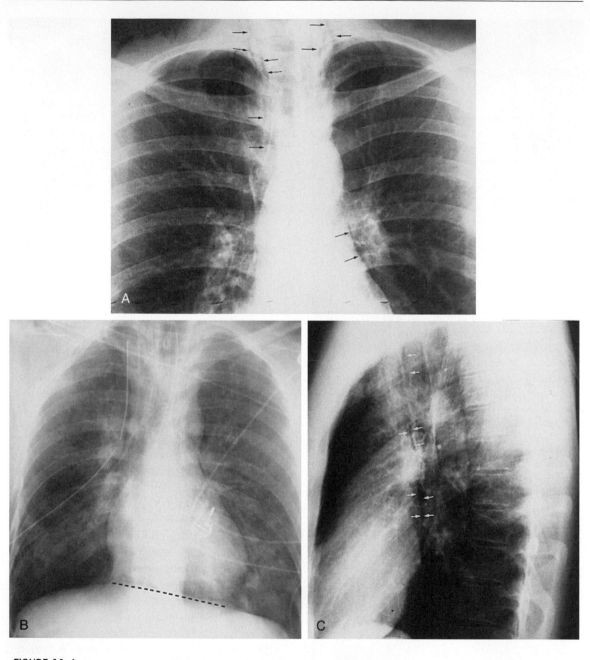

FIGURE 11-4 Posterior-anterior and lateral chest radiographs: pneumomediastinum.

A, The identification of a pneumomediastinum can be difficult. Vertically oriented lucencies at the pleural pericardial interface and in the paratracheal regions *(arrows)* can be easily missed. Note the extension of the paratracheal lucency into the neck, that is, beyond the normal lung areas.

B, Supine chest view (different patient) shows a "continuous" diaphragm sign *(dashed line)* caused by air under the heart. This sign is helpful on supine or upright studies. (See also Fig. 8-4.)

C, Lateral chest radiograph demonstrates vertically oriented lucencies adjacent to the trachea and central bronchi *(arrows)*.

anteriorly because this area is the most superior portion of the supine chest. These air collections may occur medially adjacent to the cardiac silhouette, causing the cardiac border to appear sharper than usual. Air can also collect adjacent to the lingula or middle lobe, outlining their inferior or lateral margins. If the air collection is not large, the lower lobe vessels may be seen to overlap the edge of the pneumothorax. With larger air collections, the lateral costophrenic

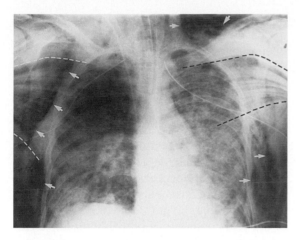

FIGURE 11-5 Anterior-posterior chest radiograph: subcutaneous emphysema. Subcutaneous air extends throughout the soft tissues of the thorax, defining the pectoral muscles bilaterally (radial lucencies inside *dashed lines*). The emphysema also extends inferolaterally into the soft tissues external to the ribs and into the supraclavicular regions *(arrows)*. Diffuse parenchymal opacities caused by acute respiratory distress syndrome are evident and bilateral chest tubes are in place.

angle deepens, and the hemidiaphragm on the affected side appears less opaque. This is the classical finding of a "deep sulcus sign" (Fig. 11-6). Like many classical findings, however, this sign does have its imposters and can be mimicked by lordotic positioning in some patients. If air can be seen outlining the anterior pleural sulcus or increased lucency is seen adjacent to the cardiac silhouette, the sign is more likely to represent a real pneumothorax.

Detection of a pneumothorax in the supine patient is most difficult in patients with diffuse lung disease, such as adult respiratory distress syndrome. The pneumothorax may be loculated, and the degree of lung collapse is limited by the stiff pulmonary parenchyma. In rare cases the diagnosis can be made using a crosstable lateral view. This works well in neonates, but the image is often inconclusive in adults. Chest computed tomography (CT) can be instrumental in detecting a pneumothorax in these cases (see Fig. 8-19).

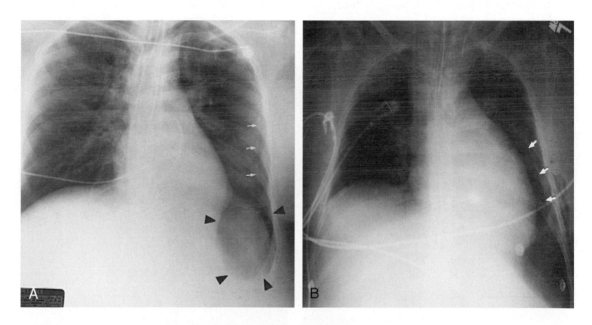

FIGURE 11-6 Anterior-posterior supine chest radiograph: deep sulcus sign of pneumothorax.

    A, The left lateral costophrenic angle is widened and blunted as the sulcus is displaced caudally by the large pneumothorax *(arrowheads)*. Note that the hemidiaphragm on the left side is less opaque than on the right side. In addition, there is a pleural line ascending along the left chest wall as the pneumothorax dissects up the lateral pleural space *(arrows)*. The latter finding is often absent.

    B, In a different patient, a deep sulcus is present in the left chest. The intrapleural air has collected adjacent to the heart, seen as a lucent band *(arrows)*. This air collection also causes the cardiac silhouette to be very sharply defined. No pleural line is seen in this case.

When a pneumothorax is detected, radiographic characteristics can influence the therapy selected, only to a limited degree. Sizing a pneumothorax, for instance, is at best inexact. If the rim of intrapleural air around the periphery of the lung averages about an inch and a half in an adult, the pneumothorax occupies roughly 30% of the hemithorax. Air is reabsorbed from the pleural space at a rate of about 1.25% of the hemithorax volume every 24 hours. Pneumothoraces that occupy 30% of the hemithorax take several weeks to resolve, and most of the pneumothoraces this size or larger are evacuated percutaneously. For most purposes, the patient's clinical situation rather than the exact percentage of collapse determines whether chest tube evacuation is warranted. Patients with marked dyspnea, those being treated with mechanical ventilation, and patients with a pneumothorax that is growing in size almost always need a chest tube placed.

The patient's clinical status (e.g., hypotension, labored breathing) is especially important in determining that a pneumothorax is under "tension." A tension pneumothorax is said to be present when intrapleural pressure within the pneumothorax exceeds atmospheric pressure throughout most of the respiratory cycle. Tension pneumothoraces are usually heralded by a sudden deterioration in the patient's cardiopulmonary status related to both the decreased cardiac output caused by impaired venous return and hypoxia caused by perfusion of unventilated lung. Classical radiographic findings of a tension pneumothorax include complete collapse of the lung, depression of the ipsilateral diaphragm, and mediastinal and tracheal shift toward the contralateral chest (Fig. 11-7). The presence of diaphragm depression on the side of the pneumothorax is probably the most reliable radiographic sign of tension. Relying on mediastinal shift alone to label a pneumothorax as a tension pneumothorax can be misleading because mild mediastinal shift is to be expected with any moderate or large pneumothorax as the more negative pressure in the unaffected hemithorax pulls structures to that side.

It is important to remember that a tension pneumothorax can be present despite only modest collapse of the lung in patients with disease that decreases the elasticity of the lung parenchyma, such as adult respiratory distress

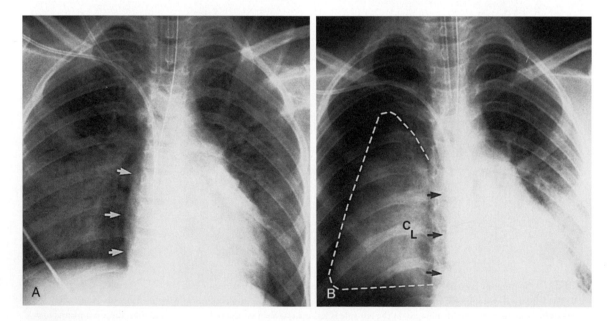

FIGURE 11-7 Serial posterior-anterior chest radiographs: tension pneumothorax.

A, Initial frontal radiograph demonstrates normal appearance of the chest following central venous pressure catheter placement. The right cardiac border shows no mediastinal shift *(arrows).*

B, Follow-up chest radiograph obtained for acute onset of dyspnea shows a large pneumothorax with the mediastinal structures and right cardiac border shifted to the left *(arrows).* The dome of the right diaphragm is depressed, and the compressed lung (CL) is now airless and collapsed inferomedially *(dashed lines).*

syndrome (see earlier discussion). Ancillary radiographic findings, such as depression and flattening of the ipsilateral diaphragm, combined with clinical findings of physiologic impairment (e.g., hypotension), may be the main indications of a tension pneumothorax in these patients.

☐ PLEURAL EFFUSIONS

General Concepts

The most frequently seen sign of pleural fluid on the posterior-anterior (PA) chest radiograph is blunting of the lateral costophrenic angle, with a meniscus-like arc at the interface between fluid and chest wall. There is considerable individual variability in the amount of fluid needed to produce this finding. Lateral views of the chest are more sensitive than PA views, and lateral decubitus radiographs are the most sensitive. Good lateral views are able to detect less than 75 mL of fluid, decubitus views possibly as little as 10 mL.

Pleural fluid collections may be overlooked or mistaken for other pathology when they have an atypical radiographic appearance. This occurs when most of the pleural fluid is subpulmonic, when the effusion is contained in the interlobar fissure ("encysted effusions"), and when radiographs are taken with the patient supine. Subpulmonic fluid collections lie entirely beneath the lung base without spilling over into the costophrenic angle. Accordingly, they do not demonstrate the usual meniscoid arc. When a subpulmonic collection is present, the apparent apex of the diaphragm may be displaced lateral to the midclavicular line and no vessels are seen below the dome of the diaphragm (Fig. 11-8). The vessels that are normally seen are part of the lower lobe vasculature and are displaced as fluid fills the posterior costophrenic sulcus and floats the lowermost lung tissue out of the way. Replacement of this aerated lung by fluid also makes the dome of the diaphragm appear more opaque. When a subpulmonic effusion is present on the left, an upright chest radiograph may show increased (>2 cm) separation of the stomach bubble from the apparent left hemidiaphragm. The increased separation represents pleural fluid between the base of the lung and the actual hemidiaphragm.

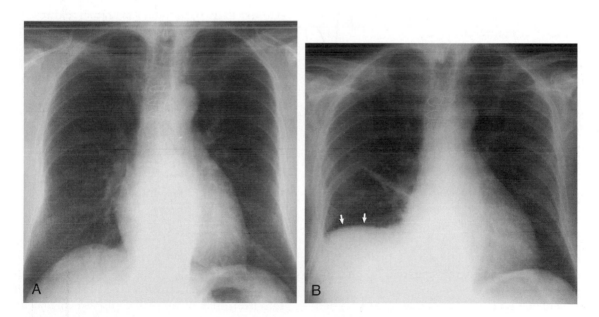

FIGURE 11-8 Posterior-anterior (PA) upright chest radiograph: subpulmonic effusion.

A, PA chest shows a normal appearance of the right hemidiaphragm. Blood vessels can be seen through the apex of the hemidiaphragm.

B, Same patient as in A after development of a subpulmonic effusion. The apex of the right hemidiaphragm has shifted laterally *(arrows)*. The hemidiaphragm has also become much more opaque because the subpulmonic fluid has floated aerated lung out of the anterior and posterior pleural sulci.

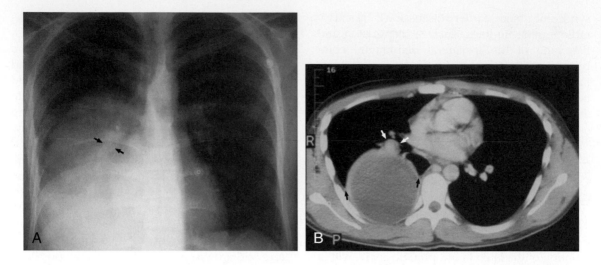

FIGURE 11-9 Posterior-anterior (PA) chest and contrast-enhanced computed tomography (CT) of loculated pleural effusion.

A, PA chest shows a large opacity occupying the inferior aspect of the right chest. No air bronchograms are present, and the lower lobe vessels are seen "through" the opacity *(arrows)*. This is evidence that the disease process may not be within the lower lobe parenchyma.

B, CT scan of the same patient. A loculated pleural effusion is present in the posterior right chest. The lower lobe vessels are displaced forward *(white arrows)* but still partially surrounded by aerated lung, causing them to be visible on the chest radiograph. Note that when loculated pleural collections become large they may form acute (rather than obtuse) angles with the chest wall *(black arrows)*.

None of these findings are highly specific for subpulmonic effusions, and lateral decubitus radiographs should be obtained to confirm the presence of pleural fluid.

The appearance of loculated pleural effusions also differs from the typical pattern of a free-flowing effusion. When loculated effusions are very large they may be mistaken for disease within the lung, such as a lobar pneumonia. Unlike the appearance of most lobar pneumonias, opacities caused by loculated effusions do not contain air bronchograms. In addition, the pulmonary vasculature can often be seen "through" the opacity (Fig. 11-9). If there are radiographic signs suggesting a loculated effusion, a chest CT scan should be obtained to confirm the diagnosis. This is important because in the setting of pneumonia all patients with large loculated pleural effusions should undergo thoracentesis.

Radiographic findings of interlobar encysted effusions are also different from those of free-flowing effusions. Interlobar encysted effusions occur in the setting of congestive heart failure. The fluid collection most often occurs within the right minor fissure and has smooth biconvex contours (Fig. 11-10). This oblong shape with

smooth tapering ends is not characteristic of most lung masses. These collections are often referred to as pseudotumors and should resolve with treatment of the underlying congestive heart failure. If no improvement is seen, the diagnosis should be questioned. Very rarely, a mass can originate from the pleura and grow along the major or minor fissure (typically a localized fibrinous tumor of the pleura). This mass can masquerade as a pseudotumor, creating what might be called a pseudo-pseudotumor (Fig. 11-11).

Large effusions in a supine patient may be clearly seen if there is enough fluid to separate the lung from the chest wall laterally. The paraspinal soft tissue shadows may also be widened. Radiographic signs are often more subtle, however, and pleural fluid in the supine patient may manifest primarily as a diffuse increase in opacity of the hemithorax. As with a large loculated effusion, the appearance differs from that of air space disease in that the pulmonary vessels are not obscured by pleural fluid and can be seen through the hazy opacity (Fig. 11-12).

If the diagnosis of pleural effusion remains uncertain after analysis of the plain radiograph, either CT or ultrasonography should be used

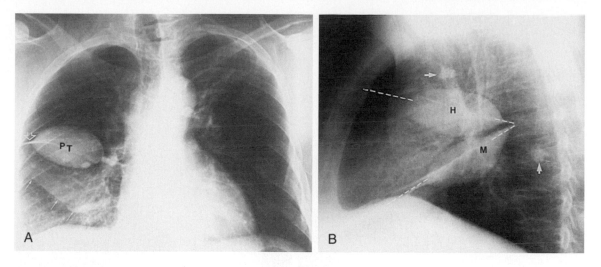

FIGURE 11-10 Posterior anterior and lateral chest radiographs: pseudotumor.

A, The frontal radiograph demonstrates the elliptical shape of the pseudotumor (PT) with the lateral margin tapering into the horizontal fissure *(open arrow)*. The margins are sharp and the opacity of the pseudotumor is homogeneous. A second, less well-defined pseudotumor is identified in the right lower lobe area. This opacity gradually decreases toward its upper border, consistent with an effusion in the oblique (major) fissure *(arrows)*.

B, Upright lateral radiograph localizes these pseudotumors within the major (M) and minor, or horizontal (H), fissures. Note the two smaller parenchymal opacities that are lung nodules *(arrows)*, not loculated effusions.

for further evaluation. Chest CT is particularly helpful in assessing loculated parapneumonic fluid (see later discussion). Ultrasonography has the advantage of being portable, and it can be used at the bedside to guide a thoracentesis. Simple effusions are hypoechoic (appear dark) on an ultrasonogram and are easy to detect. Pleural hemorrhage and empyema may produce more echoes (appear brighter) and be more difficult to differentiate from solid material with ultrasonography.

Classification of Pleural Effusions

Pleural effusions are often classified as transudates or exudates on the basis of laboratory analysis of fluid obtained by thoracentesis. CT or ultrasonography can help determine whether the pleural fluid is most likely exudative or transudative. For instance, ultrasound findings of septations or debris in the pleural fluid strongly suggest an exudate. CT scan images of most exudative pleural effusions show pleural enhancement after administration of intravenous contrast material. In contrast, the pleura adjacent to transudative effusions is rarely enhanced. Nevertheless, in most cases neither CT nor ultrasonography eliminates the

need for thoracentesis. Documentation of infection or malignancy still requires laboratory analysis of the pleural fluid. In rare circumstances, when a thoracentesis is particularly risky (e.g., a patient receiving mechanical ventilation with a small effusion), a CT or ultrasound appearance consistent with a transudate may mitigate the need for a thoracentesis.

In addition to classifying pleural effusions by their chemistries, it is useful to categorize them according to the clinical setting. These clinical categories include pleural effusions associated with cardiac or intra-abdominal disease, parapneumonic effusions, and malignant effusions.

Effusions Associated with Cardiac Disease

Congestive heart failure is a common cause of pleural effusion and the most common cause of transudative collections (Fig. 11-13). These effusions may be bilateral or unilateral. Unilateral effusions occur most commonly on the right. In a patient with other signs of congestive heart failure and an apparently unilateral left effusion, it is worthwhile to check bilateral decubitus radiographs. These may show that bilateral effusions

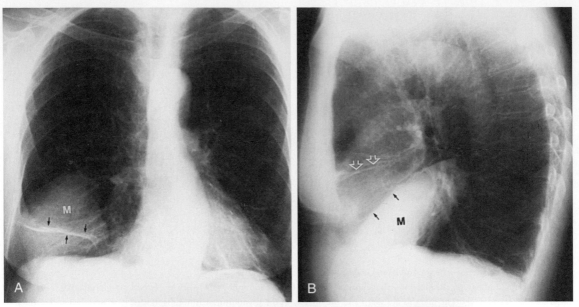

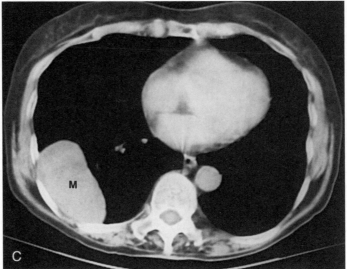

FIGURE 11-11 Posterior-anterior (PA) and lateral chest radiographs and contrast-enhanced computed tomography: localized fibrous tumor of the pleura.

A, PA chest radiograph reveals an elliptical opacity (M) that projects over a thickened horizontal fissure *(arrows)*. The margins of the mass are not well defined, and its opacity diminishes as it extends upward, similar to the appearance in Figure 11-9.

B, The lateral chest radiograph shows the oblong lobulated mass to project into the region of the anterior portion of the major fissure *(small arrows)*. *Open arrows*, minor fissure.

C, Contrast-enhanced CT in axial projection, mediastinal windows, demonstrates a large, peripheral mass (M) adjacent to the chest wall that appears more posterior and lateral in position than it appeared on the chest radiograph. Fibrous tumors of the pleura can be pedunculated and change location with a change in the patient's position. With the patient supine for the CT scan, the mass has fallen posteriorly.

are actually present. If a unilateral left-sided effusion is confirmed, a cause of the effusion other than heart failure should be entertained and a thoracentesis may be necessary.

Other diseases, such as pulmonary emboli or postcardiotomy (Dressler's) syndrome, should also be considered if an effusion associated with congestive heart failure increases in size despite clinical and radiographic improvement of pulmonary edema (Fig. 11-14). Effusions associated with pulmonary emboli are usually small (taking up less than 15% of the thorax).

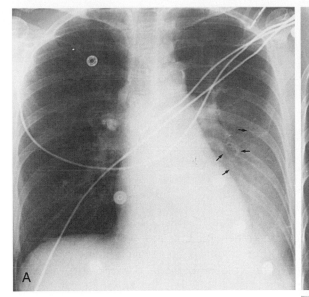

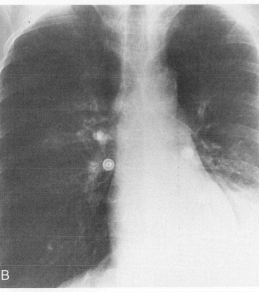

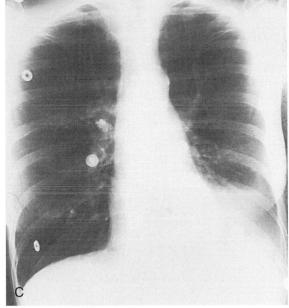

FIGURE 11-12 Anterior-posterior supine, upright and decubitus chest radiographs: left pleural effusion.

A, Supine chest view demonstrates partial opacification of the left hemithorax inferiorly. Pulmonary vessels are seen throughout this area *(arrows)*, suggesting that the opacity may not be due to consolidation. A decubitus study can confirm that the opacity is due to a free-flowing pleural effusion that has layered in the posterior aspect of the pleural cavity.

B, Left lateral decubitus chest radiograph shows the movement of the free-flowing effusion laterally along the left chest wall.

C, Upright radiograph shows effusion layering in the left base. A meniscus is visible laterally that is not present on the other radiographs.

Larger effusions occur if there is adjacent parenchymal infiltrate, probably representing a sizable infarction. Dressler's syndrome most frequently occurs following cardiac surgery but may also occur after myocardial infarction. In addition to pericarditis, pleural effusions are common. A unilateral left-sided effusion is more commonly seen with postcardiotomy syndrome than with congestive heart failure.

Effusions Associated with Intra-Abdominal Disease

A variety of intra-abdominal processes produce pleural effusions. These include subphrenic abscesses, pancreatitis (usually causing a left-sided effusion), and cirrhosis of the liver. The last condition, sometimes termed pleural ascites, may be a source of massive pleural effusion (Table 11-1). These effusions are caused by ascitic fluid traversing the diaphragm. They are usually right sided and usually, but not always, accompanied by clinically evident ascites. Characteristically, pleural ascites recurs rapidly after thoracentesis. The diagnosis can sometimes be confirmed by placing a small amount of radiopharmaceutical material intraperitoneally (by paracentesis) and documenting its passage into the chest by imaging with a gamma scintillation camera in nuclear medicine.

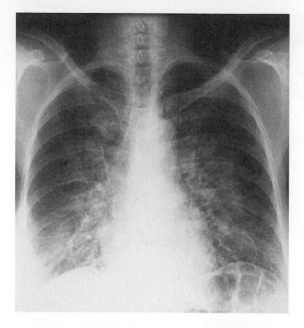

FIGURE 11-13 Posterior-anterior chest radiograph: congestive heart failure with effusion. This frontal chest view demonstrates the common findings of acute congestive failure: perihilar edema with blurring of the central pulmonary vessels, basilar interstitial edema with evident Kerley's B lines, and right cardiophrenic angle blunting secondary to small pleural effusion.

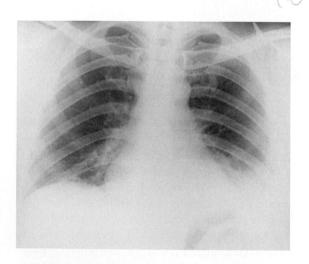

FIGURE 11-14 Posterior-anterior chest radiograph: left pleural effusion secondary to pulmonary embolus. Although the cardiac silhouette is mildly enlarged, no radiographic changes associated with pulmonary edema are evident. There is a unilateral left-sided pleural effusion secondary to pulmonary embolism.

TABLE 11-1
Causes of Massive (Entire Hemithorax) Pleural Effusion

Two thirds of cases:
  Malignancy
Remaining one third of cases:
  Cirrhosis
  Empyema
  Hemothorax
  Congestive heart failure

Small effusions occur frequently after abdominal surgery and are usually less than 10 mm thick on lateral decubitus views. Often there is accompanying postoperative atelectasis. These benign, postoperative effusions usually disappear within 2 weeks. The later appearance of an effusion raises the possibility of pulmonary emboli. Effusions related to subphrenic abscesses are also late in onset. They characteristically develop during the second postoperative week. These effusions are often accompanied by elevation of the hemidiaphragm and basilar atelectasis. In some cases, radiographs may reveal extraluminal air below the diaphragm (Fig. 11-15).

Parapneumonic Effusions

Effusions that develop adjacent to pneumonias are termed parapneumonic effusions. Thirty percent to 40% of all adults with pneumonia develop parapneumonic effusions. Most of these effusions arise from the inflamed pleura adjacent to the infection but do not contain the infectious organism itself. The effusion is an empyema if the infecting organism is seen with Gram's stain or is grown from culture of the fluid. (Other laboratory tests may predict formation of an empyema, but only the presence of active infection defines the term.)

Many of the effusions that are not empyemas resolve with treatment of the underlying pneumonia and do not require drainage with a needle or catheter. Effusions less than 11 mm thick on lateral decubitus radiographs are very likely to resolve with antibiotic therapy alone. If the effusion is greater than 11 mm thick on decubitus views, a diagnostic thoracentesis should be considered to ensure that the patient is not developing an empyema. Small effusions, those occupying less than a quarter of the hemithorax,

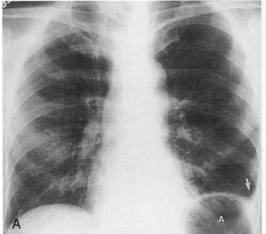

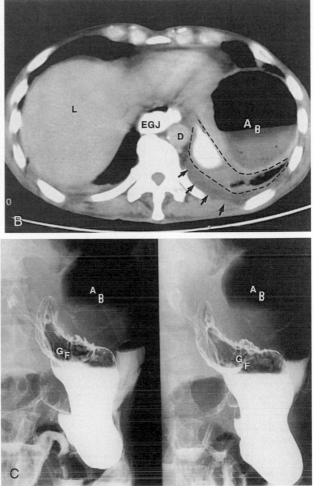

FIGURE 11-15 Posterior-anterior chest radiograph, contrast-enhanced computed tomography, and upper gastrointestinal examination: subdiaphragmatic abscess.

A, Frontal radiograph demonstrates small left cardiophrenic angle effusion *(arrow)* and slight elevation of the left hemidiaphragm. The subdiaphragmatic air collection (A) was mistaken for a gastric air bubble.

B, Contrast-enhanced CT demonstrates the left effusion *(arrows)*, a large air-filled subdiaphragmatic abscess (AB) medially and posteriorly displacing the stomach *(dashed lines)*, which is partially filled with contrast material. D, descending aorta; EGJ, esophagogastric junction; L, liver.

C, Upper gastrointestinal study with barium swallow demonstrates the displaced gastric fundus (GF) and the contiguous large subphrenic abscess (AB).

often require ultrasound guidance for safer thoracentesis. Figure 11-16 shows an algorithm for the work-up of parapneumonic effusions.

When decubitus views are obtained to assess the quantity of pleural fluid, it is always worthwhile to obtain radiographs with both right and left sides down. First, fluid that does not shift on decubitus films and remains in the nondependent portion of the chest is likely to be loculated. Second, bilateral decubitus views allow better inspection of underlying lung tissue, as the mobile portion of the pleural fluid flows to opposite sides of the chest with right and left decubitus positioning. A few infections, notably primary tuberculosis, may present with pleural effusion and little, if any, visible underlying parenchymal disease.

In most cases, CT scanning cannot replace the need for thoracentesis in the evaluation of parapneumonic effusions. The only definite CT sign of an empyema is gas within the pleural space that is found prior to instrumentation of the pleural space. Contrast-enhanced CT scans of parapneumonic effusions usually show thickened, enhancing pleura. Pleural enhancement may be present, however, whether or not the pleural fluid represents an empyema (Fig. 11-17). Lack of pleural enhancement argues strongly against the presence of an empyema.

Ultrasonography can also be used to image parapneumonic effusions. Echogenic (bright-appearing) fluid or dark fluid traversed by septations (appearing as bright bands) is more likely to represent an empyema. As with CT, however, the only definite sign of empyema is the presence of gas within the pleural space, and this finding is more easily missed with ultrasonography than it is with CT scanning.

ALGORITHM FOR PARAPNEUMONIC EFFUSION

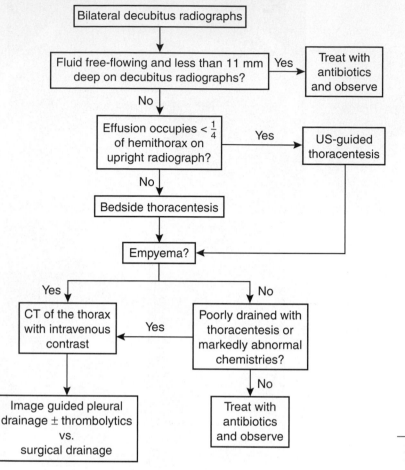

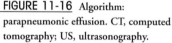

FIGURE 11-16 Algorithm: parapneumonic effusion. CT, computed tomography; US, ultrasonography.

After an empyema is diagnosed, CT scanning is particularly useful in guiding therapy. CT should be performed in almost all patients with an empyema in order to identify the size, location, and number of fluid loculations. This helps determine whether open or closed (percutaneous chest tube) drainage should be used. Ultrasonography is not as accurate in locating areas of loculated pleural fluid, particularly along the mediastinal pleura. For this reason, CT is more commonly used to examine empyemas before and after they are treated.

If closed chest tube drainage is successful, the lung should be fully expanded and the pleural space free of large air collections following tube placement. Failure to expand fully may be caused by a thick inflammatory rind covering the visceral pleura. The lung is "trapped" by this rind and cannot fully inflate to close the empyema cavity. In these cases, open decortication is often required (Fig. 11-18). If radiographs taken after tube placement show a persistent opacity but no large air collections, a repeated chest CT study should be performed. In some cases, the CT shows that the remaining opacities are secondary to coexisting parenchymal disease and pleural thickening, rather than purulent fluid that has not yet drained. Recognizing this may prevent misguided, and dangerous, attempts at draining what was thought to be residual fluid. Calcifications of both the parietal and visceral pleura occur as a late finding of empyema. These too are best evaluated by CT. Although they may occur following pyogenic infections, calcifications are classically seen following tuberculosis infections (Fig. 11-19).

Empyemas of both pyogenic and tuberculous origin can destroy enough lung parenchyma

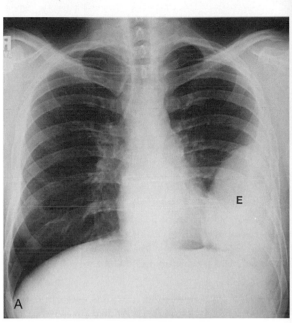

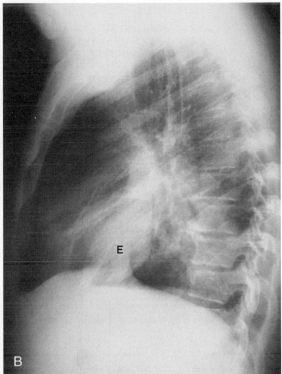

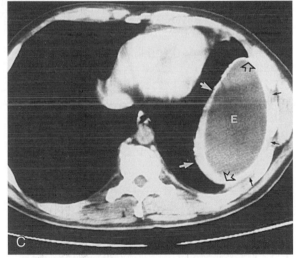

FIGURE 11-17 Posterior-anterior chest radiograph and contrast enhanced computed tomography: split pleural sign in an empyema.

Frontal (A) and lateral (B) chest examinations obtained with the patient in an upright position demonstrate a left basilar opacity with a convex medial margin. No air bronchograms are seen within the opacity. The appearance is consistent with a loculated empyema (E).

C, Contrast-enhanced CT utilizing mediastinal windows demonstrates the enhanced pleural surface. Note that the pleura splits at the level of the empyema *(open arrow)*, the visceral pleura remaining medial *(closed arrow)* and the parietal pleura lateral *(small arrows)* as it tracks around the fluid collection. E, empyema.

to produce an air leak into the pleural space. This is referred to as a bronchopleural fistula and causes an air-fluid level to be seen within the chest on radiographs (Fig. 11-20). In the clinical setting of infection, however, an intrathoracic air-fluid level can be due to either a bronchopleural fistula or a lung abscess (Fig. 11-21). Distinguishing these diagnoses is important because only a bronchopleural fistula routinely requires percutaneous drainage.

If plain films show that the cavity is distant from the pleural surface, the air-fluid level is within an abscess. If the air-fluid level appears to be adjacent to the chest wall, a chest CT scan should be obtained to determine whether an abscess or bronchopleural fistula is present. On CT, a bronchopleural fistula with empyema appears as a lenticular, smooth-walled fluid and air collection that conforms to the shape of the chest wall. Underlying parenchyma is

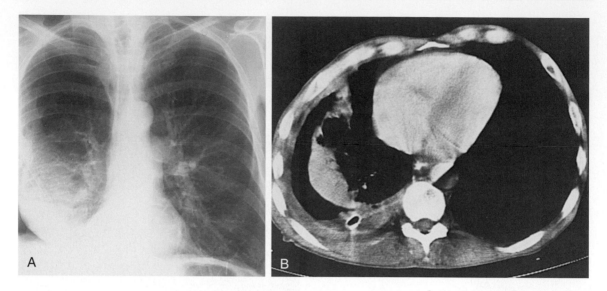

FIGURE 11-18 Posterior-anterior chest radiograph and computed tomography: trapped lung following empyema.
A and B, Despite drainage with a large-bore chest tube well positioned in the pleural space, the right lung is not fully reexpanded. Complete reexpansion is prevented by a thick visceral pleural peel. The parietal pleura is also markedly thickened.

compressed, and pulmonary vessels deviate around this fluid collection. Lung abscesses are more nearly round and do not conform to the chest wall. They have irregular inner borders and destroy rather than compress the adjacent parenchyma.

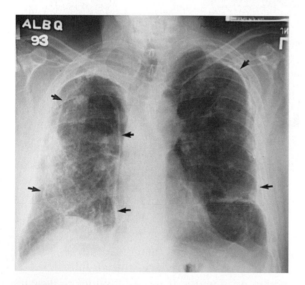

FIGURE 11-19 Posterior-anterior chest radiographs: pleural calcifications—sequelae of tuberculosis. Frontal radiograph demonstrates extensive bilateral pleural calcification (arrows) with associated parenchymal fibrosis in the right upper and lateral lung zones. The pleural calcifications are more extensive in the upper half of the thorax, in contradistinction to asbestos-related pleural disease, which is usually more extensive in the middle and lower thorax.

Malignant Pleural Disease

Malignancies can cause pleural effusion without actual tumor growth within the pleura. Involvement of mediastinal nodes can block lymphatics, and disruptions of the thoracic duct (e.g., by lymphoma) can cause chylous effusions. (Chylous effusions are usually milky and consist of the lymphatic drainage from the small bowel, called chyle.) Bronchogenic carcinoma can obstruct a central bronchus, causing a postobstructive pneumonia. Therefore, a pleural effusion ipsilateral to a bronchogenic carcinoma may not be caused by tumor involvement of the pleura but instead represent a parapneumonic effusion. Accordingly, patients with bronchogenic carcinoma should not be staged as having unresectable (stage 4) carcinoma based only on radiographic findings of an effusion.

True malignant effusions are the result of growth of tumor cells within the pleural space. This type of effusion is common, the two most frequent cell types being breast and bronchogenic carcinomas. These malignant effusions can be massive, opacifying an entire hemithorax (Fig. 11-22). Malignant pleural disease may cause nodularity and thickening (>1 cm) of the pleura. This finding can be visible on chest radiographs but is more easily detected with CT scanning when obscured by overlying pleural fluid. Compared with pleural thickening and effusion caused by inflammation, malignant

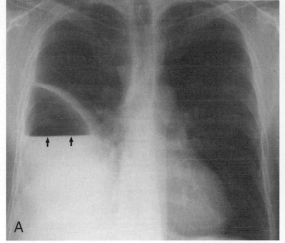

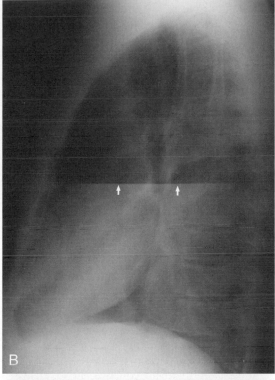

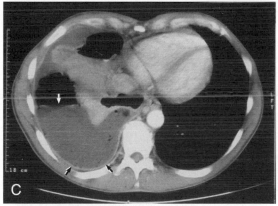

FIGURE 11-20 Posterior-anterior (PA) and lateral radiographs and contrast-enhanced computed tomography: bronchopleural fistula.

A, PA radiograph shows opacification of the inferior aspect of the right hemithorax and an easily seen air-fluid level halfway up the thorax *(arrows)*.

B, Lateral radiograph also shows opacification of the inferior aspect of the hemithorax and an air-fluid level; however, the air fluid level is much longer than that seen on the frontal radiograph *(arrows)*. The asymmetry of the air-fluid level is typical of bronchopleural fistulas. Because lung abscesses are roughly round in shape, the air-fluid levels they cause are usually about the same length in PA, lateral, or decubitus views.

C, CT with intravenous contrast confirms the presence of a bronchopleural fistula with a large air-fluid level within the pleural space *(white arrow)*. Marked pleural enhancement is present *(black arrows)*.

disease is also more likely to involve the pleura circumferentially or to involve the mediastinal pleura (Fig. 11-23). All of these findings, particularly circumferential pleural thickening, are specific for malignancy. Unfortunately, none of the findings are sensitive for the diagnosis of pleural malignancy, and their absence does not exclude the diagnosis.

If all or most of the hemithorax is opacified because of a large pleural effusion, there should be a mediastinal shift away from the opacified side. If there is evidence of volume loss with shift of the mediastinum toward the opacified side, the possibility of high-grade main bronchus obstruction or previous pneumonectomy should be considered (Fig. 11-24). Recognizing a high-grade obstruction is important. Large volume thoracentesis or catheter drainage in patients with high-grade obstruction underlying a pleural effusion may cause reexpansion pulmonary edema by generating high negative intrapleural pressures.

Malignant mesotheliomas are a far less common cause of malignant pleural effusions than bronchogenic carcinoma or pleural metastases (e.g., breast). On CT of the chest, almost

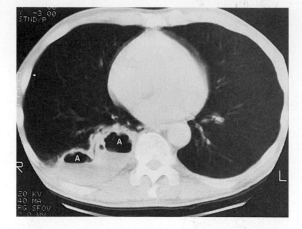

FIGURE 11-21 Contrast-enhanced computed tomography: lung abscess. A single axial image from a contrast-enhanced CT scan shown in a lung window demonstrates two large intra-parenchymal abscesses (A) in the right lower lung. Note the spherical contour with irregular walls typical for abscess. (See Figs. 7-12 and 11-20.)

all cases show pleural thickening in addition to pleural effusion. In advanced cases, the extensive pleural peel causes volume loss and tumor may be seen growing along the pleural fissures (Fig. 11-25). These patients, like those with high-grade bronchial obstruction, can show mediastinal shift toward the opacified hemithorax. Although findings of extensive pleural thickening

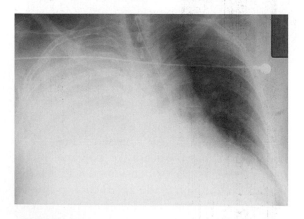

FIGURE 11-22 Posterior-anterior upright chest radiograph: massive pleural effusion. This examination shows complete opacification of the right hemithorax, a finding that could be caused by a massive effusion or parenchymal disease with an obstructed bronchus. There is tracheal deviation to the left. This indicates that in this case most of the opacity is due to a large pleural effusion rather than obstructive atelectasis from an occluded bronchus.

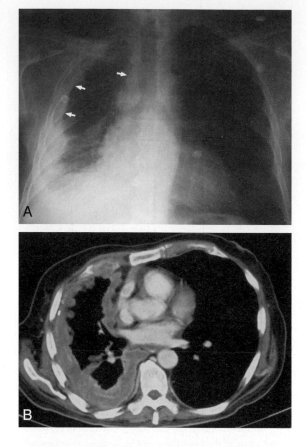

FIGURE 11-23 Posterior-anterior chest radiograph and single slice from contrast-enhanced computed tomography scan: malignant pleural disease.

A, Chest radiograph shows a pleural effusion adjacent to the right lung base, with circumferential pleural thickening *(arrows)* and volume loss in the right hemithorax.

B, CT confirms circumferential thickening of the pleura, including the mediastinal pleura. There is only modest contrast enhancement (compare with Fig. 11-20).

and effusion with volume loss ipsilateral to the pleural disease are classical for mesothelioma, they can also occur when there is extensive pleural involvement by metastatic malignancy such as adenocarcinoma (Table 11-2).

Immunologic Pleural Disease

A variety of immunologic or systemic inflammatory diseases such Dressler's syndrome, rheumatoid arthritis, systemic lupus, and drug reactions may cause pleural disease. Rheumatoid effusions occur more commonly in males and can lead to pleural fibrosis. Approximately one third of patients with rheumatoid effusions also have

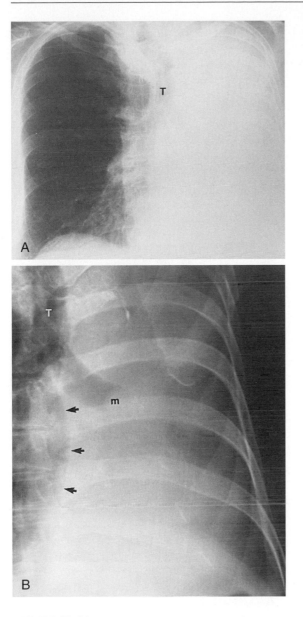

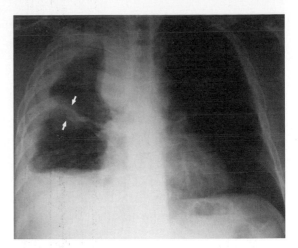

FIGURE 11-25 Posterior-anterior chest radiograph: malignant mesothelioma causing decreased volume of the hemithorax. There is volume loss in the right hemithorax, probably related to decreased chest wall compliance. In addition to right basilar pleural effusion and circumferential pleural thickening there is evident tumor invasion along the minor fissure *(arrows)*.

FIGURE 11-24 Posterior-anterior upright chest radiograph and detail: main bronchial obstruction with atelectasis.

A and B, The left hemithorax is opacified and mediastinum is shifted toward the opacified side because of loss of volume of the left hemithorax. This indicates that much of the opacity results from atelectasis, in this case caused by a left main bronchus mass (m) causing obstructive atelectasis. An associated left-sided pleural effusion may also be present but cannot be the main cause of the opacity as it is in Figure 11-22. T, trachea; *arrows*, herniated lung.

parenchymal lung disease. If a chest radiograph shows both pleural thickening and interstitial disease, either rheumatoid lung disease or asbestosis should be considered as the diagnosis.

Systemic lupus erythematosus is the most common collagen vascular disease to develop pleural disease, effusions occurring in approximately one third of the patients. Unfortunately, some of these patients also have a hypercoagulable condition, which increases their risk for pulmonary emboli that may cause a pleural effusion as well. A CT pulmonary angiogram is often the only way to sort out this conundrum.

Lastly, drug reactions may occasionally cause effusions. Some drug reactions, such as reactions to methotrexate, are probably due to a hypersensitivity reaction and may be accompanied by adjacent parenchymal opacities. Other drugs, such as hydralazine, affect the pleura by causing a lupus-like syndrome and produce pleural disease that is radiographically indistinguishable from primary systemic lupus erythematosus.

TABLE 11-2

Causes of Mediastinal Shift Toward an Opacified Hemithorax

Ipsilateral main bronchus obstruction (by secretions, mass, or foriegn body)

Pneumonectomy

Mesothelioma or other malignant pleural disease causing extensive pleural thickening and effusion

☐ PLEURAL MASSES AND PLEURAL THICKENING

Masses that are seen peripherally on plain chest film may lie within the subpleural portion of the lung parenchyma, in the pleura, or in the chest wall. The latter two sites are often indistinguishable radiographically, showing smooth tapered borders with obtuse pleural angles (Fig. 11-26; see Chapter 14). These findings are easy to identify if the lesion is seen in profile. If the lesion is seen en face, the key finding is an incomplete border, that is, lack of a discrete edge along part of the circumference of the lesion (usually its lateral aspect) because of the tapering of its margins. Confusing pictures can occur when these masses arise from the medial aspect of the pleura, making them appear to be within the mediastinum. Masses located within the interlobar fissure may appear intraparenchymal. Conversely, subpleural parenchymal lesions, including Pancoast's tumors (see later discussion), can look very much like primary pleural processes.

The differential diagnosis for pleural masses includes benign and malignant neoplasms and sequelae of trauma and inflammation (Table 11-3). Multiple apparent masses most commonly are caused by metastases, loculated effusions, or pleural plaques. Pleural plaques are often due to inflammatory changes produced by asbestos exposure. They are usually symmetric and are most commonly seen adjacent to the fifth through eighth ribs (Fig. 11-27). They sometimes occur over the central tendon of the diaphragm. Less than half calcify. Rounded atelectasis is also an asbestos-related abnormality but is difficult to categorize because it represents a hybrid of both subpleural parenchymal

TABLE 11-3
Most Common Causes of Apparent Pleural Masses

Loculated effusions

Metastases (including thymomas)

Pleural plaques

Hematomas

Lipomas

Chest wall masses (e.g., plasmacytoma)

Fibrous tumors of the pleura

Mesotheliomas

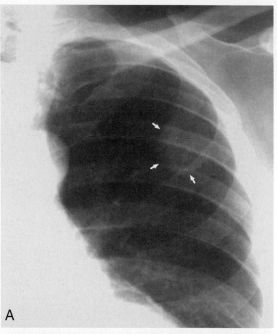

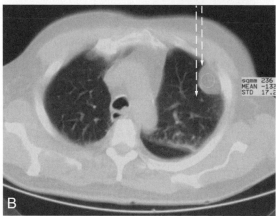

FIGURE 11-26 Detail posterior-anterior (PA) chest radiograph and contrast-enhanced computed tomography: pleural lipoma.

A, There is a nodular opacity in the left upper chest. The medial border of the opacity *(arrows)* is distinct but the lateral margin is ill defined. This combination of well-defined and poorly defined border is typical of a mass originating from the pleura or chest wall.

B, Contrast-enhanced CT scan displayed in lung parenchyma windows demonstrates a low-attenuation mass *(arrows)* with Hounsfield unit measurement of less than -100, indicating fat density. The CT demonstrates that the medial border of the mass is seen in profile when viewed in a PA projection *(dashed arrows* show the direction of the x-ray beam). The lateral border is seen en face on the PA projection and is therefore indistinct.

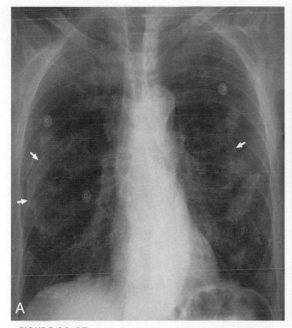

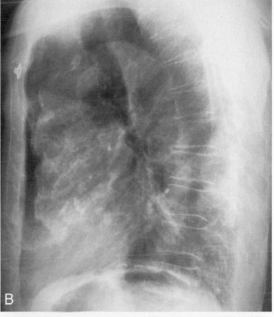

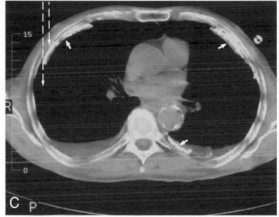

FIGURE 11-27 Posterior-anterior (PA) and lateral chest radiographs: calcified pleural plaques from asbestos exposure.

A, PA radiograph shows bilateral opacities that are well defined along the lateral border but poorly defined medially. The lateral margins *(arrows)* are better defined because the x-ray beam strikes the lateral margin of the plaques in profile. Diaphragmatic pleura calcifications are also present.

B, Lateral radiograph shows the anterior border of the plaques to be well defined because in this projection the x-ray beam strikes the anterior portion of the plaque in profile. Diaphragm calcifications are also well seen.

C, Computed tomography without intravenous contrast shows heavily calcified pleural plaques bilaterally *(solid arrows)*. *Dashed arrows* show how the PA projection x-ray beam strikes the lateral border of the right anterior pleural plaque.

disease and pleural thickening (see Fig. 9-6). Mesothelioma, the least common of asbestos-related diseases, can produce an extensive pleural mass (Fig. 11-28).

In addition to pleural plaques and mesothelioma, asbestos exposure can cause diffuse pleural thickening. Diffuse pleural thickening, however, is common in patients without asbestos exposure and is usually the result of previous infection or trauma. It is often manifested by blunting of the costophrenic angles. Modest changes in appearance may occur from radiograph to radiograph because of changes in inflation or obliquity. This can cause the apparent extent of the pleural opacity to vary and may imitate an effusion changing in size over time.

Extrapleural fat may have a similar appearance. Typically, this fat is symmetrically deposited along the midlateral chest. Differentiation of extrapleural fat or postinflammatory pleural thickening from a small pleural effusion may require decubitus views. Extrapleural fat can also be distinguished from pleural thickening by differences in attenuation measured with CT scanning.

Pleural opacities are often seen in the lung apices of older patients. Apical capping is defined as thickening of the apical pleura of more than 5 mm. It is rarely of clinical significance unless there is progressive pleural thickening or associated parenchymal disease or if the pleural border becomes convex to the lung.

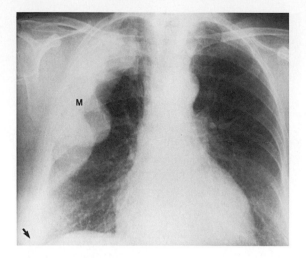

FIGURE 11-28 Posterior-anterior chest radiograph: malignant mesothelioma. Upright chest radiograph shows a multilobulated pleural mass (M) extending along the lateral pleural margin. The costophrenic angle is obscured by a small effusion *(arrow)*.

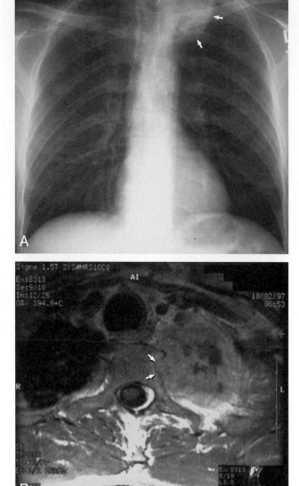

FIGURE 11-29 Posterior-anterior chest radiograph and magnetic resonance imaging (MRI): Pancoast's tumor (superior sulcus tumor).

A, There is an opacity in the left apex projecting within the contour of the first rib and above the level of the left clavicle *(arrows)*. The inferior border is convex.

B, MRI T1-weighted axial image shows a heterogeneous mass in the left apex. There is invasion of the vertebral body *(arrows)* that renders this Pancoast tumor unresectable.

Progressive apical pleural thickening with a convex lower border or adjacent osseous involvement suggests that a Pancoast tumor may be present.

Pancoast's tumor is defined by its location in the lung apex rather than cell type (although it is often a squamous cell carcinoma). Osseous destruction of ribs is often present but does not prohibit resection. Vertebral body involvement, however, is a contraindication to surgery. Clinical findings such as Horner's syndrome and shoulder pain may be present. Magnetic resonance imaging may be the best method of determining the extent of this neoplasm, especially with regard to involvement of the brachial plexus, spine, great vessels, or other vital structures (Fig. 11-29).

☐ DIAPHRAGM

Many processes that affect the pleura commonly occur along its diaphragmatic surface. Pleural processes such as loculated or subpulmonic pleural fluid and pleura-based masses can distort the diaphragmatic contour. Other contour abnormalities of the diaphragm relate to pathology of the diaphragmatic muscle.

Both pleural disease and diaphragmatic pathology can present as apparent elevation of a hemidiaphragm on chest radiograph. The right diaphragm is usually half an intercostal space higher than the left. In less than 10% of patients, the left is higher, often accompanied by a gas-filled colonic loop in the left upper quadrant. New or increasing elevation of either hemidiaphragm may be a sign of disease. Common causes of abnormal diaphragmatic contour are given in Table 11-4.

Diaphragmatic Elevation

The first step in evaluating apparent elevation of the hemidiaphragm is to review previous radiographs or reports. If these cannot be found or the elevation is new, one should look carefully for radiographic signs of lobar atelectasis, such as shift of a pleural fissure. Signs of a subpulmonic effusion should also be sought and decubitus views obtained if the initial radiographs suggest that diagnosis. Most of the time, decubitus view are sufficient to confirm or exclude the presence of a subpulmonic effusion and neither CT or ultrasonography is needed.

If both subpulmonic effusion and lobar atelectasis are excluded, there is usually either an abnormality of the diaphragm itself or disease in the upper abdomen (e.g., subdiaphragmatic abscess; see Fig. 11-15). Diaphragmatic paralysis is a relatively common abnormality of the diaphragm. It is can be caused by a variety of conditions including mediastinal neoplasm, cervical spine disease (e.g., spondylosis), and various neuropathies (including that caused by herpes zoster) and can be seen as a postsurgical complication of open heart surgery. Even after exhaustive evaluation, the underlying causes of many cases of diaphragmatic paralysis remain idiopathic.

Diaphragmatic paralysis can be confirmed with a low-technology method that is performed in seconds. The patient's diaphragms are observed under fluoroscopy or ultrasonography while he or she inhales quickly (sniffs). Normally, the diaphragms move downward. Upward diaphragmatic movement with this maneuver is paradoxical and is evidence of diaphragmatic paralysis. If paralysis is present, some physicians advise CT of the mediastinum to exclude a mediastinal mass. This is reasonable if there is no history of trauma or surgery. It is uncommon, however, for the CT to discover mediastinal pathology as a cause for

diaphragm paralysis if PA and lateral chest radiographs shows no abnormality other than the elevated hemidiaphragm (Fig. 11-30).

Eventration of the diaphragm can also cause elevation of a hemidiaphragm. It is a congenital absence of all or part of the diaphragmatic muscle. When complete, eventration may be indistinguishable from diaphragmatic paralysis. More commonly, eventrations are partial and cause a lobulated diaphragm contour and occur anteromedially on the right (Fig. 11-31). In this instance, the liver usually fills in the space beneath the diaphragm. If the clinical and radiographic picture is confusing, the presence of liver tissue, rather than a mass, beneath the diaphragm can be confirmed with ultrasonography or CT.

Diaphragmatic Hernias and Ruptures

Congenital diaphragmatic hernias can mimic elevation of the hemidiaphragm. These hernias result from failure of normal closure of the pleuroperitoneal canal in utero, causing a defect in the posteromedial diaphragm known as Bochdalek's hernia or in the anteromedial or retrosternal diaphragm known as Morgagni's hernia. Both Bochdalek's and Morgagni's hernias can mimic elevation of the hemidiaphragm. Bochdalek's hernias are much more common than Morgagni's hernias during infancy and, when large, can be fatal. Asymptomatic, small Bochdalek's hernias are occasionally seen as incidental findings in adults and usually contain only fat (Fig. 11-32). Morgagni's hernias are also most often asymptomatic and are most commonly diagnosed in adulthood. They usually occur anteriorly on the right and manifest as a smooth, well-defined opacity in the right cardiophrenic angle. Differentiation from an eventration may be difficult, but it is usually not an important distinction to make. Although strangulation and obstruction of the gastrointestinal tract can occur if the hernia sac contains gut, this rarely happens. Most Morgagni's hernias contain only omentum, and the patients remain asymptomatic. Colonic interpositions, done after esophageal resections, are usually placed anteriorly in the chest and may have a radiographic appearance similar to that of Morgagni's hernias. Either diagnosis can be confirmed with CT scanning or, if the hernia sac contains gut, with barium studies of the gastrointestinal tract (Fig. 11-33). The major

ALGORITHM FOR ELEVATED HEMIDIAPHRAGM

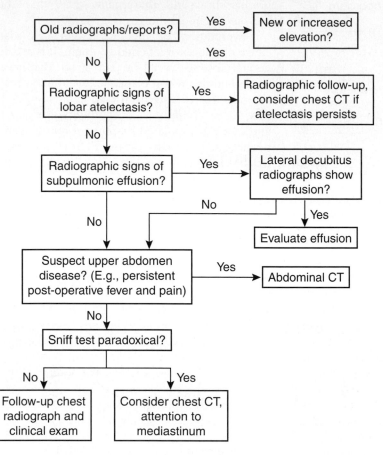

FIGURE 11-30 Algorithm: elevated hemidiaphragm. CT, computed tomography.

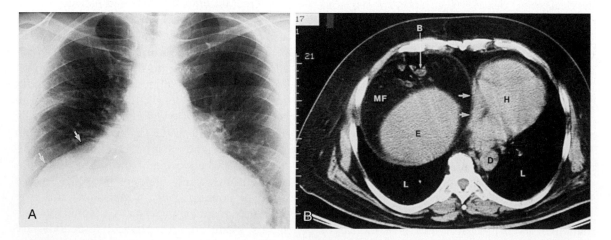

FIGURE 11-31 Posterior-anterior chest radiograph and computed tomography scan of the liver and spleen: eventration of the diaphragm.

A, PA chest radiograph demonstrates a mass that is convex to the right *(arrows)* and appears to be contiguous with the cardiac silhouette.

B, CT utilizing mediastinal windows demonstrates marked elevation of the anterior and middle portion of the right diaphragm (E) with mesenteric fat (MF) and bowel loops (B) beneath it. D, descending aorta; H, heart; L, lung. *Arrows* indicate diaphragm.

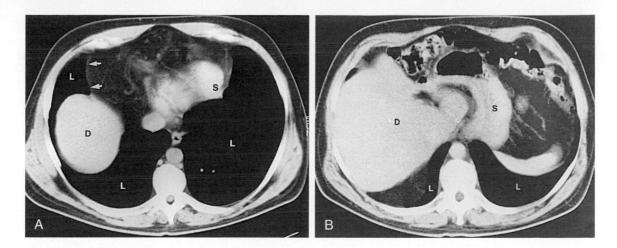

FIGURE 11-32 Contrast-enhanced computed tomography: Morgagni's hernia and Bochdalek's hernia.

A, Morgagni's hernia: contrast-enhanced CT utilizing mediastinal windows demonstrates heterogeneous, mostly fatty attenuation structure extending into the region of the anteromedial right chest cavity, displacing the lung *(arrows)*. The hernia contains mesenteric fat, a few vessels, and a portion of the stomach (S). D, right diaphragm and liver; L, lung.

B, Bochdalek's hernia: contrast-enhanced CT, same patient. Lower CT section shows a mass of fat density projecting through the posterior diaphragm on the right, just lateral to lung tissue (L). Although Bochdalek's hernias seen in infants are typically on the left, CT studies in adults may reveal small Bochdalek's hernias on either side.

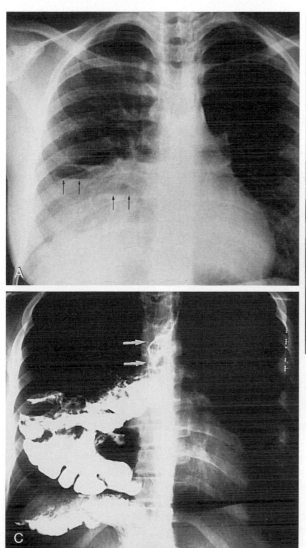

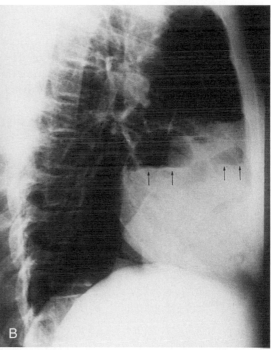

FIGURE 11-33 Posterior-anterior and lateral chest radiographs and barium swallow study: colonic interposition.

A, Frontal chest radiograph shows that the right heart border is obscured. There is heterogeneous opacification of right lower hemithorax with multiple air-fluid levels *(arrows)*.

B, Left lateral chest view shows the multiple air-fluid levels to be located anteriorly. The appearance suggests a differential diagnosis of Morgagni's hernia, multiple lung abscesses, or, as in this instance, colonic interposition.

C, Barium swallow study demonstrates obvious colonic mucosa with haustra, matching the air fluid levels seen on plain radiographs.

benefit in recognizing colonic interpositions or Morgagni's hernias is avoiding further diagnostic studies (e.g., biopsy or thoracentesis) to evaluate what appears to be an unusual pleural or mediastinal mass.

Hiatal hernias are caused by gastric herniation through the esophageal hiatus of the diaphragm. They are by far the most common diaphragmatic hernias. Hiatal hernias, however, usually appear to be in the mediastinum and are therefore discussed in Chapter 13. Only when very large do they affect the diaphragmatic contour, as do the other hernias already discussed.

Like diaphragmatic hernias, diaphragmatic injuries can allow intra-abdominal contents to pass into the thorax. Diaphragmatic injuries occur with penetrating or blunt trauma. When they are caused by the latter, there is almost always associated pneumothorax or rib fractures and more than half the time other major intra-abdominal injuries (such liver or spleen laceration). Because diaphragmatic injuries typically occur in the setting of major multiple trauma, there may a delay in diagnosis. The diaphragm defects caused by traumatic diaphragmatic ruptures tend to be narrower than the defects caused by Morgagni's or Bochdalek's hernias. Bowel herniation through

these narrow-mouthed defects is more likely to lead to complications such as bowel obstruction and strangulation than is herniation caused by congenital hernias (Fig. 11-34). Traumatic diaphragm ruptures are typically repaired surgically because of this risk.

Under The Diaphragm

Intra-abdominal processes can also affect the diaphragmatic contour. Some of these, such as subdiaphragmatic abscesses, have already been discussed. Even if the diaphragm appears normal, it is worthwhile to pay attention to the upper abdomen when examining a chest radiograph. Occasionally, lung nodules hidden deep in the posterior costophrenic sulcus project in this area on a PA chest radiograph. Gallstones, although calcified in only 15% of cases, may also be visible (Fig. 11-35). Clues to the patient's surgical history are sometimes present. Surgical clips in the area of the gastroesophageal junction may be from an antireflux procedure; those in the left upper quadrant may signify a prior splenectomy.

Free intraperitoneal gas should be carefully sought in the right clinical setting (e.g., the septic patient in the intensive care unit). With the correct technique, as little as a few milliliters of

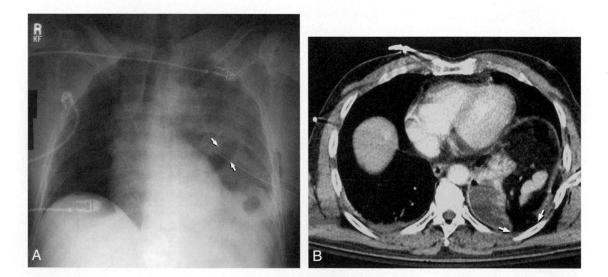

FIGURE 11-34 Portable chest radiograph and computed tomography of traumatic diaphragmatic rupture.

A, Portable radiograph shows an unusual gas pattern in the left lower hemithorax *(arrows)*. The left hemidiaphragm contour is not seen. A left pleural tube and subcutaneous emphysema is also present.

B, CT section from the same patient shows that the stomach is abnormally situated, fallen back against the posterior chest wall (sometimes called the dependent viscera sign). There is a break in the posterior aspect of the diaphragm *(arrows)*. Unprotected by the liver, the left diaphragm is more commonly injured than the right.

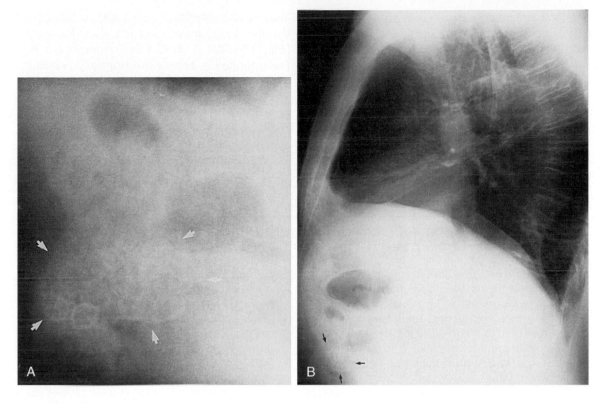

FIGURE 11-35 Lateral chest radiograph and close-up: gallstones.

A, Close-up of the lateral film demonstrates a gallbladder packed with small calculi *(arrows)*.

B, These can be detected only with close inspection of the standard lateral view *(arrows)*.

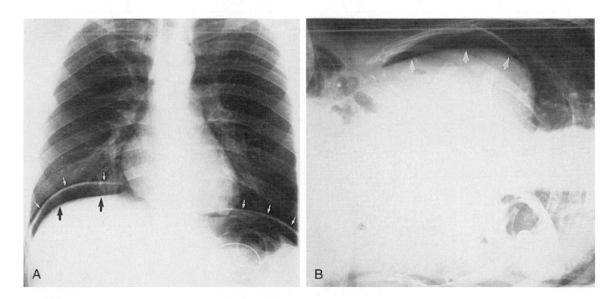

FIGURE 11-36 Upright chest and left lateral decubitus abdomen views: pneumoperitoneum.

A, Upright chest radiograph in the postoperative patient demonstrates sickle-shaped lucencies shaped by the inferior contour of the diaphragms *(white arrows)*. Usually, free intraperitoneal air is best seen above the liver edge *(black arrows)* beneath the diaphragm on the right side.

B, The left lateral decubitus abdomen study (named for side down) demonstrates typical appearance of free intraperitoneal gas *(arrows)* above the margin of the liver. This is the best examination for identifying small amounts of pneumoperitoneum in patients who cannot be positioned upright.

free intraperitoneal gas may be visible on the chest radiograph. On an upright chest radiograph, the presence of intraperitoneal air is easiest to recognize on the right, appearing as a sickle-shaped lucency beneath the diaphragm and above the homogeneous opacity of the liver (Fig. 11-36A). (The lateral view may be more sensitive than the PA projection.) Optimal visualization requires that the patient be upright for 10 minutes, sometimes a difficult task in the intensive care unit. A left lateral decubitus abdominal view is a good alternative (Fig. 11-36B). It should be remembered that postoperatively free air can normally persist for many days, especially in thin individuals. The vast majority of postoperative free intraperitoneal air, however, clears within a week. An *increasing* amount of free intraperitoneal air is abnormal at *any* time postoperatively and should be investigated further.

Pearls for Clinicians—Pleura and Diaphragm

1. The most reliable sign of a pneumothorax is a thin, curved white line that parallels the curvature of the inner thoracic cage. Most pneumothorax imposters either do not produce a white line (skin folds) or do not parallel the curvature of the thoracic cage (companion shadows).
2. Most parapneumonic pleural effusions enhance, whether they are infected or not. The only way an imaging study (including CT) can definitely diagnose an empyema is if it shows gas within pleural fluid that has not been instrumented.
3. CT findings, such as circumferential pleural thickening, are specific but not sensitive for the diagnosis of malignant pleural effusions. Even absence of contrast enhancement of the pleura does not exclude the possibility of neoplasm.
4. When chest radiographs show a large "mass" adjacent to the diaphragm, consider the possibility that the abnormality is caused by a diaphragmatic hernia (or diaphragmatic rupture).
5. On a radiograph, a chest mass that does not obscure the overlying pulmonary vasculature and is sharply marginated along only one segment of its circumference, may lie in the pleural space or within the chest wall rather than within the lung.

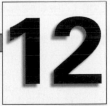

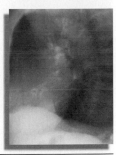

Cardiovascular Disease

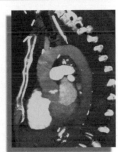

Although there have been many technological advances in noninvasive cardiac imaging over the past decade, the chest radiograph remains an important means of initially assessing the heart and the intrathoracic vasculature. Key observations on radiographs can guide the selection of additional imaging studies. When evaluating the chest radiograph for evidence of cardiac disease, it is important to look at structures in addition to the heart. Observations about the pulmonary vasculature, the lung interstitium, and the great vessels may aid in diagnosis and treatment more than observations about the cardiac silhouette. The chest radiograph is also useful in assessing the placement of various intracardiac and intravascular devices.

Numerous advanced imaging methods are available to define cardiac anatomy and function. Echocardiography, angiography, radionuclide ventriculography, and myocardial perfusion scans have been performed for decades. The role of computed tomography (CT) in cardiovascular imaging has greatly expanded because of the availability of multidetector scanners that make possible marked reductions in both section thickness and scan time. CT scanning can now also be gated to the electrocardiography (ECG) signal, allowing images to be obtained primarily during diastole so that cardiac motion is minimized (Fig. 12-1). Although technically more complex than CT, magnetic resonance imaging (MRI) is also being used with increasing frequency for cardiovascular imaging. MRI is better than CT at distinguishing normal myocardium from other types of soft tissues (e.g., tumor or myocardium scar) (Fig. 12-2). Magnetic resonance angiography (MRA), angiography performed with MRI, is also very effective in depicting the aortic arch and its vessels, without using radiation or nephrotoxic intravenous contrast material (Fig. 12-3 and Table 12-1). Despite these advances, in this chapter we discuss only the most common uses of CT and MR in cardiovascular imaging and focus on using chest radiography as the initial step in evaluating the cardiovascular system.

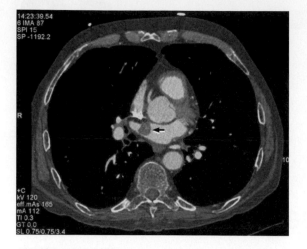

FIGURE 12-1 Computed tomography (CT) of the chest: atrial myxoma. CT section obtained using a multidetector CT scanner with cardiac gating. This technique uses only the imaging data acquired during diastole in order to minimize cardiac motion. A small mass is seen attached to the interatrial septum *(arrow)*. The right coronary artery is also seen originating from the ascending aorta.

☐ PULMONARY VASCULATURE

Pulmonary Venous Hypertension

Evaluation of the chest radiograph for cardiovascular disease is best begun by a search for signs of pulmonary venous and pulmonary arterial hypertension. Pulmonary venous hypertension is most commonly caused by increased left ventricular end-diastolic pressure related to left ventricular dysfunction, although it can be caused by an obstructive lesion at or proximal to the mitral valve and by mitral regurgitation (Table 12-2). The key radiographic changes of pulmonary venous hypertension are vascular redistribution, interstitial edema, and alveolar edema. There is a rough correlation between radiographic findings and the degree of pulmonary hypertension as measured with a Swan-Ganz catheter, the pulmonary capillary wedge pressure (PCWP). Some textbooks describe an orderly progression from one sign to the next as venous hypertension worsens, but this is rarely seen in the clinical practice.

The sign associated with the mildest level of pulmonary venous hypertension is vascular redistribution. This means that upper lobe vessels become wider and more opaque than lower lobe vessels. The sign is most accurate if the upper lobe vessels are increased in diameter (e.g., larger than the adjacent bronchus) *and* the lower lobe vessels are diminished in size. Prior radiographs for comparison are sometimes crucial to confirm this change.

Often the best place to compare bronchus and pulmonary artery is the anterior segment of the upper lobe because the artery is seen on

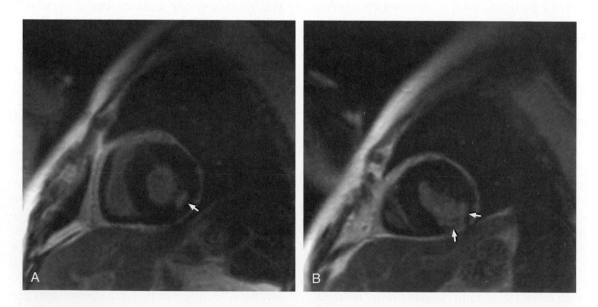

FIGURE 12-2 Magnetic resonance (MR) images of the heart: postinfarction scar. Two MR images of the left and right ventricles obtained 10 minutes after intravenous contrast material (gadolinium) was administered. The high signal (bright area) in the left ventricular wall *(arrows)* is an area of scar formed as a result of myocardial infarction. This area will not regain function if a coronary artery bypass is performed.

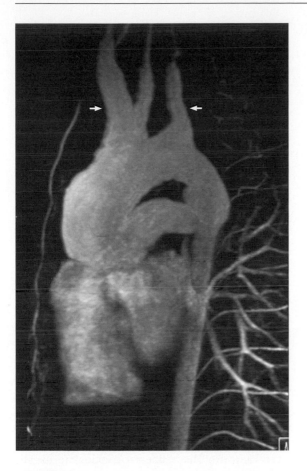

FIGURE 12-3 Magnetic resonance angiography of the thoracic aorta: Takayasu's disease (a large vessel vasculitis). The vessel lumens are high in signal (bright) because of enhancement by intravenous gadolinium. The ascending aorta lumen is irregular and dilated. The brachiocephalic and left subclavian arteries *(arrows)* are also dilated as they originate from the aorta.

end in the frontal projection. Increase in both upper and lower lung vessel size is not indicative of venous hypertension but may be present in conditions that cause increased pulmonary blood volume, such as right-to-left shunts (e.g., an atrial septal defect), or renal failure with volume overload. In patients with normal volume and cardiac status the upper lobe vessels enlarge slightly, matching the size of the adjacent bronchus, when the patient lies supine. This is seen daily on radiographs from the intensive care unit (ICU) and should not be mistaken as a sign of disease.

Redistribution is more commonly seen in patients with chronic recurrent heart failure than in patients with acute disease (Fig. 12-4). This is probably because redistribution is not caused by simple increases in intravascular volume but depends in part on pulmonary vascular tone. Even in the setting of recurrent heart failure, however, radiographic findings may be obscured in patients with upper lobe disease, such as emphysema and tuberculosis.

The azygous vein can also be used as a barometer of intravascular volume. Unfortunately, it reflects primarily right atrial pressures and is related to pulmonary venous hypertension only indirectly. This is similar to many physical findings (including jugular venous distention and pedal edema). The vein is seen in over half of anterior-posterior (AP) chest radiographs and lies just above the takeoff of the right main stem bronchus. An azygous diameter greater than 9 mm in an upright patient is abnormal; however, it may be as large as 14 mm on AP

TABLE 12-1

Current Uses of Magnetic Resonance Imaging and Computed Tomography in Evaluation of Cardiovascular Disease

	MRI	Single-Detector CT	Multidetector CT
Coronary artery calcifications (quantify)	No	No	Yes
Coronary artery angiography	Limited	No	Yes*
Aortic traumatic injury	No	Yes	Yes
Aortic dissection	Yes	Yes	Yes
Pericardial calcifications	No	Yes	Yes
Pericardiac effusion/thickening	Yes	Yes	Yes
Cardiac function	Yes	No	Limited

*If multidetector CT has 16 detectors or more.

TABLE 12-2
Causes of Pulmonary Venous Hypertension

Increased left ventricular end-diastolic pressure
  Decreased contractility (e.g., ischemic
    cardiomyopathy)
  Increased preload (e.g., massive fluid resuscitation)
  Diastolic dysfunction
Mitral valve disease
  Mitral stenosis
  Mitral insufficiency
Other obstructive lesions (all rare)
  Left atrial myxomas
  Veno-occlusive disease

supine radiographs of normal individuals. Rather than using any absolute measurements, it is best to compare the appearance of the azygous vein between radiographs of the same patient over time. Used in this way, the azygous vein can be a good clue to the patient's volume status. Note that we use the term volume status, not cardiac status, here. In patients with heart failure who have been treated with diuretics, the azygous vein may return to normal size despite continued poor cardiac function. Conversely, patients with a normal heart show an enlarged azygous vein when given very large amounts of intravenous fluids. Engorgement of the azygous vein can be differentiated from azygous node adenopathy by the vein's change in size with changes in the patient's position or respiration. The azygous vein decreases in size when the patient is upright or performs a Valsalva maneuver. A lymph node does not (Fig. 12-5).

As the PCWP rises further, usually above 19 to 20 mm Hg, interstitial edema develops. Bronchial cuffing, Kerley's B lines, and thickening of lung fissures are the most easily detected radiographic signs of interstitial edema (see Figs. 5-6 and 11-13). Normal bronchial walls appear pencil-point thin when seen end on. Interstitial edema widens the bronchial walls and makes their margins appear indistinct (termed bronchial cuffing) (Fig. 12-6). Kerley's B lines are caused by accumulation of fluid in the interlobular septa (see Chapter 5). They appear as short horizontal lines that usually make contact with the pleura. (Lines caused by normal pulmonary vessels are not visible within 2 cm of the chest wall.) Kerley's B lines are best seen near the costophrenic angles on frontal projections and adjacent to the sternum on lateral views (see Fig. 5-5). These linear opacities are usually

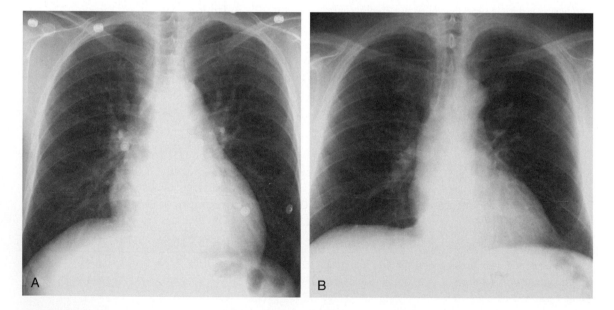

FIGURE 12-4 Posterior-anterior (PA) views of the chest: a patient with vascular redistribution and a patient with normal pulmonary vasculature.

A, PA chest of a patient with vasculature redistribution. The upper lung vessels are enlarged and are greater in diameter than lower lobe blood vessels at a similar distance from the hilum. The cardiac silhouette size is also enlarged.

B, PA chest of a normal patient for comparison. Upper lung blood vessels are smaller in caliber than the lower lung vessels.

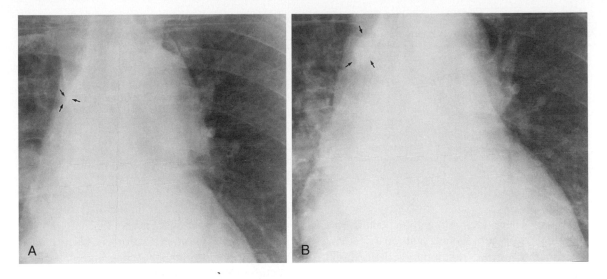

FIGURE 12-5 Posterior-anterior upright and anterior-posterior supine radiographs: radiographs from the same patient illustrating changes in appearance of the azygous vein.

A, When the patient is upright, the azygous vein is flat and barely perceptible *(arrows).*

B, Supine radiograph shows the azygous vein to be much wider in diameter *(arrows).*

due to interstitial edema but can be caused by other conditions as well, such as inflammation or neoplastic processes (Table 12-3). Just as interstitial edema accumulates in the interlobular septa to cause Kerley's B lines, edema can also accumulate in the lung adjacent to the pleural surfaces. This causes the interlobar fissures to appear thicker and at times may be a more noticeable sign than Kerley's B lines because the fissures are bigger structures than the interlobular septa (see Fig. 5-6).

If the pulmonary venous pressures rise still higher, usually above PCWP values of 25 mm Hg, alveolar opacities (air space disease) begin to

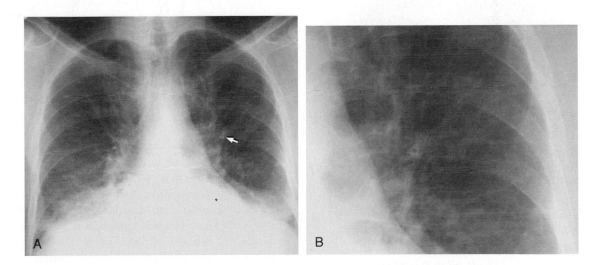

FIGURE 12-6 Posterior-anterior chest radiograph: peribronchial cuffing.

A, Upright chest radiograph shows evidence of interstitial edema, including Kerley's B lines, indistinct hila, and peribronchial cuffing *(arrow).* Basilar alveolar edema is also present.

B, Detail from radiograph shows left upper lobe bronchus wall to be markedly thickened and indistinct compared with its normal thin, well-defined appearance.

TABLE 12-3
Causes of Extensive Kerley's B Lines

Congestive heart failure*
Lymphangitic carcinoma*
Infection
   Mycoplasma
   Hantavirus
Acute hypersensitivity reactions (includes acute
   eosinophilic pneumonia)

*Most common.

be visible. There are radiographic criteria for separating this cardiogenic pulmonary edema from noncardiogenic pulmonary edema (adult respiratory distress syndrome). If the air space disease is perihilar or bibasilar, symmetric, and responds to diureses, the diagnosis of cardiogenic pulmonary edema is easy (Fig. 12-7). More often, it is difficult to make a clear distinction between cardiogenic and noncardiogenic pulmonary edema on radiographs. The radiographic signs listed in Table 8-4 are most accurate in early or less severe cases of pulmonary edema.

Typically, the air space disease caused by cardiogenic edema is symmetric; however, in

occasional cases the edema may have an atypical, asymmetric pattern that mimics pneumonia. Asymmetric pulmonary edema can be caused by gravitational changes (e.g., the patient preferentially lying on one side) and by pulmonary vascular obstruction by tumor or emboli. Perhaps the most common cause of atypical pulmonary edema is the presence of preexisting parenchymal lung disease, such as large bullae that distort the pattern of pulmonary blood flow.

Radiographic findings in patients with chronic congestive heart failure also differ from those in patients with acute disease. Among patients with chronic or recurrent heart failure, radiographic findings of interstitial edema, including Kerley's B lines, do not seem to occur until venous pressures have reached higher levels than those needed to cause edema in patients with acute congestive heart failure. This appears to be due to the development of increased lung lymphatic drainage in response to prolonged exposure to pulmonary venous hypertension. Thus, radiographs of patients with chronic heart failure are more likely to show vascular redistribution and less likely to show interstitial edema than those of patients with acute congestive heart failure.

Pulmonary Arterial Hypertension

In addition to evaluating the chest radiograph for signs of pulmonary venous hypertension, it is important to search for evidence of pulmonary arterial hypertension. Unlike pulmonary venous hypertension, pulmonary arterial hypertension is rarely evident on the chest radiograph unless it has been long standing. Pulmonary arterial hypertension can be caused by chronic pulmonary venous hypertension related to left-sided heart failure (postcapillary pulmonary hypertension). The degree of pulmonary arterial hypertension is usually not severe, however, unless the left-sided heart failure is accompanied by significant mitral valve disease (see later). If radiographic signs of both pulmonary arterial and pulmonary venous hypertension are evident on the chest radiograph, further evaluation of the mitral valve (e.g., with echocardiography) should be considered if that has not been done in the past.

Pulmonary arterial hypertension unrelated to venous hypertension is caused by increased pulmonary blood flow or by increased vascular resistance (precapillary pulmonary hypertension).

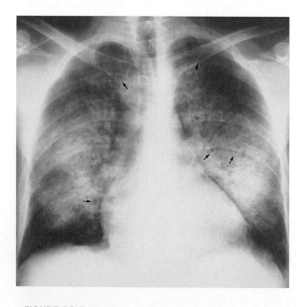

FIGURE 12-7 Posterior-anterior upright radiograph: pulmonary edema—butterfly pattern and peribronchial cuffing. This frontal radiograph demonstrates the perihilar distribution of acute pulmonary edema (butterfly or bat wing pattern) that is more commonly seen with volume overload than congestive heart failure. Note the blurring of the hilar vessels. Extensive peribronchial cuffing is present *(arrows)*.

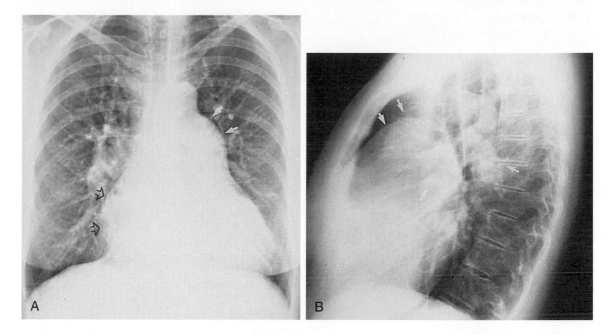

FIGURE 12-8 Posterior-anterior and lateral chest radiographs: atrial septal defect.

A, This frontal chest radiograph shows diffusely increased pulmonary blood flow (i.e., pulmonary plethora). The right heart border is more convex than normal *(open arrows)*, and the pulmonary trunk is huge *(solid arrows)*. Note the lack of enlargement of the ascending aorta or aortic arch.

B, On the lateral view, there is partial opacification of the retrosternal clear space by an enlarged right ventricle and pulmonary trunk *(retrosternal arrows)*. Right and left descending pulmonary arteries are also markedly enlarged *(hilar arrows)*.

Increased pulmonary blood flow can be caused by congenital heart diseases that produce a left-to-right shunt. Atrial septal defects are the most common congenital heart disease to cause increased left-to-right flow in adults. Before developing increased pulmonary resistance, these patients show evidence of increased pulmonary arterial flow. This causes "pulmonary plethora," an increase in the caliber of both pulmonary arteries and veins (Fig. 12-8). It can be difficult to differentiate an increase in pulmonary blood flow from the effects of venous hypertension on chest radiographs. The engorged vessels from overcirculation usually appear more distinct than those enlarged by pulmonary venous hypertension because interstitial edema is absent. In addition, blood flow is increased throughout the lung parenchyma without preferential increase in blood flow to the upper lobes. These radiographic changes can be subtle, and pulmonary arterial overcirculation is not apparent on chest radiographs until the ratio of shunt blood flow to systemic blood flow is about 2:1 or greater. Noninvasive radionuclide studies can detect smaller shunts, probably as small as 1.2:1.

With time, persistent pulmonary overcirculation can cause pulmonary arteriopathy that raises pulmonary vascular resistance. Radiographically, this appears as well-defined enlargement of the central pulmonary arteries with rapid tapering of vessels in the middle and distal thirds of the lung. This disparity in the size of central and peripheral vasculature is a clue that pulmonary vascular resistance is increased. Pulmonary artery calcification can develop in severe cases (Fig. 12-9). This denotes long-standing severe pulmonary hypertension and suggests that the pulmonary artery pressure is very high (e.g., comparable to systemic pressures). If pulmonary vascular resistance is high enough to decrease the amount of right-to-left shunting across an atrial septal defect, radiographic evidence of pulmonary plethora diminishes.

Vascular abnormalities such as pulmonary emboli and primary pulmonary hypertension cause pulmonary arterial hypertension by increasing precapillary resistance. In these disease states, radiographs show central pulmonary arterial enlargement. The peripheral vasculature has a pruned-tree appearance, similar

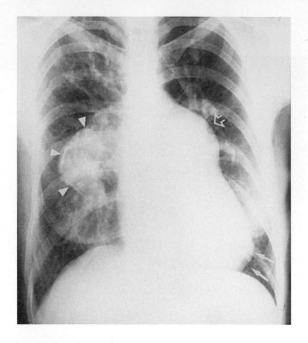

FIGURE 12-9 Posterior-anterior chest radiograph: atrial septal defect with pulmonary artery calcifications. This frontal chest radiograph demonstrates aneurysmal dilatation of the pulmonary trunk *(open arrow)* and enlargement of the right pulmonary artery. Intramural calcifications are also seen in the right pulmonary artery *(arrowheads)*. These occur when the pulmonary arterial pressures approximate systemic arterial pressures.

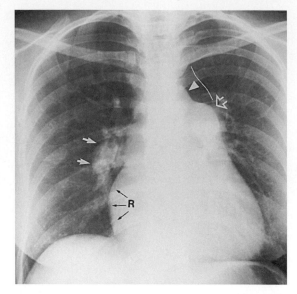

FIGURE 12-10 Posterior-anterior chest radiograph: primary pulmonary hypertension. Frontal radiograph shows features of advanced pulmonary arterial hypertension with increased convexity of right heart border *(black arrows and R)*, dilated pulmonary trunk *(open arrow)*, and enlarged central pulmonary arteries *(white arrows)*. The aortic arch is diminutive *(arrowhead)*.

to that seen in patients with a long-standing left-to-right shunt (Fig. 12-10). Often there is accompanying right heart enlargement (see "Right Heart Enlargement" later). Radionuclide lung scanning can differentiate chronic emboli from primary pulmonary hypertension but is now used less commonly than CT pulmonary angiography. Radionuclide scans in patients with chronic thromboemboli usually reveal multiple segmental perfusion defects, whereas scans in patients with primary pulmonary hypertension show only nonspecific inhomogeneity of perfusion without obstruction of the blood flow to discrete lung segments. CT pulmonary angiography in patients with chronic emboli often shows evidence of thrombus adherent to the walls of pulmonary arteries (see Chapter 10).

Chronic lung disease related to chronic obstructive pulmonary disease (COPD) and pulmonary fibrosis is the most common cause of precapillary pulmonary arterial hypertension (Table 12-4). The radiographic findings are similar to those of primary pulmonary vascular

disease except that parenchymal lung disease is also apparent. In the setting of COPD, a descending right pulmonary artery diameter (on frontal view) greater than 16 mm or a left descending pulmonary artery diameter (on lateral view) greater than 18 mm is strongly associated with increased pulmonary arterial pressures (Fig. 12-11).

The convexity caused by the main pulmonary artery on the frontal radiographs is also

TABLE 12-4
Causes of Pulmonary Arterial Hypertension

Postcapillary
   Congestive heart failure with mitral insufficiency*
   Mitral stenosis
Overcirculation
   Atrial septal defect
   Patent ductus arteriosus
Precapillary
   Chronic thromboemboli*
   Primary pulmonary hypertension
   Chronic lung disease*
      Chronic obstructive lung disease
      Idiopathic pulmonary fibrosis

*Most common.

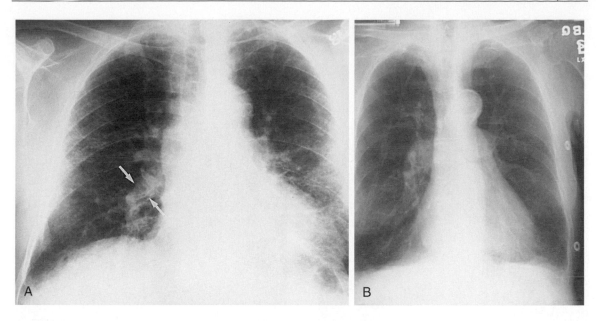

FIGURE 12-11 Posterior-anterior chest: cor pulmonale.

A, Frontal radiograph of a patient with interstitial fibrosis. The right descending pulmonary artery is greater than 16 mm in diameter *(arrows)*, which is consistent with pulmonary arterial hypertension secondary to chronic lung disease.

B, Frontal view of patient with chronic obstructive pulmonary disease and secondary pulmonary hypertension. The central pulmonary arteries are dilated and the cardial silhouette is large for this degree of lung hyperinflation.

enlarged in patients with pulmonary hypertension. Often this enlargement of the pulmonary trunk is more evident than the enlargement of the descending pulmonary arteries. This may caused by the effects of Laplace's law, which states that larger structures experience greater increases in wall strain as arterial pressure rises. Unfortunately, an exact measurement of the main pulmonary artery is difficult because only part of its border is seen on radiographs; however, if its diameter appears larger than the aortic arch, pulmonary hypertension is likely to be present. The main pulmonary artery is easily identified and measured on most CT scans, including those performed without intravenous contrast or thin sections. If the width of the pulmonary artery is greater than 3.0 cm or greater than the width of the ascending aorta, pulmonary hypertension is probably present (Fig. 12-12).

☐ **AORTA**

Routine evaluation of the thoracic aorta, like analysis of the pulmonary vasculature, is central to the effective use of the chest radiograph

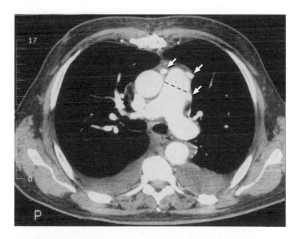

FIGURE 12-12 Contrast-enhanced computed tomography: mild pulmonary hypertension. CT section at the level used for measuring the diameter of the main pulmonary artery *(dashed line)*. In this case the diameter is measured as 3 cm and is approximately the same as that of the ascending aorta.

If pulmonary hypertension is suspected, it is helpful to look for other signs of elevated right heart pressures, such as dilatation of the inferior vena cava. Note also that the patient has undergone coronary artery bypass and three grafts are seen traveling around the pulmonary artery *(arrows)*.

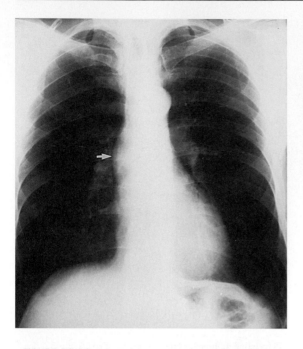

FIGURE 12-13 Posterior-anterior chest radiograph of a young adult male: aortic stenosis. The ascending aorta is enlarged and makes up the right mediastinal border *(arrow)*. Overall heart size is normal.

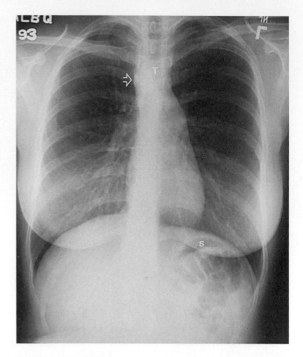

FIGURE 12-14 Posterior-anterior chest radiograph: right arch. In this frontal projection, the aortic arch is on the right *(arrow)*, and the trachea (T) is slightly displaced to the left. Cardiac contour is otherwise normal, and the gastric bubble (B) is normally located, on the left.

in assessment of the cardiovascular system. Abnormalities of the aorta can reflect underlying cardiac disease or be caused by primary disease of this vessel. In young and middle-aged adults the superior vena cava makes up the superior portion of the right cardiomediastinal shadow, but with increasing age the ascending aorta may widen and extend farther to the right than the vena cava. If the ascending aorta is large enough to extend to the right of the superior vena cava in a young patient, the diagnosis of aortic stenosis, systemic hypertension, or aortic insufficiency should be considered (Fig. 12-13). The size and location of the aortic arch and the size and course of the descending aorta should also be checked for abnormal enlargement. The latter may be ectatic in older patients and may appear even larger on frontal views when it follows a tortuous course. The lateral view is often helpful in determining whether true dilatation is present.

Congenital Aortic Disease

A right aortic arch is a congenital anomaly that is seen in about 1 out of 2500 individuals (Fig. 12-14). The pattern of origin of the great

vessels from the aorta indicates the likelihood of associated congenital heart disease. In most adults with a right arch, the left subclavian artery is the last vessel to leave the arch, crossing from the right to the left side behind the trachea and esophagus (termed an aberrant left subclavian artery). This is associated with congenital heart disease in about 2% of cases. A few patients with an aberrant left subclavian artery may develop dysphagia from vascular impingement on the esophagus.

Coarctation of the aorta is a congenital narrowing of the aortic arch, which usually occurs just distal to the origin of the last of the great vessels (normally the left subclavian artery). This aortic malformation is often associated with other congenital cardiac anomalies, such as a bicuspid aortic valve. Plain radiographic findings include a notch in the descending aorta and more distal poststenotic dilatation. This can give that portion of the aorta a 3-shaped contour. Alternatively, the aortic arch may be inconspicuous. Notching of the fourth to the eighth ribs is usually present in adults and sometimes more easily seen than the abnormalities of the aorta. These notches are small erosions along the inferior border of the posterolateral aspect of the rib caused by enlarged intercostal arteries. (The inferior borders of these ribs may normally be indistinct, but true notches have well-defined sclerotic borders.) When coarctation is suspected because of physical examination or plain radiograph findings, the diagnosis can be confirmed noninvasively by MRI (Fig. 12-15).

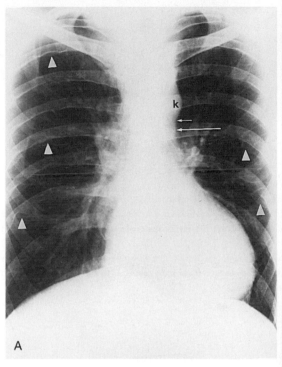

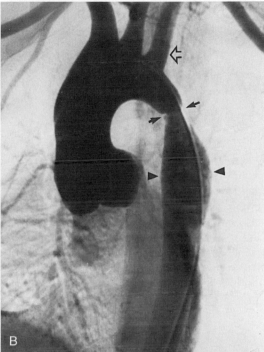

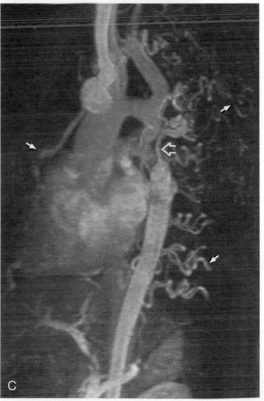

<u>FIGURE 12-15</u> Posterior-anterior chest radiograph, arch aortogram, and magnetic resonance angiography: aortic coarctation.

A, The frontal radiograph shows a small aortic arch/knob (k). The slight indentation that represents the coarctation *(short arrow)* and the poststenotic dilatation *(long arrow)* are difficult to see. There is associated bilateral rib notching *(arrowheads)*.

B, Arch angiography in left anterior oblique view shows classical findings of adult coarctation. The coarctation *(solid arrows)* occurs after the origin of the left subclavian artery *(open arrow)*. There is marked poststenotic dilatation *(arrowheads)* of the descending aorta.

C, Magnetic resonance angiography performed with gadolinium in a different patient. The area of narrowing distal to the left subclavian is easily seen *(open arrow)*. The internal mammary and intercostal blood vessels are enlarged because of collateral blood flow around the coarctation *(small solid arrows)*.

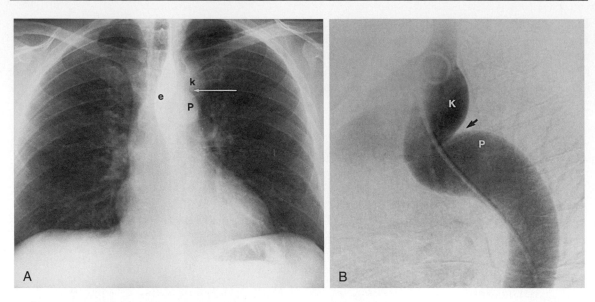

FIGURE 12-16 Posterior-anterior chest radiograph and arch aortogram: pseudocoarctation.

A, The frontal chest radiograph demonstrates a very high aortic "knob" (k) and a lobulated contour of the superior portion of the descending aorta *(arrow)*. The descending aorta below the "kink" is slightly dilated. e, contrast material within the esophagus; p, "postkink" segment of descending aorta.

B, Aortic arch angiogram in left anterior oblique projection shows the pseudocoarctation kink *(arrow)* caused by elongation of the aorta. This accounts for the lobulated appearance of the lateral border of the aorta on plain radiographs. k, distal portion of the aortic arch, the radiographic aortic knob; p, postkink mildly dilated descending aorta.

In adults, chest radiographic findings similar to those seen in a coarctation may be caused by a condition known as a pseudocoarctation. This condition is caused by elongation and tortuosity of the posterior arch and proximal descending aorta, with secondary kinking of the aorta (Fig. 12-16). A pseudocoarctation causes the contour of the aortic arch and proximal descending aorta to appear lobulated, similar to a coarctation, but no rib notching is present. The aortic arch also appears higher than normal and may be mistaken for a mass in the upper left mediastinum. No significant arterial gradient is present across the area of kinking, and no treatment is necessary.

Acquired Aortic Disease

Life-threatening acquired aortic diseases include traumatic aortic injuries, aortic dissections and their variants (intramural hematomas and penetrating ulcers), and aortic aneurysms. Traumatic aortic injuries are commonly caused by severe deceleration injuries such as high-speed motor vehicle accidents and are responsible for 20% of fatalities in this setting. Most patients with traumatic aortic injuries (80% to 90%) do not survive to reach the hospital. Of those who reach medical care, most die without rapid diagnosis and treatment. In the past, mediastinal widening on chest radiography was used as an indicator of traumatic aortic injury (TAI); however, this sign is nonspecific. Patients at risk for TAI often have multiple injuries and are unable to sit upright or take a deep inspiration. The resulting supine position and hypoinflation may both cause the mediastinum to appear widened on a chest radiograph. Loss of the contour of the aortic arch is a more specific sign of TAI, but its sensitivity is low.

In the past, angiography was used to evaluate patients in whom radiographic findings or the mechanism of injury suggested TAI. Over the past decade, however, CT has become the study of choice. CT studies often document the injury by showing either an abnormal contour of the aorta or a thin sheet of tissue within the aortic lumen (an intimal flap) at the junction between the aortic arch and descending aorta (Fig. 12-17). Patients with a definite contour abnormality or intimal flap undergo surgery without further imaging. Patients without a

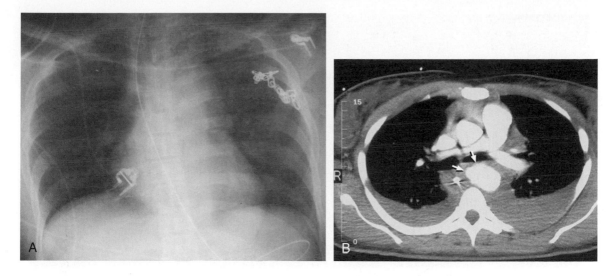

FIGURE 12-17 Anterior-posterior (AP) chest and computed tomography (CT): traumatic aortic injury.

A, AP chest shows a widened mediastinum. More specific findings are also present, including loss of the contour of the aortic arch and deviation of the nasogastric tube to the right.

B, CT image from the same patient. The lumen of the descending aorta is asymmetric and irregular *(arrows).* A hematoma surrounds the area of aortic injury.

periaortic hematoma or an abnormality of the aortic contour or lumen are usually observed. Occasionally (in 2% to 5% of cases), a TAI escapes detection yet the patient still survives. These patient may later present with a calcified pseudoaneurysm of the distal aortic arch.

The most deadly nontraumatic abnormality of the aortic arch is an aortic dissection. Predisposing factors include hypertension, aortic valve disease, Marfan's syndrome, and pregnancy. Dissections that occur in the ascending aorta within several centimeters of the aortic valve are termed type A and are associated with a high mortality rate if not treated surgically. Dissections that begin distal to the origin of the left subclavian artery are termed type B and can often be managed medically.

About a quarter of the chest radiographs of patients with aortic dissection are normal. Mediastinal widening on the frontal projection occurs in approximately half of the patients. Obliteration of the aortic arch and *left*-sided hemothorax may also occur (Fig. 12-18). One often mentioned sign, displacement of calcifications within the aortic wall, is rarely seen. This occurs when calcification in an intimal plaque is displaced inward by the dissection and is seen more than 4 mm medial to the outer aortic wall. Unfortunately, this sign is

best applied to the descending aorta, where the x-ray beam is perpendicular to the blood vessel. Calcifications, on the other hand, occur most commonly in the aortic arch, where the sign can be misleading because the aorta is seen obliquely at this level. Plain radiographic findings of aortic dissection are, in short, unreliable.

In order to direct therapy for an aortic dissection, a diagnostic study must detect the presence of a false aortic lumen, which is separated

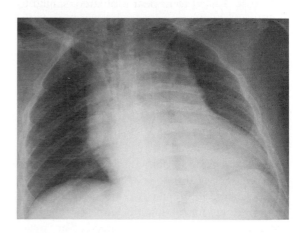

FIGURE 12-18 Anterior-posterior chest: type A aortic dissection. The mediastinum is markedly widened and the aortic arch is obscured. The trachea is shifted to the right.

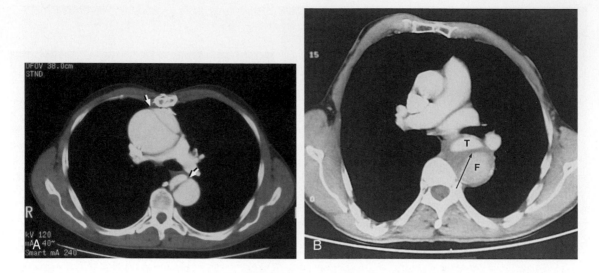

FIGURE 12-19 Contrast-enhanced computed tomography sections: type A and type B aortic dissections.

A, CT section shows widened ascending aorta and the presence of a dissection flap in both the ascending and descending aorta *(arrows)*.

B, Contrast-enhanced CT scan obtained with mediastinal windows shows dissection confined to the descending aorta. The ascending aorta is normal. There is contrast material in both the false lumen (F) and the true lumen (T), and the intimal flap *(arrow)* between them is well defined. The false lumen may fill more slowly with intravenous contrast material and therefore appear less dense.

from the true lumen by an intimal flap. The study must also determine where the dissection originates (differentiating a type A from a type B dissection). Fortunately, we now have several accurate and noninvasive methods of obtaining this information: CT angiography, MRI, and transesophageal echocardiography (TEE).

All three methods are excellent at detecting aortic dissection, with sensitivities greater than 95% (Fig. 12-19). MRI and TEE may be slightly more specific than single-slice CT scanners in the detection of aortic dissections, but direct comparisons between MRI and TEE and the newest multislice CT scanners have not yet been done. For practical purposes, all three methods of imaging have comparable accuracy and the decision to use one instead of another often rests on other factors. MRI can be problematic because of the limits it places on the ability to monitor the patient, particularly during the early management of the dissection, when control of hypertension is crucial. Contrast-enhanced CT can be done more quickly than MRI, and the patient can be easily monitored. The major advantage of TEE is that it can be done at the bedside. In most cases, a negative TEE, MRI, or CT examination is adequate to exclude the

presence of an aortic dissection. Once the "gold standard," catheter-directed aortography may actually be less sensitive than CT angiograms and is rarely performed to make the diagnosis of aortic dissection.

Two other diseases are related to aortic dissections: intramural hematomas and penetrating aortic ulcers. Intramural hematomas may be due to thrombosis of the false lumen of an aortic dissection or spontaneous rupture of the vasa vasorum in the aortic wall. CT of the chest shows smooth, eccentric thickening of the aortic wall (Fig. 12-20). Scanning before administration of intravenous contrast material often shows that the thickening of the wall is high in attenuation, consistent with acute hemorrhage rather than chronic thrombus. Penetrating ulcers occur when an ulcerated aortic plaque burrows through the intima into the aortic media. These can progress to form an intramural hematoma or progress to complete rupture of the aorta. Although not as well worked out, the management of intramural hematomas and penetrating ulcers is usually similar to the treatment of aortic dissections. Ascending aortic disease usually requires surgery, whereas descending aortic disease is typically medically managed.

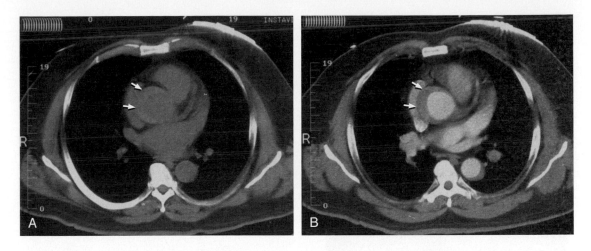

FIGURE 12-20 Computed tomography sections without and with intravenous contrast: intramural hemorrhage.

A, On the CT scan performed without intravenous contrast there is a "crescent" of high attenuation around part of the ascending aorta *(arrows)*. This is hemorrhage in the aortic wall.

B, CT scan of the same patient after intravenous contrast. The thickening of the wall of the ascending aorta is still evident *(arrows)*, but it is no longer apparent that the hemorrhage is high in attenuation compared with the rest of the aortic wall.

Thoracic aortic aneurysms are the third category of life-threatening acquired aortic disease. These are discussed at length in Chapter 13. The aneurysms may be saccular (focal) or fusiform (long and tapered) but in general extend over a shorter segment of aorta than dissections (Figs. 12-21 and 12-22). Occasionally, an aneurysm with an intramural thrombus may appear similar to an area of dissection in which thrombosis of the false lumen has occurred. Mural thrombus within an aneurysm is usually concentrically distributed and, unlike thrombus within a dissection, it is seen on the inside of intimal calcifications.

☐ CARDIAC SILHOUETTE

Visual inspection of the cardiac silhouette starts with gauging its size. Most radiologists define an enlarged cardiac silhouette as one in which the cardiothoracic ratio exceeds 0.55. This ratio is determined by a measurement from the farthest left extent (the apex) to the farthest right extent of the cardiac shadow. (Note that these are not on the same horizontal plane. The most rightward point of the cardiac silhouette is usually slightly superior to the cardiac apex.) This distance is divided by the thoracic diameter as measured from inner rib to inner rib at the level of the top of the right hemidiaphragm. A common

mistake is to assume that enlargement of the cardiac silhouette is equivalent to cardiomegaly. Remember that pericardial disease is often indistinguishable from enlargement of the cardiac chambers on radiographs (Table 12-5).

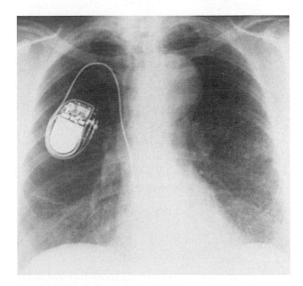

FIGURE 12-21 Posterior-anterior chest radiograph: aortic arch aneurysm without calcification of the wall. Frontal radiograph demonstrates hugely dilated aortic arch consistent with an aneurysm of the aorta. This aneurysm involved a shorter segment of the aorta than is usually involved by the dissection.

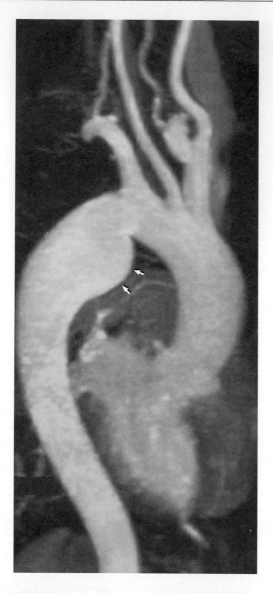

FIGURE 12-22 Magnetic resonance angiogram: aortic aneurysm. Magnetic resonance angiogram shows focal dilatation of the descending aorta *(arrows)* just distal to the takeoff of the left subclavian artery. In this location, saccular dilatation of the aorta may represent a true aneurysm or a post-traumatic false aneurysm. A false aneurysm forms when a traumatic aortic tear is contained by the intact portion of the aortic wall and surrounding tissues.

Less commonly, a mediastinal mass can also masquerade as cardiomegaly on frontal views. When this occurs, the cardiac silhouette appears to project lateral to the hilum (Fig. 12-23). This almost never happens in true cardiac enlargement.

After the size of the cardiac silhouette is gauged, its margins should be examined.

TABLE 12-5
Common Causes of Enlargement of the Cardiac Silhouette

Abnormal (left ventricular) preload
    Chronic volume overload (chronic renal failure)
    Aortic insufficiency
    Mitral insufficiency
Abnormal (left ventricular) contractility
    Dilated cardiomyopathy
    Ischemic cardiomyopathy
Cor pulmonale (severe)
Pericardial effusion

The superior vena cava begins in the area of the right first rib costochondral junction and descends to form the superior border of the right mediastinum (its shadow overlies that of the ascending aorta). The right atrium forms the inferior portion of the right cardiac border, starting below the intersection of the right main bronchus with the trachea (right tracheobronchial angle). The left subclavian artery forms the left superior mediastinal border. Below the subclavian artery, the left cardiac border is composed primarily of three structures. From superior to inferior, these structures are the aortic arch, the pulmonary trunk, and the left ventricle. The left atrial appendage forms only a very small part of the cardiac border of a normal heart and is situated between the pulmonary trunk and the left ventricle (Fig. 12-24). When enlarged, both pulmonary trunk and left atrial appendage can cause a focal bulge (or "mogul") along the left cardiac border. If the bulge is formed by the pulmonary trunk, at least part of its silhouette projects above the left main bronchus. If the bulge is caused by left atrial appendage enlargement, it lies below the bronchus.

On lateral radiographs, the right ventricle forms the anterior cardiac border, which abuts the lower sternum. More superiorly, the anterior border is formed by the pulmonary outflow tract and, above that, the ascending aorta. The posterior cardiac border is formed by the left ventricle near the diaphragm and by the left atrium beginning several centimeters higher (Fig. 12-25). A very small portion of the right atrium may also be seen posteriorly just above the diaphragm, at its junction with the inferior vena cava.

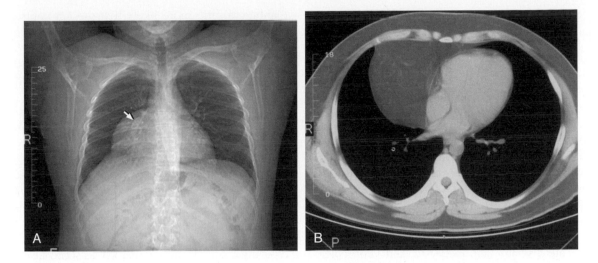

FIGURE 12-23 Posterior-anterior chest radiograph and computed tomography: apparent cardiac enlargement in a patient with a Morgagni hernia.

A, Frontal digital radiograph shows a soft tissue opacity that projects adjacent to the heart, causing the cardiac silhouette to appear globular. The pulmonary vessels are visible "within" this mass *(arrow)*. The mass, therefore, overlies but does not originate from the vascular hilum. This observation, termed the hilum overlay sign, indicates that the mass is unlikely to be cardiac in origin.

B, CT section shows large fat-containing mass adjacent to the heart. CT sections performed more caudally confirmed this mass to be a Morgagni hernia.

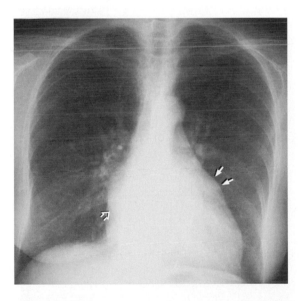

FIGURE 12-24 Posterior-anterior chest: mitral stenosis and insufficiency. The cardiac silhouette size is enlarged. The left cardiac border is straightened and there is a convex bump in the contour *(arrows)* caused by the enlarged left atrial appendage. The enlarged atria also caused a subtle double density overlying the right side of the cardiac silhouette *(open arrow)*.

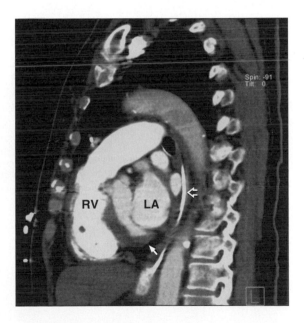

FIGURE 12-25 Sagittal computed tomography section through the heart: normal anatomy. CT section reconstructed in the sagittal plane, just to the left of the spine. The right ventricle (RV) is anterior against the sternum and is contiguous with the pulmonary artery exiting from its superior margin. The left atrium (LA) makes up the posterior portion of the heart, near the esophagus, which contains a nasogastric tube *(open arrow)*. Only a small amount of the left ventricle is seen *(solid arrow)*.

Left Ventricular Dilatation and Hypertrophy

When cardiac chamber enlargement causes an enlarged cardiac silhouette, it is most often the result of left ventricular dilatation. Left ventricular dilatation suggests that either left ventricular preload is increased or there is decreased contractility of the left ventricle. On the frontal views of the chest, the dilated left ventricle causes the apex of the cardiac silhouette to project more inferior and farther to the left than usual. While assessing left ventricular size, the clinician should also pay attention to the contour of the left ventricle. An abnormal contour could indicate a ventricular aneurysm. Left ventricular aneurysms are most common at the apex and in the anterior wall and are associated with high 5-year mortality. About half of the aneurysms detected by echocardiography or MRI are evident on chest radiographs (Fig. 12-26). Left ventricular size can also be assessed on lateral radiographs. The farther the cardiac silhouette extends back toward the spine and behind the inferior vena cava (seen where it crosses the diaphragm), the more likely that the left ventricle is enlarged. Rather than making specific measurements of the heart on a lateral view, it is probably best to use the observations here to support or refute one's impressions of left ventricular size on a frontal view (Fig. 12-27).

Left ventricular hypertrophy results in thickening of the ventricle wall (to over 1.1 cm). Often this occurs at the expense of the volume of the ventricular lumen, and unless hypertrophy is accompanied by dilatation the cardiac silhouette is not enlarged. Hypertrophy may be caused by a cardiomyopathy but more commonly is due to increased afterload (increased resistance to flow out from the left ventricle typically related to hypertension). In some cases, plain radiographs may also reveal dilatation of the ascending aorta and aortic arch. Although dilatation and increased convexity of the ascending aorta is commonly seen with normal aging, its presence in an adolescent or young adult raises the possibility of increased afterload (e.g., hypertension, aortic stenosis, coarctation) even if the overall size of the cardiac silhouette is normal.

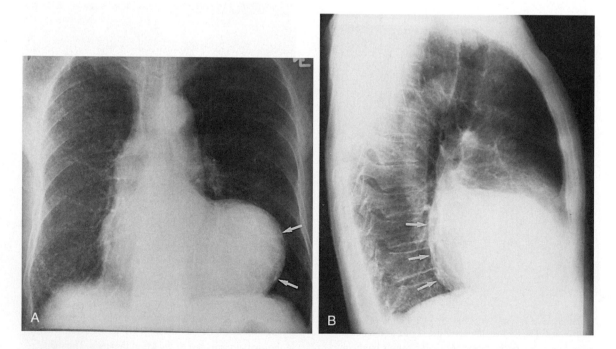

FIGURE 12-26 Posterior-anterior (PA) and lateral chest radiographs: left ventricular aneurysm.

A, On the PA film, the left ventricular apex has a squared off appearance, a large bulge extending laterally from the apex. A calcified rim *(arrows)* indicates that this is an area of old infarction with aneurysm formation. (Mural thrombus can also calcify.)

B, The lateral chest radiograph shows the cardiac silhouette to extend beyond the anterior margin of the vertebral body *(arrows),* indicating marked left ventricular dilatation. The aneurysm itself is located in the more anterior portion of the left ventricle.

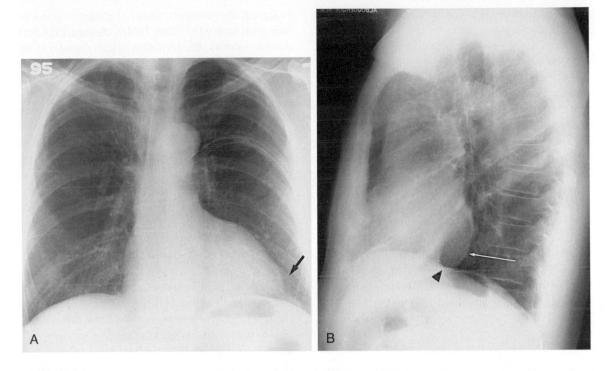

FIGURE 12-27 Posterior-anterior (PA) and lateral chest radiographs: left ventricular enlargement.

A, PA chest radiograph demonstrates a cardiac apex that is displaced laterally and downward *(arrow)*.

B, The lateral radiograph shows that the left ventricle projects well posterior to the inferior vena cava intercept with the diaphragm *(arrowhead)*, nearly as far posterior as the vertebral bodies *(arrow)*. Taken together, the findings in A and B suggest left ventricular enlargement.

Other adult cardiac diseases may also arise with normal heart size (Table 12-6). In other conditions such as severe COPD, hyperinflation of the lungs and depression of the diaphragms can cause an enlarged heart to appear of normal size on posterior-anterior (PA) views.

Right Heart Enlargement

Some cardiovascular radiologists hold that right atrial and right ventricular enlargement cannot

TABLE 12-6
Cardiac Disease without Enlargement of the Cardiac Silhouette

Aortic stenosis

Arterial hypertension

Hypertrophic cardiomyopathy

Acute myocardial infarction

Mitral stenosis

Restrictive cardiomyopathy

Constrictive pericarditis

be differentiated from each other on plain radiographs. Moreover, with most adult conditions, right atrium and right ventricle dilatation tend to coexist. (Exceptions such as Ebstein's anomaly are rare in adults.) As a result, it is practical to think of the radiographic findings discussed next as signs of generalized *right heart* enlargement.

Right heart enlargement may appear similar to left ventricular enlargement on a PA chest radiograph. Unless the right ventricle is massively dilated, it does not form any of the borders of the cardiac silhouette. Instead, it pushes the left ventricle farther laterally. Uplifting of the cardiac apex causing a boot-shaped heart is seen in childhood congenital heart disease, possibly because of dilatation of the ventricular inflow. It is almost never seen in adults with cor pulmonale. Other signs of right heart enlargement are increased convexity of the right cardiac silhouette, sometimes accompanied by upward displacement of the intersection between the right heart border and the superior vena cava (Fig. 12-8). These findings are apparent only in extreme cases. Rotation of the patient to the right accentuates right heart structures and can mimic these findings.

The lateral projection can help to confirm the presence of right heart enlargement. On the lateral view, the right ventricle is located anteriorly, where it makes contact with the inferior aspect of the sternum. Superior to the cardiac silhouette is a retrosternal clear space (which is normally about as opaque as the aerated lung behind the heart). Most textbooks state that if the anterior heart border makes contact with the sternum for greater than a third of its length, there is probably enlargement of the right ventricle, the right atrial appendage, or both (Fig. 12-28). The textbooks usually do not mention that this finding is dependent on the shape of the chest wall. For instance, in patients with obstructive lung disease and a barrel-shaped chest, only a truly gargantuan right ventricle can

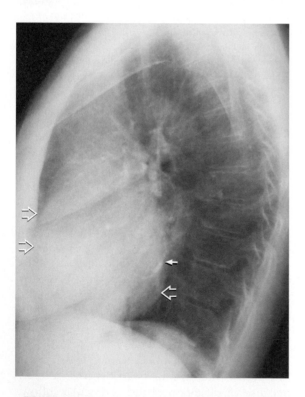

FIGURE 12-28 Lateral chest radiograph: mitral stenosis and mitral insufficiency with resulting pulmonary hypertension. The right ventricle is enlarged and in contact with about half of the sternum *(anterior open arrows)*. The left atrial wall is partially calcified *(arrow)* because of high left atrial pressures. Below the left atrium, a small portion of the left ventricular contour is seen *(posterior open arrow)*. The left ventricle is mildly dilated because of the effects of mitral insufficiency (see Fig. 12-25 for demonstration of anatomy).

creep up the sternum. In other patients, particularly patients who have had a sternotomy and cardiac bypass, the retrosternal clear space is no longer clear and the upper margin of the right ventricle is very difficult to identify with certainty.

Left Atrial Enlargement

Left atrial enlargement is typically the result of either left ventricular failure or primary mitral valvular disease. When left atrial enlargement is evident on the chest radiograph, it is useful to determine whether left ventricular enlargement is also present. Isolated mitral stenosis enlarges the left atrium but does not affect the left ventricle. The overall size of the cardiac silhouette is usually normal (unless pulmonary hypertension causes right heart enlargement). In contrast, hemodynamically significant mitral insufficiency causes both the left atrium and the left ventricle to dilate, the ventricle dilating in response to increased diastolic filling from regurgitant blood flow across the mitral valve. In diseases in which myocardial disease is the primary event (e.g., ischemic cardiomyopathy), dilatation of the left ventricle occurs first and results in dilatation of the mitral valve ring that causes secondary valve insufficiency. As with mitral insufficiency from primary valve disease, both the left atrium and ventricle are enlarged.

Although the cardiothoracic ratio may remain normal, many signs of left atrial enlargement are visible on plain radiographs. On a frontal view, left atrial enlargement can create a "double density" just inside the right heart border. Unfortunately, a similar shadow is also seen in some normal subjects. The sign is more specific for atrial enlargement if the distance from the midborder of the double density to the left main bronchus is greater than 7 cm (measured on frontal view). Elevation of the left main stem bronchus with an increase in the carinal angle (to greater than 80 degrees) is easier to see; however, the sensitivity and specificity of this sign are relatively low, about 60% (Fig. 12-29). Remember that left atrial enlargement is commonly accompanied by evidence of vascular redistribution caused by chronic elevation of left atrial pressure. In the setting of completely normal pulmonary vasculature, all of the radiographic signs discussed here should be reevaluated.

Enlargement of the left atrial appendage is more likely to occur with mitral stenosis than

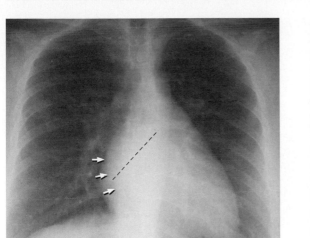

FIGURE 12-29 Posterior-anterior chest radiograph: mitral valve disease. The radiograph demonstrates straightening of the left heart border and splaying of the main carina caused by elevation of the left main stem bronchus. The carinal angle is almost 90 degrees. A double density is also seen along the right aspect of the cardiac silhouette *(arrows)*. A measurement of greater than 7 cm *(dashed line)* from the border of the double density (right wall of the left atrium) to the left main bronchus suggests left atrial enlargement.

with mitral regurgitation. As noted earlier, marked enlargement of the atrial appendage can cause a bulge along the left cardiac silhouette border. Lesser degrees of enlargement cause straightening of the cardiac silhouette. In day-to-day practice, however, a straightened left heart border is more likely to be due to left lower lobe atelectasis than an enlarged atrial appendage. Left lower lobe atelectasis causes the heart to rotate clockwise, shifting the pulmonary outflow tract to the left so that more of it contributes to the left cardiac silhouette. This finding is seen daily on radiographs of ICU patients.

☐ PERICARDIAL DISEASE

As mentioned previously, it is important to consider the possibility of pericardial effusion whenever there is enlargement of the cardiac silhouette. The classical "water bottle" shape of the cardiac silhouette is not specific to pericardial effusion and may be seen in dilated cardiomyopathies as well. On lateral radiographs, increased pericardial fluid or pericardial thickening can appear as a gray stripe separating

darker (more lucent) stripes caused by the retrosternal and epicardial fat. This sign is more specific for pericardial disease than is the shape of the cardiac silhouette and is sometimes called the "Oreo sign." Unfortunately, the "Oreo sign" is present on less than 15% of chest radiographs of patients with pericardial effusions (Fig. 12-30). The single best clue to the presence of a pericardial effusion may be a change in heart size, especially if there are not concurrent pulmonary vascular changes associated with congestive failure (Fig. 12-31). Although venous hypertension is notably absent in these patients, often the azygous vein is dilated because of increasing right atrial filling pressures.

Constrictive pericarditis is equally difficult to diagnose on chest radiographs. The cardiac shadow may be normal or minimally enlarged, and changes in appearance of the vasculature depend on the chronicity and severity of the disease. Pericardial calcifications may be present, but these are much easier to appreciate with CT than plain radiographs. On routine chest radiographs, the calcifications are usually seen best on the lateral image and appear overlying the right ventricle, in the interventricular groove, and in the atrioventricular groove (Fig. 12-32). Pericardial calcifications are most commonly

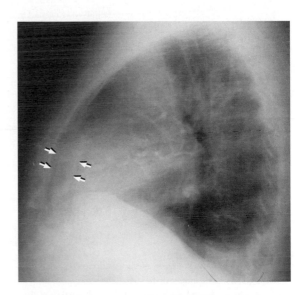

FIGURE 12-30 Lateral chest radiograph: pericardial effusion. The radiolucent (dark) pericardial fat stripe and epicardial fat stripe outline the pericardial space *(arrows)*. A large pericardial effusion is indicated by the wide separation of the pericardial fat from the epicardial fat. Unfortunately, this radiographic sign helps to diagnosis few cases of pericardial effusion.

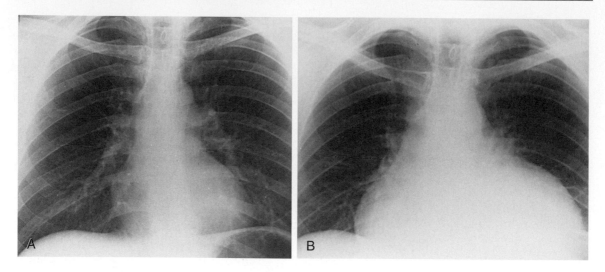

FIGURE 12-31 Serial chest radiographs: viral pericarditis.

A, Admission radiograph demonstrates a normal cardiomediastinal silhouette.

B, Follow-up radiograph taken 72 hours later shows marked increase in cardiac silhouette size. The rapid change in the silhouette without the development of abnormal pulmonary vasculature suggests acute pericardial effusion. This was confirmed by echocardiography.

caused by tuberculous pericarditis and therefore are less helpful in the diagnosis of constrictive pericarditis in countries where tuberculosis is well controlled. In addition, visually impressive pericardial calcification does not signify that the pericardial thickening impairs cardiac function. Significant hemodynamic changes of constriction may or may not be present.

Several different imaging techniques are useful for evaluation of pericardial disease when

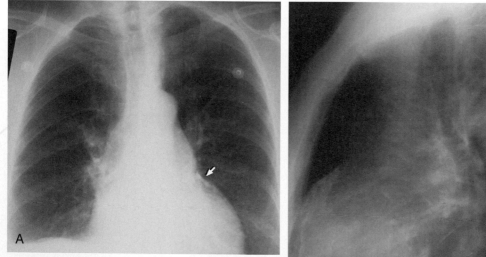

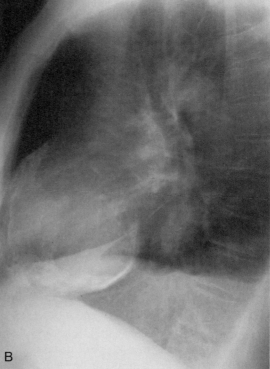

FIGURE 12-32 Posterior-anterior and lateral chest radiographs: pericardial calcifications.

A, On the frontal projection only a small portion of the pericardial calcifications is visible, seen best along the left border of the cardiac silhouette *(arrow)*.

B, On the lateral view curvilinear calcifications are easily seen. Calcifications extend along the anterior wall of the right ventricle under the inferior aspect of the heart and cover the posterior wall of the left ventricle.

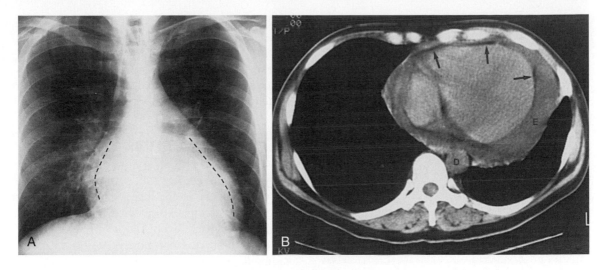

FIGURE 12-33 Posterior-anterior chest radiograph and contrast-enhanced computed tomography: pericardial effusion.

A, Chest view shows enlargement of the cardiac silhouette. There is a slightly radiolucent (darker) "halo" around the outer cardiac border *(dashed lines)* caused by effusion outside the more opaque heart muscle. Unfortunately, this radiographic sign is very difficult to detect.

B, Contrast-enhanced axial CT scan using mediastinal windows shows a moderate-sized pericardial effusion (E), separated from the heart by epicardial fat *(arrows)*. D, descending aorta.

it is suspected on the basis of radiographic or clinical findings. Echocardiography is usually the first imaging technique performed. It is very accurate in detecting pericardial effusion but is more limited in detecting pericardial thickening. CT and MRI are more sensitive than echocardiography in detecting pericardial thickening and are occasionally ordered for that purpose. More commonly, pericardial disease is seen on CT studies done for other reasons (e.g., staging of malignancy, evaluation of pleural effusion). On cross-sectional imaging with CT (or MRI), the normal pericardium is outlined by pericardial and epicardial fat. Average pericardial width is about 2 mm but increases to 4 mm near the diaphragm. If the soft tissue or fluid interposed between the two fat planes is greater than these measurements, pericardial thickening or pericardial fluid is present (Fig. 12-33).

Single-detector spiral CT imaging can detect the presence of pericardial thickening, calcifications, or fluid but is not as accurate as echocardiography or MRI in determining whether pericardial disease impairs cardiac function. In some cases, static CT images can detect evidence that ventricular filling is impaired, such as enlargement of the atria and dilatation of the inferior vena cava and hepatic veins caused by elevated right atrial pressures (Fig. 12-34).

MRI is more accurate than CT at differentiating pericardial thickening from pericardial fluid (Fig. 12-35). MRI is also able to perform dynamic imaging of the heart that can detect abnormalities in chamber wall motion during the cardiac cycle. These abnormalities in wall motion,

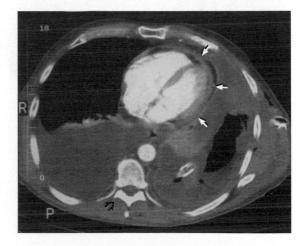

FIGURE 12-34 Contrast-enhanced computed tomography: constrictive pericarditis. The pericardium is diffusely thickened *(arrows)* and obliterates the epicardial fat adjacent to the left ventricle. The ventricles are small and tubular, suggesting pericardial constriction. (Bilateral pleural effusions and a left-sided chest tube are also present.)

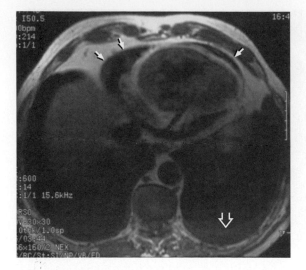

FIGURE 12-35 Magnetic resonance imaging: pericardial effusion. Section from an MRI study performed with cardiac gating and a "black blood" technique. Imaged with this MRI technique, moving fluid does not emit measurable radiofrequency signal and therefore appears black. Pericardial fluid appears black because it moves with cardiac pulsation *(arrows)*. The small amount of pleural fluid that is present moved little during the scan. It therefore produces some signal and appears gray *(open arrow)*.

such as right ventricular (outflow tract) collapse during diastole, are signs that the pericardial disease is causing hemodynamic compromise. Unlike CT, MRI cannot detect pericardial calcifications, but this is usually not an important limitation (see earlier).

☐ CARDIAC VALVES

Analysis of the cardiac silhouette should include an examination of the cardiac valve areas for postsurgical changes or calcifications (Fig. 12-36). Prosthetic valves, even bioprostheses, usually have a radiopaque component visible on chest radiographs. Sometimes, instead of a prosthetic valve, a radiopaque annuloplasty ring is used to constrict a dilated valve ring and the valve itself is not replaced. On portable radiographs, valve prosthesis and annuloplasty rings can be difficult to see because of poor penetration of the mediastinum by x-rays and blurring from motion during the long exposure time.

Mitral and aortic valves are the most common sites of prosthetic valves. On frontal projection, the aortic valve is located at the base of the

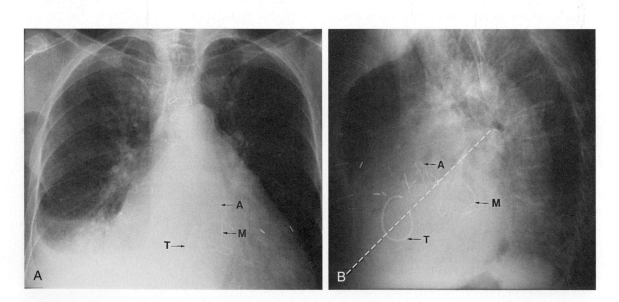

FIGURE 12-36 Posterior-anterior and lateral chest examination: three prosthetic valves.

A, Frontal radiograph demonstrates three valves: aortic (A), mitral (M), and tricuspid (T). There is also generalized cardiomegaly with vascular cephalization and a right pleural effusion.

B, Lateral radiograph demonstrates the valves and relative size of each (see text). The line from the hila to the anterior costophrenic angle transects the tricuspid valve plane. The aortic valve projects anterior and superior to this line and the mitral valve posterior and inferior to it.

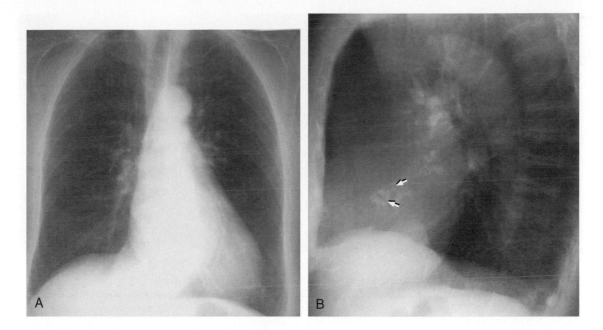

FIGURE 12-37 Posterior-anterior and lateral chest radiographs: aortic stenosis.

A, Frontal projection shows the overall cardiac silhouette to be within normal limits but the cardiac apex to be displaced downward, suggesting mild left ventricular enlargement.

B, Lateral projection shows thick amorphous calcifications in the area of the aortic valve *(arrows)*. Aortic valvular calcification that is visible on a chest radiograph is associated with a significant pressure gradient across the valve.

ascending aortic shadow in the upper middle third of the cardiac silhouette. Frequently it overlies the spine. The mitral valve usually lies to the left of the spine, often below a line drawn from the left hilum to the right cardiophrenic angle. On the lateral projection, the aortic valve lies above a line drawn from the carina to the anterior costophrenic angle. The mitral valve is located below this line.

These anatomic points can be useful in identifying valvular calcifications as well. Calcifications of the aortic valve are best seen on the lateral view because they are often obscured by the spine on the PA radiograph (Fig. 12-37). If aortic calcifications are visible on plain radiographs, aortic stenosis is almost certainly present and it is likely to be hemodynamically significant. Aortic calcifications seen in patients in their 40s and 50s most likely have formed on a bicuspid aortic valve. Calcifications seen in older patients are more opaque and clump-like on chest radiographs and usually represent senile aortic stenosis. Aortic calcifications are also readily seen on CT imaging. The amount of calcium within the valve as measured by (cardiac-gated) multidetector CT predicts the severity of the stenosis (Fig. 12-38).

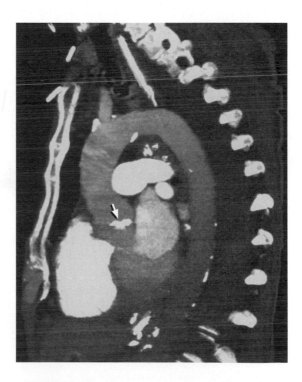

FIGURE 12-38 Contrast-enhanced computed tomography sagittal reconstruction: aortic valve calcifications. Sagittal CT image shows dense calcifications in the area of the aortic valve *(arrow)*. Large amounts of valvular calcification suggest hemodynamically significant aortic stenosis.

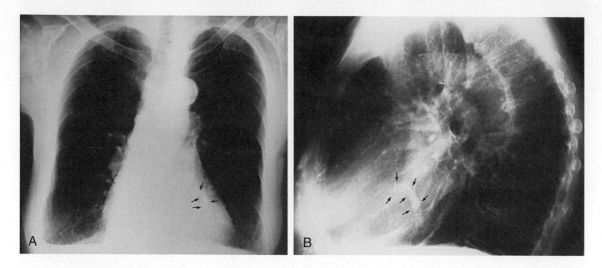

FIGURE 12-39 Posterior-anterior and lateral chest radiographs: mitral valve/annulus calcification.

A, Frontal radiograph demonstrates an area of thick linear calcification peripherally over the left aspect of the cardiac silhouette *(arrows)*.

B, Lateral film with thick curvilinear calcification of the mitral annulus *(arrows)*.

Mitral valve calcifications are seen much less commonly than aortic valve calcifications. Mitral annulus calcification, however, is relatively common. Annulus calcification is typically very opaque and often forms a reverse C shape. It is seen in elderly people and is usually not physiologically significant (Fig. 12-39).

In patients with prosthetic valves, assessing the valve diameter on chest radiographs can help determine which valve has been replaced. Valve orifice size is inversely proportional to the driving pressure across that valve. Therefore, the prosthetic valves can roughly be ranked from the smallest to the largest size: aortic, pulmonic, mitral, and tricuspid.

The specific radiographic appearances of the different brands of prosthetic valves or annuloplasty rings are of interest primarily to specialists. For the most part, patients with prosthetic heart valves and annuloplasty rings can safely be placed in an MRI scanner (with magnetic field strength up to 1.5 tesla) for diagnostic imaging. Although some types of valves or rings may also be affected by the magnetic field, the force placed on the prosthesis is generally less than that applied by the normal beating of the heart muscle.

☐ CORONARY ARTERY CALCIFICATIONS

Coronary artery calcifications can occasionally be seen on the PA view where they overlie the left atrial appendage. Usually, the calcifications are seen more clearly on the lateral radiograph (Fig. 12-40). Coronary artery calcifications can appear as lines, or "tram tracks," most commonly in the area of the left anterior descending coronary artery.

Coronary calcifications are much more easily seen with CT than with routine radiographs. Over the past several years there has been intense interest in using CT scanning as a screening test for coronary artery disease. We now understand that acute cardiac events (e.g., unstable angina, myocardial infarction, coronary death) are probably caused by the rupture of the fibrous portion of a "vulnerable," usually noncalcified, plaque. Often these areas of plaque rupture are found at sites free of high-grade (>75% narrowing) stenosis. The quantity of coronary artery calcification correlates with the total plaque burden in the heart but does not specifically identify vulnerable plaque.

Coronary calcifications therefore indicate that coronary disease is definitely present but do not identify impending myocardial infarction. The calcifications are best viewed as a long-term risk factor for myocardial infarction or death from coronary disease, similar to diabetes and hypertension. Coronary calcifications are quantified in terms of calcium mass (in milligrams) or an Agatston score, a calculation based on the cross-sectional area of the calcifications and their HU values on axial CT slices (Fig. 12-41). In general, Agatston scores above 300 are associated with double the risk for

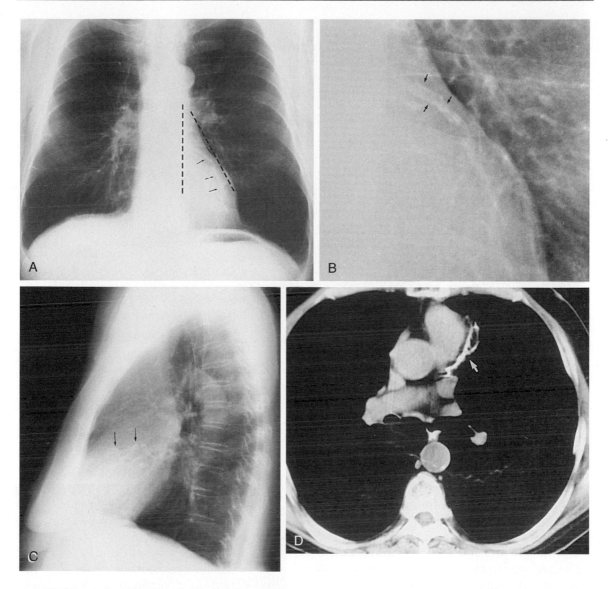

FIGURE 12-40 Posterior-anterior and lateral chest radiographs and computed tomography: coronary artery calcifications.

A, The frontal radiograph demonstrates prominent coronary artery calcifications *(arrows)* of the left anterior descending artery, within the coronary artery triangle *(dashed lines)*.

B, Detail from A shows coronary calcifications more clearly *(arrows)*.

C, A lateral radiograph demonstrates calcified vessels with a tram track appearance. Calcification extending anteriorly *(arrows)* is probably within the left anterior descending artery.

D, Routine CT section showing coronary artery calcification *(arrow)* of the left anterior descending artery.

nonfatal myocardial infarction or coronary death over the next several years. The complete absence of coronary artery calcification predicts a low likelihood (usually less than 5%) of either.

Although coronary artery calcifications are commonly seen on standard CT of the chest, there is enough motion artifact that it is difficult to quantify their extent. Accordingly, CT techniques used for quantification of coronary artery calcium have employed technology able to obtain CT sections through the heart very quickly.

These methods include electron beam CT scanners that obtain each cross section in 50 milliseconds and, much more commonly, multidetector CT scanners. These scanners use the ECG signal to guide data processing so that each cross section is constructed with data obtained during diastole, usually over 250 milliseconds or less. The newest generation CT scanners with 16 to 64 detectors are able to image extremely rapidly and still create very thin sections, allowing them to perform coronary artery angiography.

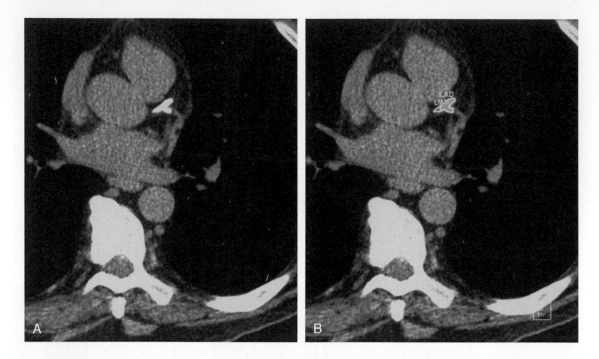

FIGURE 12-41 Non–contrast-enhanced multidetector computed tomography sections: coronary artery calcifications.

A, Axial CT shows dense calcifications in the left anterior descending coronary artery.

B, Same image as in A with computer-generated measurement of the area of calcification to be used in calculation of the Agatston score for quantification of the calcifications.

These CT angiograms can reliably visualize the proximal portions of the coronary vasculature (Fig. 12-42). The most effective use of CT coronary angiography is yet to be worked out, but the technique will probably be most useful in excluding significant disease in patients with relatively low pretest probabilities.

☐ CATHETERS AND ELECTRODES

As part of the radiographic evaluation of the cardiovascular system, it is important to examine all intravascular catheters and pacemaker electrodes for malpositions and other abnormalities. This is especially true immediately after cardiac surgery. In addition to intravascular catheters, endotracheal, pleural, and mediastinal tubes are placed. These frequently overlap and sometimes produce confusing shadows (Fig. 12-43).

Venous Catheters

Central venous lines are best positioned in the distal 2.5 cm of the brachiocephalic veins or in

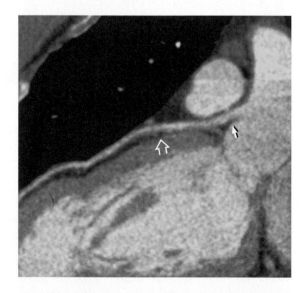

FIGURE 12-42 Reconstructed image from contrast-enhanced computed tomography: left coronary artery. Image constructed from data obtained with a multidetector CT scanner shows the course of the left main (arrow) and left anterior descending coronary artery (open arrow). Imaging was performed with simultaneous electrocardiographic tracing so that only the data acquired during diastole were used to make this image, minimizing motion artifact.

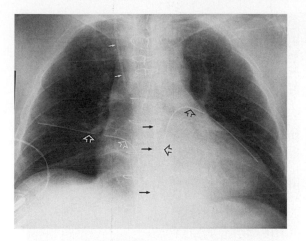

FIGURE 12-43 Anterior-posterior chest radiograph: status shortly after cardiac bypass grafting. Lines and tubes include central venous pressure catheter *(white arrows)*, pleural tubes *(open arrows)*, and mediastinal drain *(black arrows)*. (Nasogastric and endotracheal tubes are not labeled.)

the superior vena cava to avoid venous valves. On plain radiographs, the tip of the central venous pressure line should then lie medial or inferior to the anterior portion of the first right rib. Placement of the catheter tip in the right atrium (usually below the third costochondral junction) may increase the risk of atrial thrombus formation and the risk of arrhythmias. Tunneled dialysis catheters, however, are sometimes placed with their distal ports in the atrium in order to maintain adequate blood flow.

Many possible catheter malpositions can and do occur. It is easy to recognize some common malpositions, such as retrograde cannulation of the internal jugular vein from the subclavian vein. Other malpositions are more subtle and often require a lateral view to diagnose (Table 12-7). These can represent cannulation of smaller venous tributaries, including the azygous venous system,

and may result in catheter occlusion or venous thrombosis (Fig. 12-44). Venous anomalies can also be responsible for unusual catheter configurations. Duplicated or left-sided superior vena cavae are the most common of these anomalies, occurring in about 0.5% of the population (Fig. 12-45). Although a left-sided superior vena cava can account for the location of the tip of the central venous pressure line on the left side of the mediastinum, this can also be due to accidental arterial cannulation. The latter is more common (Fig. 12-46).

Malposition of a pulmonary artery catheter (e.g., Swan-Ganz) is also common. The tip of this catheter is optimally placed in the central right or left pulmonary artery, no farther distal than about 2 cm lateral to the hilum. More distal placement of the catheter tip often occurs within 24 to 48 hours after placement as the intracardiac loop of the catheter tightens. Distal placement increases the risk of catheter-induced thrombosis and pulmonary infarction (Fig. 12-47).

Intra-Aortic Balloon Pumps and Pacemakers

Intra-aortic balloon pumps are frequently used to support unstable cardiac patients. The intravascular balloons require careful placement to avoid major complications. On radiographs, a cylindrical radiopaque marker is visible at the catheter tip, and the balloon itself may be seen if the radiograph is taken during diastole when the balloon is filled with carbon dioxide (Fig. 12-48). The catheter tip is meant to lie just distal to the origin of the left subclavian artery, in the proximal descending aorta. More proximal placement can result in left common carotid occlusion and stroke, and more distal placement decreases the efficiency of the balloon and

TABLE 12-7
Possible Venous Catheter Malpositions

Location of Catheter Tip	Position on Posterior-Anterior View	Position on Lateral View
Azygous vein	Above junction of trachea and right main bronchus	At or posterior to trachea
Pericardiophrenic vein	Left side of mediastinum	Far anterior under sternum
Left internal mammary vein	Left side of mediastinum	Far anterior under sternum
Right internal mammary vein	Normal or deviates to right	Far anterior under sternum
Aorta	Deviates to left of superior vena cava	Ascending or descending aorta

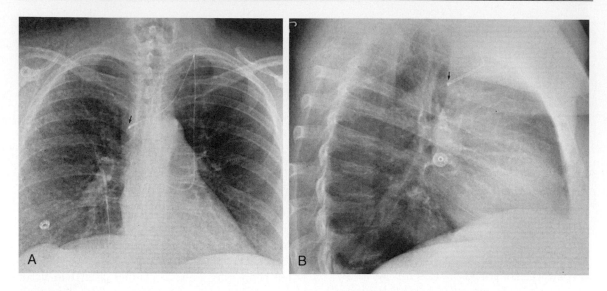

FIGURE 12-44 Posterior-anterior and lateral chest radiographs: central venous pressure catheter with tip near junction of the azygous vein and vena cava.

A, Frontal radiograph shows a central venous pressure catheter that appears foreshortened *(arrow)*.

B, Lateral chest radiograph shows the tip of the catheter to curve in a posterior direction. This is the normal course of the left brachiocephalic vein as it travels in front of the other mediastinal blood vessels and then turns back toward the spine to enter the superior vena cava. The catheter is not likely to be within the azygous vein unless the tip overlies the trachea or projects posterior to it on lateral view.

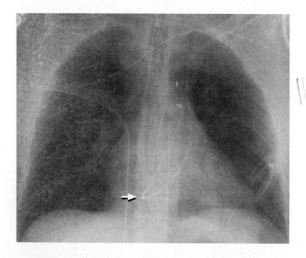

FIGURE 12-45 PA chest left superior vena cava. Radiograph taken after cardiac surgery shows a Swan-Ganz catheter descending on the left side of the mediastinum via the left superior vena cava. The catheter enters the right atrium *(arrow)* via the coronary sinus and then travels upward passing through the tricuspid valve and right ventricle outflow tract.

risks intra-abdominal ischemia from occlusion of visceral vessels.

Pacemaker electrode placement can also be assessed on plain chest radiographs. The distal ends of right atrial leads are usually J shaped to facilitate placement in the right atrium. The ventricular electrode of the pacemaker should lie in the right ventricular apex. This is seen slightly to the left of midline on PA or AP views. On the lateral view, the tip should lie in the anterior-inferior aspect of the cardiac silhouette, 3 to 4 mm behind the epicardial fat line (Fig. 12-49). If malpositioned, an electrode tip can perforate the myocardium. In the past, lead placement in the coronary sinus also represented lead malposition. Current pacing systems that provide biventricular pacing do so by using a third lead purposely placed through the coronary sinus into one of the cardiac veins. On PA projection the coronary sinus electrode appears to be in the right ventricle or pulmonary outflow tract but is seen to be far posterior on lateral radiograph (Fig. 12-50). Electrode lead breakage is now uncommon but can occur at the connection of the electrodes to the generator, within a loop, or as the electrode passes between the clavicle and first rib.

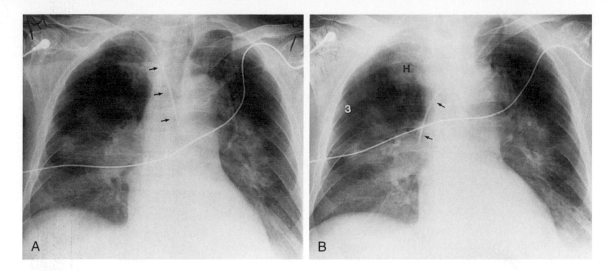

FIGURE 12-46 Serial posterior-anterior (PA) chest radiographs: central venous pressure catheter tip in ascending segment of the aortic arch and normal superior vena cava position.

A, PA chest radiograph demonstrates the central venous pressure catheter heading to the left side of the mediastinum *(arrows)*. The catheter initially enters the right subclavian artery, then proceeds through the brachiocephalic artery and into the ascending segment of the arch.

B, Follow-up radiograph after reinsertion of the catheter into the normal location, the proximal superior vena cava. This catheter has been placed through the internal jugular vein into the superior vena cava. Normal position should be between the first and third costochondral junction (anterior ribs). H marks a hematoma from initial attempt at catheter placement (see part A).

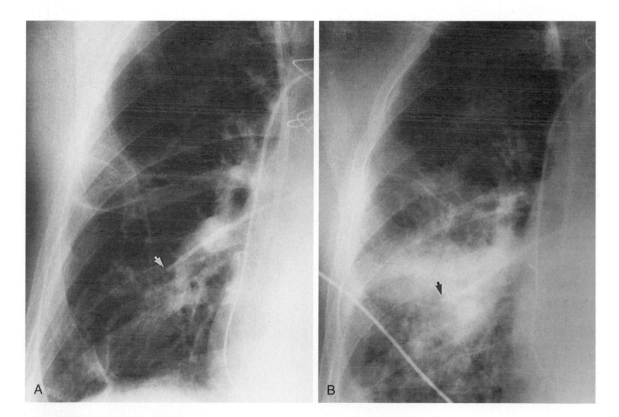

FIGURE 12-47 Serial close-up posterior-anterior (PA) chest radiographs: distal Swan-Ganz catheter placement with subsequent infarction.

A, PA chest radiograph taken to document the initial position of the Swan-Ganz catheter demonstrates the position of the tip *(arrow)*, within the right lower lobe artery.

B, Follow-up film at 24 hours demonstrates the slightly more distal position of the catheter *(arrow)*. There is an ill-defined wedge-shaped region of air space disease centered around the catheter tip, representing an infarction.

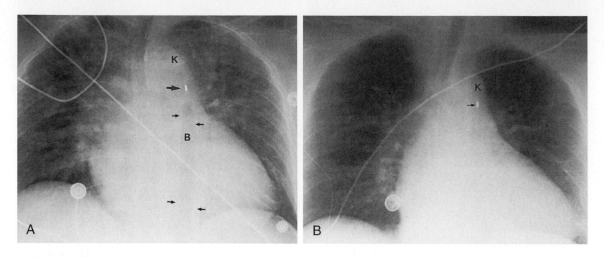

<u>FIGURE 12-48</u> Serial chest examinations: intra-aortic balloon pump—inflated and deflated.

A, The intra-aortic balloon pump is inflated (*small arrows*) during diastole. The tip of the catheter is positioned in the proximal descending thoracic aorta indicated by the radiodense tip *(large arrow)*. B, balloon; K, aortic knob.

B, Same patient demonstrating collapsed intra-aortic balloon pump during systole. The position of the catheter tip is maintained.

Implantable cardioverter defibrillators differ from standard pacemakers in appearance. Usually two parts of the defibrillator electrode appear thicker than the rest of the lead, one within the superior vena cava, the other within the right ventricle. These thicker areas are in fact shock coils, used to dissipate heat from high-voltage discharges. Implantable cardioverter defibrillators are often combined with univentricular or biventricular pacemakers (Fig. 12-51).

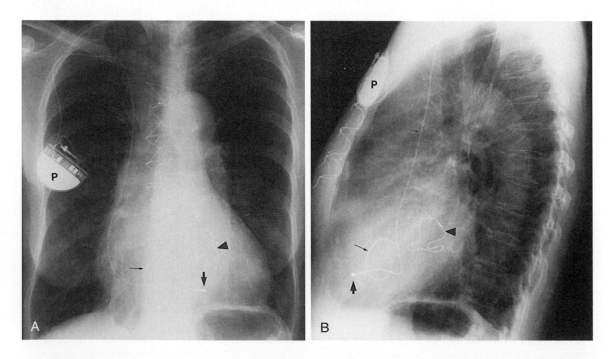

<u>FIGURE 12-49</u> Anterior-posterior (AP) and lateral chest radiographs: normal appearance and position of cardiac right ventricular pacemaker. AP (A) and lateral (B) views of the chest show the tip *(large arrow)* of the pacemaker wire to the left of midline, having crossed through the superior vena cava, right atrium, and tricuspid annuloplasty ring into the anterior portion of the right ventricle. P, pacemaker; *arrowhead*, mitral valve bioprosthesis; *small arrow*, tricuspid annuloplasty ring.

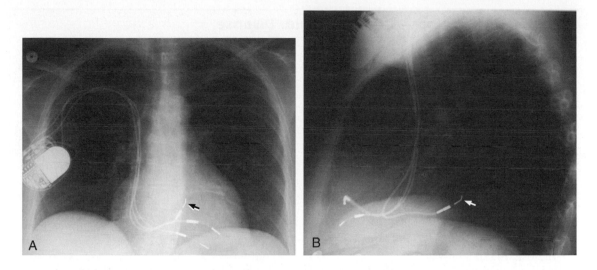

FIGURE 12-50 Posterior-anterior and lateral chest radiographs: biventricular pacemaker.

A, Frontal projection shows two right ventricular electrodes and a third electrode that is placed slightly more cephalad *(black arrow)*.

B, Lateral projection shows that one electrode *(arrow)* is positioned along the posterior aspect of the heart, consistent with location within the coronary sinus/cardiac venous system.

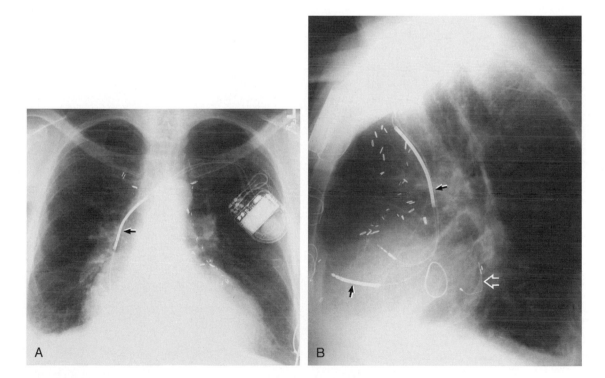

FIGURE 12-51 Posterior-anterior and lateral radiographs: implanted cardioverter defibrillator and atrial biventricular pacemaker.

A, Frontal projection shows the proximal shock coil *(arrow)* of the cardioverter defibrillator. The cardiac silhouette is enlarged and there are signs of mild congestive heart failure.

B, Lateral projection demonstrates proximal and distal shock coils *(arrows)*, atrial pacing lead, mitral valve prosthesis, and electrode within a cardiac vein for left ventricular pacing *(open arrow)*.

Pearls for Clinicians—Cardiovascular Disease

1. The cardiothoracic ratio is a rough estimate of cardiac size and can be altered easily with changes in the patient's position and inspiration. Obtain an upright inspiratory radiograph whenever possible and rely on changes in vascular redistribution, interstitial edema, and the width of the vascular pedicle for assessing changes in the patient's intravascular volume status.

2. Left atrial and left ventricular enlargements have characteristic findings on chest radiographs and can be useful in reaching a diagnosis. For instance, left atrial enlargement without left ventricular enlargement suggests mitral stenosis.

3. Right ventricular and right atrial enlargements are difficult to confirm on the basis of the cardiac silhouette but are rarely present if the central pulmonary arteries are normal in size. If the frontal radiograph shows the convex opacity of the main pulmonary artery/pulmonary outflow tract to be larger than the aortic arch, pulmonary hypertension and right heart enlargement are very likely.

4. Spiral CT of the aorta, particularly with multidetector scanners, is very sensitive for both traumatic and nontraumatic aortic disease (e.g., dissections). Angiography rarely alters the diagnosis after a good-quality CT scan has been performed.

5. Static CT and MR images are very sensitive in detecting pericardial thickening or pericardial fluid but can detect constriction or tamponade only if there are secondary signs. Dynamic MR techniques (showing cardiac wall and blood motion), echocardiography, or cardiac catheterization is needed to determine whether there is physiologic impairment.

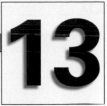

Hilum and Mediastinum

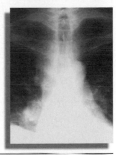

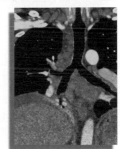

□ HILAR ANATOMY

Analyzing the hila on plain radiographs is the most challenging task in chest radiology, made difficult by the large degree of variability between individuals. Fortunately, there are a few helpful anatomic landmarks. (See figures in Chapter 1.)

The right pulmonary artery first becomes visible on plain radiographs when it emerges from the pericardium. At that point, it has already bifurcated into a right upper lobe branch and a branch to the right middle and lower lobes (right interlobar or descending pulmonary artery). The right interlobar artery descends lateral to the intermediate bronchus and forms most of the inferior aspect of the right hilum.

Most of the superior portion of the right hilum is formed by the superior pulmonary vein. The vein lies just medial to the upper lobe artery and becomes larger and more easily seen in patients with congestive heart failure. The superior pulmonary vein and the interlobar artery intersect at the hilum (Fig. 13-1). The angle formed between these two vessels is sometimes called the hilar angle. It appears as a shallow "V" turned on its side.

Hilar pathology can blunt the apex of that angle (see later discussion). On lateral radiographs, the bulk of the right hilar arterial vessels project anterior to the airway. The proximal right interlobar pulmonary artery combines with portions of the right upper lobe veins to form an oval opacity about the size of one's thumb distal to its last joint. This is a good anatomic landmark but not the best place to assess the size of central pulmonary arteries because the opacity is formed by overlying shadows of both arteries and veins.

The left pulmonary artery exits the pericardium undivided and therefore appears slightly larger than the right. The left pulmonary artery then passes *over* the left upper lobe bronchus (seen end on as a black circle on lateral projection). Descending, it follows the left lower lobe bronchus posterolaterally. This course accounts for the left hilum being higher than the right. On lateral views of the chest, it also gives the left pulmonary artery the appearance

233

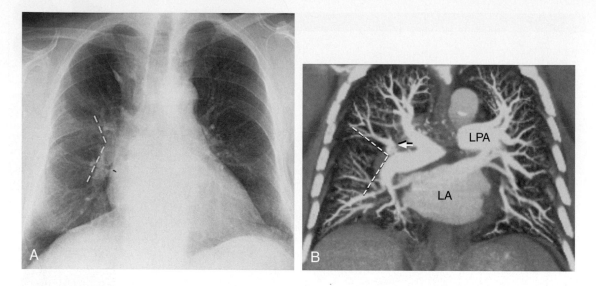

FIGURE 13-1 Posterior-anterior chest radiograph and computed tomography coronal reconstruction: outline of hilar angle.

A, The right superior pulmonary vein and right interlobar pulmonary artery cross, forming a shallow V *(dashed lines)*, sometimes called the hilar angle. Masses or lymphadenopathy can blunt the apex of the V. Pulmonary edema can blur its outline.

B, CT image from a different patient than in A, reconstructed in the coronal plane, shows the right upper lobe and descending pulmonary arteries converging. The right superior pulmonary vein is situated just below the upper lobe pulmonary artery *(arrow)* and therefore makes up the upper border of the V actually seen on frontal radiographs *(dashed lines)*. Note that the upper lobe arteries on the left originate directly from the left main pulmonary artery (LPA) instead of arising from a main upper lobe branch, making the hilar V less well defined. LA, left atrium.

of a mini-arch, located just beneath the actual aortic arch (Fig. 13-2).

The left superior pulmonary vein and the inferior veins do not contribute much to the hilar contours on frontal radiographs. The left superior pulmonary vein is usually superimposed on the shadow of the left pulmonary artery or mediastinal fat. Both right and left lower lobe pulmonary veins run horizontally and enter the left atria at the inferior margin of the hilum. They are best seen posteroinferiorly to the hilum on the lateral views of the chest. It is important to recognize the course of these vessels because they cause ill-defined opacities that novices sometimes confuse for lower lobe pneumonias on lateral radiographs. On occasion the confluence of the inferior pulmonary veins, seen end on, can be mistaken for a nodule.

☐ HILAR ABNORMALITIES

Using these landmarks, there are two steps in evaluating the hila. The first step is to determine whether the hila appear abnormal. If the hila

are abnormal, the second step is to determine whether the abnormality is caused by vascular structures or is due to other tissue, such as enlarged lymph nodes. Distinguishing vascular structures from pathologic adenopathy is a common problem, especially in patients with chronic obstructive pulmonary disease. These patients often have enlarged central pulmonary arteries as a result of pulmonary hypertension but are also at increased risk for having enlarged hilar lymph nodes from metastatic bronchogenic carcinoma.

The hila appear abnormal if they are abnormally opaque, abnormally large or small, or have an abnormal contour. The evaluation of hilar opacity is subjective. It is helpful to compare the degree of opacity of one hilum with the other. Better yet, prior radiographs should be examined to determine whether there has been a change.

The hilar size appears abnormal if the hila are both too small, too large, or markedly asymmetric in size. Small hila are usually caused by vascular abnormalities. It is uncommon for both hila to be small, but the finding can be

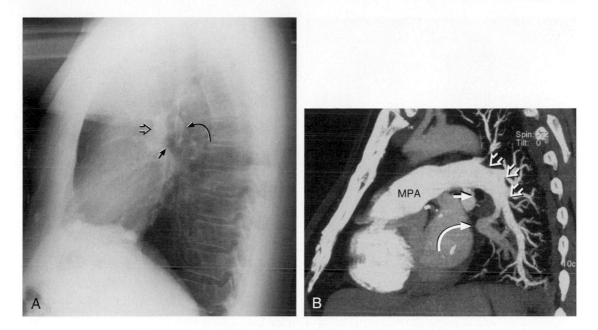

FIGURE 13-2 Lateral chest radiograph and computed tomography sagittal reconstruction: identification of right and left pulmonary arteries and inferior pulmonary veins.

A, On the lateral chest view, left upper lobe bronchus is seen end on projecting below the lower tracheal air column *(arrow)*. The right and left interlobar pulmonary arteries form opacities anterior and posterior to the bronchi, respectively *(open arrow and curved solid arrow)*.

B, CT image from a different patient than in A, reconstructed in the sagittal plane, performed to the left of midline. Image shows the left pulmonary artery originating from the main pulmonary artery (MPA). The lower lobe artery *(open arrows)* arches posteriorly over the left upper lobe bronchus *(solid arrow)*. Pulmonary veins are seen end on *(curved arrow)*.

associated with diminished pulmonary vascularity in pediatric patients with cyanotic heart disease. Congenital hypoplasia of a pulmonary artery and Swyer-James syndrome may give rise to a unilaterally small hilum. (In Swyer-James syndrome bronchiolitis causes unilateral air trapping that results in decreased blood flow to one lung; see Chapter 4.)

Modest asymmetry in hilar size is normal and can be accentuated if the patient is rotated when the film is taken. Marked asymmetry, or increasing size of one hilum, is usually caused by a mass or adenopathy rather than a vascular abnormality. Rare vascular abnormalities such as pulmonary artery aneurysm and pulmonary valvular stenosis (with poststenotic pulmonary artery dilatation) can also cause unilateral enlargement.

Both adenopathy (see later discussion of sarcoid) and dilatation of the central pulmonary arteries from pulmonary hypertension are common causes of bilateral hilar enlargement. Often, when the central pulmonary arteries are enlarged enough to appear mass-like, the pulmonary outflow tract/main pulmonary artery also appears enlarged on the frontal radiograph (see Fig. 12-9).

When the hilar contour is normal, the pulmonary veins and arteries converge, forming the hilar angle just lateral to the cardiomediastinal border. If an enlarged hilum is caused by a dilated central pulmonary artery, the vessels are pushed laterally but still converge at or lateral to the margin of the widened cardiomediastinal silhouette (Fig. 13-3).

If a nonvascular mass causes hilar enlargement, the pulmonary vessels are not displaced laterally and can converge medial to the margin of the mass. Nonvascular hilar masses may also blunt the apex of the hilar angle. They form convex shadows with more sharply curving borders (shorter arcs) than those formed by pulmonary vasculature (Fig. 13-4).

The contours of nonvascular masses caused by adenopathy also appear different from pulmonary vasculature on a lateral view. Extensive hilar adenopathy produces lobulated opacities

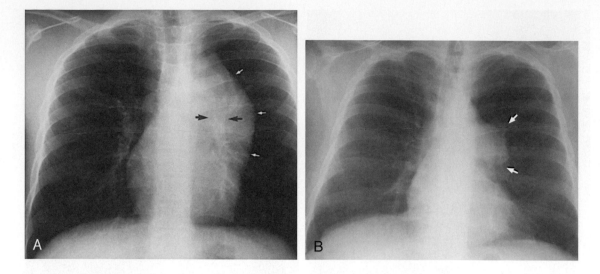

FIGURE 13-3 Posterior-anterior chest radiographs: hilar overlay sign and hilar convergence sign.

A, The left hilar vessels *(black arrows)* converge medial to the border of mass *(white arrows)*. They are easily visible through the mass, indicating that the mass overlies the hilum but is not part of it (hilar overlay sign).

B, Left hilar mass representing an enlarged main and left pulmonary artery, both caused by pulmonic valve stenosis. Pulmonary artery branches are visible up the margin of the mass where they converge *(arrows)*. Vessels are not visible medial to the mass. This is termed the hilar convergence sign. The sign confirms that the mass is in the hilum and suggests it is of vascular origin.

that appear to encircle the central bronchi, sometimes called a hilar "rosette" (Fig. 13-5). On lateral radiographs, enlarged pulmonary arteries do not project around the entire circumference of the central bronchi but instead spare the inferior-posterior portion of the apparent ring.

Although the position of the hila does not help distinguish vascular shadows from masses, changes in the relative height of the two hila can be an important sign of other chest pathology. Specifically, abnormalities in hilar position can be caused by parenchymal volume loss (see Chapter 5). The left hilum is nearly always

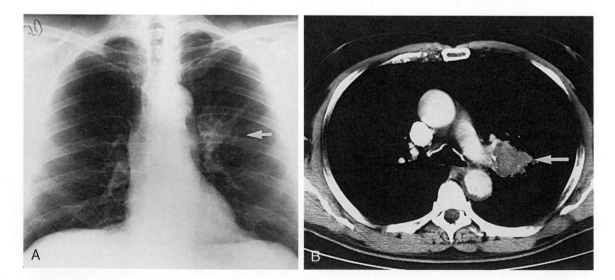

FIGURE 13-4 Posterior-anterior chest radiographs and computed tomography: bronchogenic carcinoma with left hilar mass.

A, This frontal radiograph demonstrates a convex (outward) left hilar opacity adjacent to the hilar vasculature *(arrow)*. The curve of its margin has a shorter arc and a different orientation than the usual vascular shadows. Note also that the inferior pulmonary vessels enter the hilum medial to the (nonvascular) mass.

B, Contrast-enhanced CT shows a low-density left hilar mass *(arrow)* adjacent to the pulmonary artery.

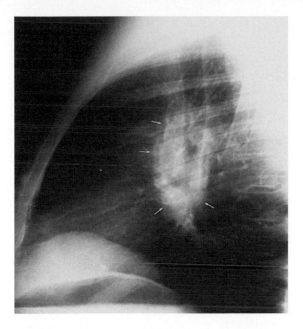

FIGURE 13-5 Lateral chest radiograph: sarcoidosis with hilar adenopathy. The lateral radiograph of a patient with stage 1 sarcoidosis demonstrates marked hilar lymphadenopathy. The central airways appear to be encased by paratracheal, hilar, and subcarinal lymph nodes.

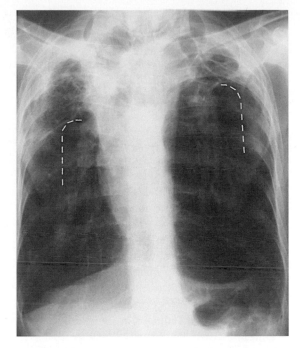

FIGURE 13-6 Posterior-anterior chest radiograph: bilateral hilar retraction–waterfall sign. This study demonstrates cephalad retraction of both hila and parenchymal fibrosis associated with an old tuberculosis infection. The loss in lung volume elongates the lower lobe pulmonary arteries and causes them to course more vertically than usual. This produces the waterfall sign *(dashed lines)*.

higher than the right. If the right is higher than the left or if the left is more than 3 cm above the right, volume loss should be suspected. Volume loss in the upper lobe elevates the ipsilateral hilum; volume loss in the lower lobe pulls it down. Granulomatous disease can cause volume loss in both the upper lobes with bilateral hilar retraction. This causes pulmonary vessels to course downward more vertically than normal, sometimes called the "waterfall sign" (Fig. 13-6).

Review of the plain radiographs *and* comparison with prior studies is the first step in evaluating the hila. After this, if there is still doubt about whether the hilum is normal or whether the abnormal appearance is caused by vessels or a mass, computed tomography (CT) of the chest should be performed.

Intravenous contrast is helpful in CT studies obtained to evaluate the hilum because contrast material increases the attenuation (whiteness) of blood vessels and helps distinguish them from adjacent lymph nodes. As scanning times decrease with more advanced CT scanners, the timing of the intravenous contrast bolus must be tailored to the patient. For instance, the movement of contrast material to the lungs may be slowed in patients with a slow circulation time related to poor cardiac output. Unless proper adjustments are made, the x-ray beam may pass through the hila before the contrast agent has reached the hilar blood vessels.

In cases in which intravenous contrast is contraindicated, noncontrast CT can sometimes provide useful information about the hila. Several anatomic landmarks are clearly seen without contrast. For instance, the intermediate bronchus is easily identified as the large bronchus heading inferiorly after the right upper lobe splits off from the main bronchus. The superior pulmonary veins and descending pulmonary artery lie anterior and lateral, respectively, to this bronchus. Posteriorly, the wall of the intermediate bronchus should be in contact with the lung parenchyma. The bronchial wall should be no more than 2 to 3 mm thick (see Fig. 1-18D). Increased soft tissue density behind the bronchus is abnormal and may represent mass or adenopathy.

The anatomy is similar, but not identical, on the left side of the chest. Below the left upper lobe orifice, the descending (interlobar) left pulmonary artery lies posterior and lateral to the left lower lobe bronchus. This leaves open a small window posteriorly between the descending aorta and left descending pulmonary artery where lung tissue abuts the bronchial wall. This area of contact is called the retrobronchial stripe and is present in 90% of normal people. If it is absent, it may have been filled in by adenopathy (see Fig. 1-18D).

Despite these and other landmarks, sometimes it is not possible to differentiate between mass and vessel on a non–contrast-enhanced CT scan. If the patient cannot receive iodine-based intravenous contrast material, magnetic resonance imaging (MRI) can be useful. Because of the profound effect of moving blood on the magnetic field, MR images are very effective in identifying vascular structures (Fig. 13-7). In addition, gadolinium-based intravenous contrast material can be used to enhance MRI images of blood vessels. This material does not contain iodine and carries a very low risk of causing renal insufficiency or a contrast reaction. Unfortunately, the spatial resolution of MRI (its ability to identify small objects) is not as good as that of CT. Although it is less of a problem with current faster scanning techniques, MRI examinations are also more likely than CT to be compromised by respiratory motion (see Chapter 2).

Causes of Hilar Adenopathy

Most conditions that cause bilateral hilar adenopathy also involve the mediastinal nodes and are discussed later in the chapter. The differential diagnosis of bilateral hilar adenopathy is dominated by neoplasm and sarcoid. Both Hodgkin's and non-Hodgkin's lymphoma can cause bilateral hilar adenopathy, almost always with concurrent mediastinal involvement. Bronchogenic neoplasms, most commonly small cell and aggressive adenocarcinomas, can also produce extensive mediastinal and bilateral hilar adenopathy. Metastases from other sites (e.g., breast carcinoma) are less common causes.

Sarcoidosis classically arises as bilateral hilar adenopathy in asymptomatic young women. Unilateral adenopathy is an uncommon manifestation (5% of cases). Sarcoidosis, however, is a common disease and should still be considered in patients with unilateral hilar adenopathy, particularly in populations with a high prevalence of that disease. Other causes of unilateral hilar adenopathy include bronchogenic carcinoma (all types), lymphoma, granulomatous infections, and, in acutely ill patients, tularemia and plague (Table 13-1). Note that although

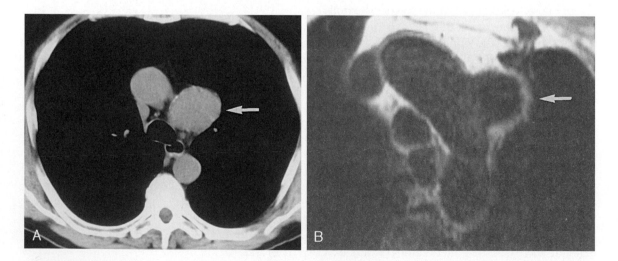

FIGURE 13-7 Computed tomography and magnetic resonance imaging: pseudoaneurysm. MRI can identify vascular masses in the hila and mediastinum.

A, This patient's non–contrast-enhanced CT scan shows a mass in the area of the aorticopulmonary window *(arrow)*. Iodinated contrast medium could not be given because of a severe contrast allergy.

B, MRI was performed and shows that the interior of the mass has very low signal *(arrow)*, consistent with flowing blood. Findings are consistent with post-traumatic aortic pseudoaneurysm.

TABLE 13-1

Causes of Unilateral or Bilateral Hilar Adenopathy

Bronchogenic carcinoma

Lymphoma/leukemia

Sarcoidosis

Metastases from nonthoracic tumors

Infections

    Tuberculosis/*Mycobacterium avium* complex

    Histoplasmosis/coccidioidomycosis

    Tularemia, plague

mycobacterial infections cause adenopathy in some settings, in normal hosts reactivation tuberculosis does not cause enough enlargement of lymph nodes to be detected on chest radiography (see Chapter 7).

In most cases, neither plain radiographs nor CT can differentiate one type of adenopathy from another. On CT, tubercular nodes with active disease may have a low-attenuation center and show peripheral enhancement with intravenous contrast. Necrotic tumors, however, can produce a similar picture. Densely calcified

nodes are usually the residual of a granulomatous infection (e.g., tuberculosis or histoplasmosis; Fig. 13-8). Dense calcifications are also seen in cases of mediastinal fibrosis caused by histoplasmosis. Eggshell-like calcifications are characteristic of silicosis but can also be seen in a few other diseases (Table 13-2). An algorithm that simplifies the work-up of an uncalcified hilar mass is presented in Figure 13-9.

☐ MEDIASTINAL ANATOMY

Like the hila, a few anatomic landmarks are helpful in analyzing the mediastinum. The area around the azygous vein is one of these landmarks. On upright radiographs, a soft tissue opacity in this location that is greater than 9 mm in diameter is abnormal. It may represent an abnormally large azygous vein or a lymph node. If the opacity changes in size with changes in position or a Valsalva maneuver (becomes smaller), it is most likely a vein. Rarely, the azygous vein is enlarged because the inferior vena cava is occluded or congenitally absent and venous return is diverted to the azygous system.

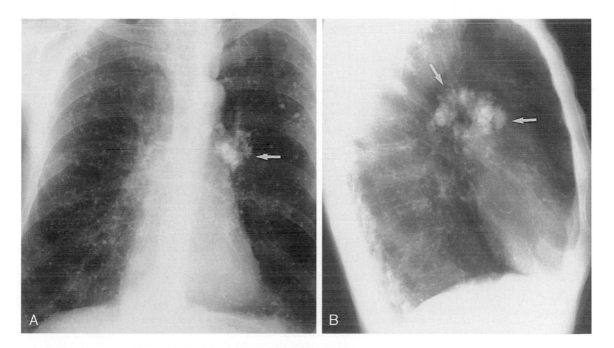

FIGURE 13-8 Posterior-anterior and lateral chest radiographs: histoplasmosis.

    A and B, Uncountable small calcified nodules are present in the lung parenchyma, characteristic of healed histoplasmosis. (Although healed varicella can also leave behind calcified lung nodules, calcified hilar nodes would be rare.) Calcified left hilar nodes are present bilaterally *(arrows)* but are better seen on the left.

TABLE 13-2
Causes of Eggshell Calcifications

Silicosis*
Hodgkin's postirradiation
Coal workers' pneumoconiosis
Sarcoidosis
Histoplasmosis

*Most common.

Between the azygous vein and the diaphragm, the mediastinal soft tissues are in contact with the right lung (azygoesophageal recess). This interface between lungs and mediastinum is seen on radiographs as a curved area of increased opacity, its border normally concave to the right (Fig. 13-10; see Fig. 1-19H). There is a similar border to the left of the spine (left paraspinal line), which lies medial to the shadow formed by the left wall of the descending aorta. Both the azygoesophageal recess and the left paraspinal border are seen only on well-exposed radiographs. Outward convexity of either contour can indicate the presence of mediastinal pathology (Fig. 13-11).

The aorticopulmonary window and the right tracheal wall are also good places to look for mediastinal disease on the posterior-anterior view. The aorticopulmonary window is the space between the aortic arch and the main pulmonary artery. Any convex opacity in this area is probably abnormal. Among other possibilities, convexity here may represent enlarged

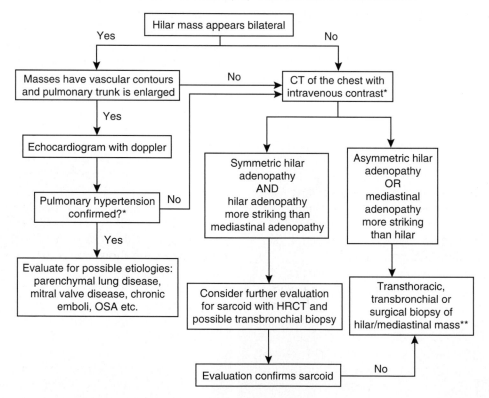

ALGORITHM FOR HILAR MASS(ES) SEEN ON CHEST RADIOGRAPH

*If echocardiogram is normal but CT shows enlarged pulmonary arteries ± dilated right heart or IVC consider repeating echocardiogram or using MR or nuclear medicine techniques to assess RV function
**In acutely/sub-acutely ill patients also consider evaluation for infectious agents, e.g., tularemia

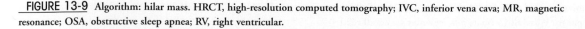

FIGURE 13-9 Algorithm: hilar mass. HRCT, high-resolution computed tomography; IVC, inferior vena cava; MR, magnetic resonance; OSA, obstructive sleep apnea; RV, right ventricular.

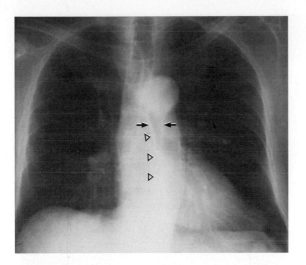

FIGURE 13-10 Posterior-anterior chest radiograph: normal azygoesophageal recess. The azygoesophageal recess is visible as a slightly concave interface between the right wall of the esophagus and the right lung *(arrowheads)*. The patient is slightly rotated to the left, causing the azygoesophageal recess to project off the spine and making it easier to see than on most radiographs. A small amount of air in the esophagus causes the triangular lucency seen just inferior to the aortic arch *(arrows)*.

aorticopulmonary lymph nodes, the nodes through which the left upper lobe drains. The right tracheal wall is normally well defined because it is outlined by air inside the trachea (medially) and by the aerated lung that lies against the tracheal wall laterally. The superior vena cava overlies the right tracheal wall on chest radiographs but usually does not obscure the outer silhouette of the tracheal wall because it lies anterior to the trachea and is not directly in contact with the outer wall (see "Silhouette Sign," Chapter 1).

Normally, the linear opacity caused by the right tracheal wall and adjacent pleura, sometimes called the right paratracheal stripe, should be less than 4 mm wide. The right tracheal wall appears wide when lymph nodes or other masses are in contact with the trachea and their shadows merge with that of the tracheal wall (Fig. 13-12). Unfortunately, on chest radiographs taken in the supine position the right tracheal wall may appear ill defined when no pathology is present.

On the lateral view, anterior mediastinal pathology can cause increased opacity behind the sternum (Fig. 13-13). Middle mediastinal masses cause increased opacity in the aorticopulmonary window and in the area between the trachea and spine above the level of the

aortic arch (Raider's angle). Opacities in the latter, roughly triangular region may be caused by lymphadenopathy, mass, or esophageal disease (Fig. 13-14). Posterior mediastinal masses are located even farther posterior and can project behind the vertebral bodies (see following discussion).

Most of these landmarks are not discernible on portable radiographs because lower energy x-rays are used, resulting in fewer photons that penetrate the mediastinum. The patient's positioning further hampers interpretation. For instance, a supine, anterior-posterior portable chest radiograph often makes a normal mediastinum appear abnormally wide.

All the mediastinal landmarks are easier to discern on CT of the chest, including the right paratracheal area, azygoesophageal recess, and aorticopulmonary window. CT makes it possible to better determine the exact location of pathologic node groups in the pericardiac, subcarinal, or prevascular areas. This is important because the location of the nodes can determine the best means of biopsy. For instance, subcarinal nodes are easily approached by bronchoscopic transbronchial needle aspiration. Right paratracheal adenopathy (e.g., that seen between the superior vena cava and the trachea) can be approached by mediastinoscopy or transbronchial needle aspiration. Both right paratracheal and subcarinal nodes are important in the setting of lung cancer because malignancies in either lung may drain to these node groups (Fig. 13-15).

CT images also make it possible to examine lymph node size and shape. Lymph nodes are usually oval in cross section and the shortest diameter, the short axis, is used when measuring them. In general, the larger the lymph node, the more likely it is to harbor disease. Lymph nodes with a short axis greater than 2 cm usually indicate pathology. Smaller nodes can represent disease in the setting of lung cancer. In the past, a node with a short axis greater than 1 cm was considered a potential metastasis and necessitated pathologic evaluation. Categorization of nodes solely by size, however, has proved nonspecific and insensitive in staging lung cancer (see Chapter 9).

As discussed in the hilar section, MRI is useful in problem cases in which contrast cannot be used but the vasculature needs to be seen more clearly. MRI is most frequently used in the evaluation of mediastinal disease related to the aorta (see later discussion in this chapter).

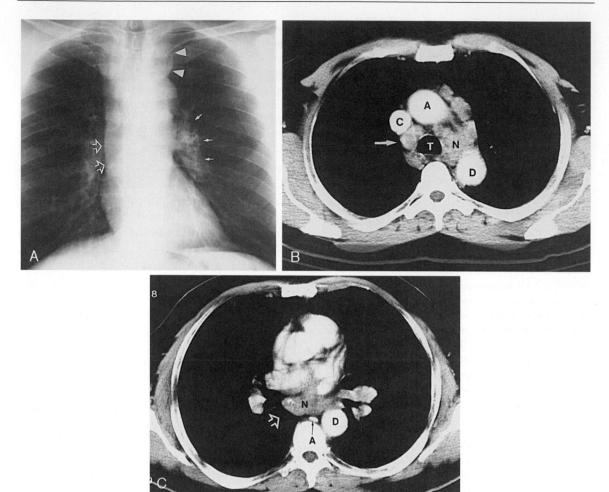

FIGURE 13-11 Posterior-anterior chest radiograph and contrast-enhanced computed tomography: diffuse mediastinal adenopathy involving azygoesophageal recess.

A, Chest examination shows left hilar adenopathy *(short arrows)*, azygoesophageal recess adenopathy *(open arrows)*, and left paratracheal mass *(arrowheads)*. The right outer border of the right tracheal wall is obscured.

B, Contrast-enhanced CT at level above carina shows right paratracheal lymph nodes *(arrow)* and adenopathy in the AP windows (N). A, ascending aorta; C, superior vena cava; D, descending aorta; T, trachea.

C, Extensive subcarinal nodes (N) with encroachment into the azygoesophageal recess *(open arrow)*. Anterior to the nodes are the confluence of pulmonary veins and the left atrium. A, azygous vein; D, descending aorta.

☐ MEDIASTINAL MASSES

Most discussions of the mediastinum divide it into compartments. Unfortunately, there is more than one nomenclature for these compartments. Felson's method is widely used and easy to understand. This method is based on the lateral chest radiograph. It defines the anterior mediastinum as including the heart and everything anterior to it. The posterior mediastinum encompasses the majority of the spine and the paravertebral gutters. The middle mediastinum consists of all structures in between, including the trachea and proximal bronchial tree, esophagus, mediastinal nodes, and portions of the central pulmonary vasculature.

These divisions are helpful because they help refine the differential diagnosis of a mediastinal mass. Although there are standard lists of these diagnoses (which can be memorized), common sense can also help. First, one decides where the epicenter of the mass is located. Then the parent structures normally found in that compartment are considered.

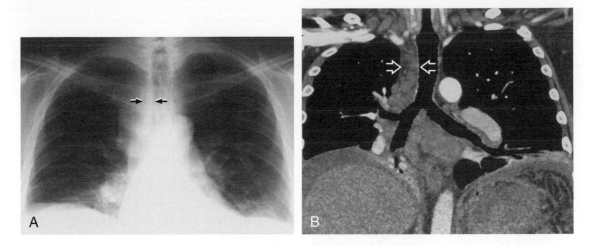

FIGURE 13-12 Posterior-anterior chest radiograph and computed tomography: paratracheal mass.

A, The frontal radiograph shows that the lungs are hypoinflated and the mediastinal contour is wide. Although a degree of mediastinal widening can be attributed to the hypoinflation, hypoinflation should not obscure the outer border of the tracheal wall *(arrows)*. Abnormalities on the left paratracheal area are more difficult to detect than on the right because adjacent vascular structures usually make the left tracheal margin indistinct.

B, CT coronal image shows a conglomeration of smaller nodes extending along the right wall of the trachea *(open arrows)*. These lymph nodes displace the lung away from the trachea so that the outer contour of the wall cannot be seen on the frontal chest radiograph.

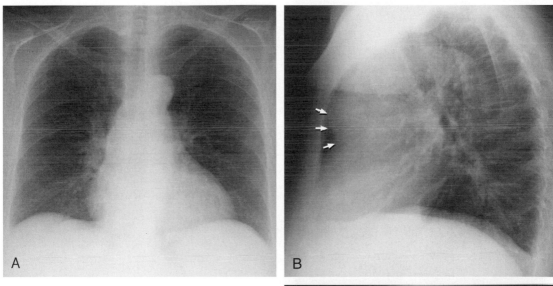

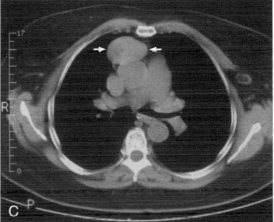

FIGURE 13-13 Posterior-anterior and lateral chest radiographs and non–contrast-enhanced computed tomography: thymoma.

A, On the frontal radiograph there is no evident mass. The mass probably projects over the area of the ascending aorta.

B, The lateral chest radiograph shows the well-defined anterior border of an anterior mediastinal mass *(arrows)*. These findings were sufficient to prompt CT scanning of the chest.

C, CT scan shows a well-defined oval homogenous mass *(arrows)*, a thymoma that was later resected.

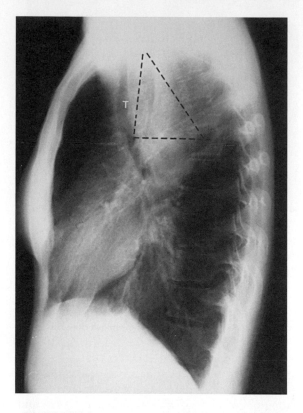

FIGURE 13-14 Lateral chest radiograph: achalasia. The area between the trachea and spine *(dashed lines)* is normally less opaque (darker) than seen in this radiograph. Increased opacity here suggests a mediastinal mass. In this case, the mass was a dilated fluid-filled esophagus that bows the trachea (T) anteriorly.

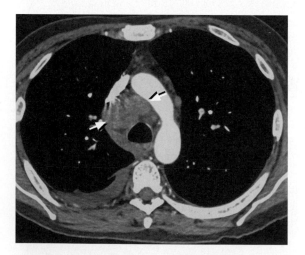

FIGURE 13-15 Contrast-enhanced computed tomography: enlarged paratracheal nodes caused by spread of bronchogenic carcinoma. Two very large right paratracheal lymph nodes are present, each with a short diameter of approximately 2 cm *(arrows)*. The paratracheal nodes are the common pathway of lymphatic drainage from much of the lung and are often involved by spread of lung carcinoma.

For instance, if the abnormality is in the posterior compartment, adjacent to the spine, neoplasms of nerve sheath origin (e.g., neurofibromas) should always be included in the differential diagnosis.

Anterior Mediastinum (Table 13-3)

Thymus

The radiologic appearance of the thymus gland changes markedly with age. The gland plays an important role in the development of the immune system and in infancy is very large compared with other mediastinal structures. The gland continues to grow during puberty, but not as rapidly as other components of the mediastinum, so that its relative size decreases.

Chest CT scans of children show the thymus to have convex outward borders and tissue density equal to or greater than that of muscle. During late adolescence and early adulthood the gland can still be seen on CT as a bilobed structure that lies just anterior to the great vessels below the level of the horizontal portion of the left brachiocephalic vein (Fig. 13-16). With increasing age, the lobes of the gland gradually become concave outward and are replaced with fat. The normal thymus is not seen on chest radiographs of adults.

TABLE 13-3
Anterior Mediastinal Masses

Thyroid masses
Goiter*
Carcinoma

Lymphoma
Hodgkin's*
Non-Hodgkin's

Germ cell tumors
Teratoma*
Malignant germ cell tumor

Thymic masses
Thymic hyperplasia
Thymoma*

Cardiophrenic angle masses
Pericardial fat*
Pericardial cysts
Metastatic lymphadenopathy
Morgagni's hernias

*Most common within subset.

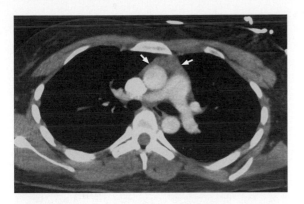

FIGURE 13-16 Computed tomography: normal thymus gland in young adult. CT shows the normal thymus gland anterior to the ascending aorta in the prevascular triangle *(arrows)*. In adolescents and adults younger than 25 years, the lobes of the thymus gland are not yet fully fatty replaced. They normally have flat or concave outer borders. Convex outer borders suggest pathology.

Thymic neoplasms are associated with a number of syndromes, including hypogammaglobulinemia and aplastic anemia. Myasthenia gravis is the most common disease associated with thymic abnormalities. Fifty percent of patients with thymomas have myasthenia.

Conversely, about 10% to 15% of patients with myasthenia gravis have a thymoma. More commonly, patients with myasthenia, about 50%, have thymic hyperplasia.

A thymoma is suggested by CT imaging if a portion of the thymus appears globular or if one lobe is much larger than the other (Fig. 13-17). These masses are characteristically outlined by fat and may contain calcium. Up to 35% of thymomas may be invasive (usually locally). Unfortunately, neither biopsy nor imaging is sufficiently accurate in predicting tissue invasion by the tumor and therefore all thymomas should be resected.

It is difficult to differentiate between normal thymus and thymic hyperplasia with CT or MRI. The size of the thymus on CT correlates only moderately well with the presence of hyperplasia. Fortunately, in the setting of myasthenia gravis the decision to remove the thymus is a clinical one, based on the patient's response to therapy for myasthenia rather than radiologic proof of thymic hyperplasia.

Other thymic tumors are less common than thymomas. These include thymic cysts and thymolipoma. The latter can grow quite large without symptoms because of its fatty content and resultant plasticity.

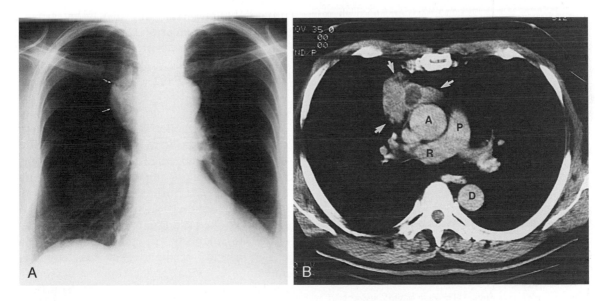

FIGURE 13-17 Posterior-anterior chest radiograph and contrast-enhanced computed tomography: thymoma.

A, The frontal chest radiograph demonstrates a large mass distorting the right upper mediastinal border with a smooth well-defined convex border *(arrows)*.

B, Contrast-enhanced CT at the level of the horizontal portion of the right pulmonary artery shows a large, asymmetric, lobular, 4 by 6 cm thymic mass *(arrows)* with a central area of low attenuation. Asymmetric extension into one side of the chest, usually the right, is typical of thymomas. A, ascending aorta; D, descending aorta; P, main pulmonary artery; R, right pulmonary artery.

Germ Cell Tumors

Germ cell tumors can arise in several extragonadal sites in the body. One of those sites is the mediastinum, usually the anterior compartment. Most often these tumors are teratomas, and the majority are benign. Males are more likely to have a malignant tumor.

Teratomas may appear similar to thymomas on imaging studies. Both may be large and contain calcifications (Fig. 13-18). Teratomas, however, are much more common in children and

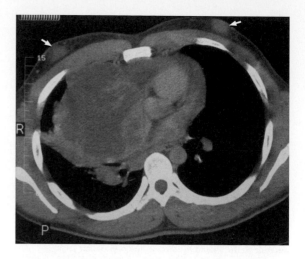

FIGURE 13-19 Contrast-enhanced computed tomography of the chest: malignant germ cell tumor. CT shows a very large anterior mediastinal mass that contains low attenuation areas, indicating cystic component. Fat planes are obliterated by this mass, suggesting its malignant nature. Also note the presence of gynecomastia *(arrows)* caused by secretion of human chorionic gonadotropin by this tumor.

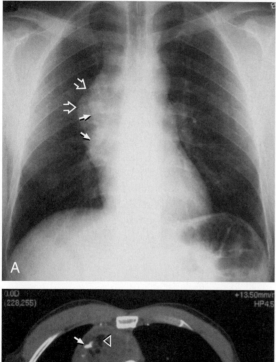

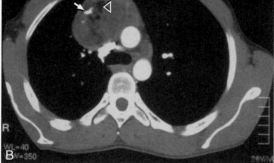

FIGURE 13-18 Posterior-anterior chest radiograph and contrast-enhanced computed tomography: mediastinal teratoma.

A, PA radiograph shows a large mediastinal mass with smooth margins *(open arrows)*. The right hilum *(solid arrows)* is visible through the mass, suggesting that the mass is neither of vascular origin nor engulfing the hilar vessels.

B, Contrast-enhanced CT confirms the anterior mediastinal location of the mass and also reveals the presence of calcifications *(arrow)* and fat *(arrowhead)*. The presence of both fat and calcium indicates that the mass is probably a benign teratoma.

young adults, and thymomas are more common in people older than 40. The presence of fat density on CT is the most important clue to the diagnosis of a benign teratoma. Malignant germ cell tumors are less likely to have fat or calcifications within them. They may grow rapidly, have large cystic areas on CT, and be associated with increased levels of serum markers such as human chorionic gonadotropin and alphafetoprotein (Fig. 13-19).

Thyroid Masses

An intrathoracic goiter is a relatively common cause of an anterior mediastinal mass. Other masses of thyroid origin, such as carcinoma, are less common. Goiters commonly cause the trachea to deviate posteriorly, laterally, or both. Rarely, they extend to the posterior aspect of the middle mediastinum and cause the trachea to deviate anteriorly. On chest radiographs, the upper margins of the opacity caused by an anterior mediastinal goiter fade out above the clavicles. This finding is termed the cervicothoracic sign. The sign occurs because the margins of the goiter above the trachea lie adjacent to the soft tissues of the neck and are no longer bordered by the lungs (see Chapter 1, "Silhouette Sign"). (Masses in the posterior mediastinum are still marginated by lung tissue above the level of the clavicles and therefore maintain distinct margins on radiographs.) Coarse soft tissue calcifications on plain radiographs are also a clue to the presence of a goiter (Fig. 13-20).

A radionuclide thyroid scan can diagnose a substernal goiter. Unfortunately, some substernal goiters are poorly functional so that the amount of radionuclide material taken up by the intrathoracic portion of the goiter may be difficult to detect. The thyroid origin of these masses can be confirmed by demonstrating that the mass is continuous with the thyroid gland on contiguous CT sections. Intrathoracic goiters are usually of heterogeneous density, the higher density portions caused by the presence of iodine within thyroid tissue. Although thyroid tissue is characteristically enhanced strongly when imaged after the administration

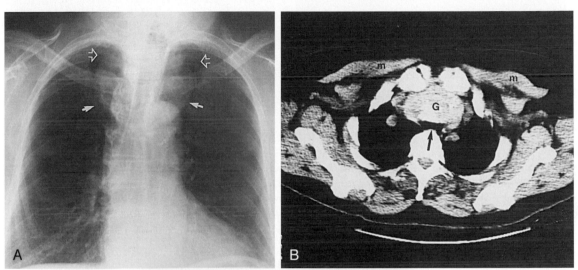

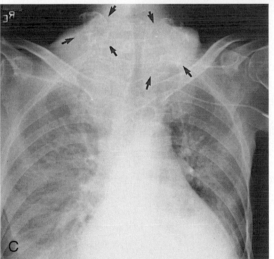

FIGURE 13-20 Posterior-anterior chest radiograph and non–contrast-enhanced computed tomography: goiter.

A, PA chest view demonstrates a large superior mediastinal mass. Extension into the anterior neck produces the cervicothoracic sign; that is, as the homogeneous mass *(solid arrows)* extends cephalad, the lateral margins fade out above the level of the clavicles *(open arrows)*. This indicates that the mass is in the anterior mediastinum. Masses in the middle and posterior mediastinum have distinct borders above the level of the clavicles because they are still outlined by adjacent lung tissue at that level.

B, Non–contrast-enhanced CT section at the level of the thyroid shows the goiter (G) with homogeneous increased attenuation (higher than adjacent muscle [m]) because of iodine content. The mass compresses the trachea *(arrow)*.

C, Chest radiograph showing calcified goiter in a different patient. There is marked thyromegaly with scattered calcification *(arrows)*. The trachea is significantly narrowed above the thoracic inlet.

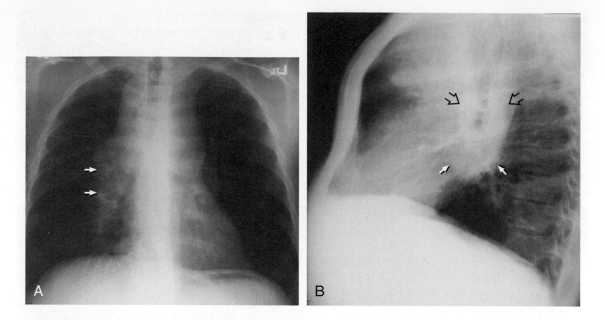

FIGURE 13-21 Posterior-anterior and lateral chest radiographs: Hodgkin's lymphoma.

A, PA radiograph of a patient with nodular sclerosing Hodgkin's lymphoma shows a diffusely widened superior mediastinum. Although there is increased opacity overlying the trachea, the outer border of right tracheal wall is still visible because the mass lies anterior to the trachea. Extensive right hilar adenopathy is also present *(arrows)*.

B, Lateral radiograph shows the large anterior mediastinal mass *(arrows)*. There is also extensive hilar adenopathy. The enlarged lymph nodes *(solid arrows)* combine with the opacities caused by the pulmonary vessels *(open arrows)* to form a doughnut-shaped opacity *(arrows)*, termed a hilar rosette.

of intravenous contrast material, contrast is usually not needed to determine that the tissue is of thyroid origin and the iodine contained in the contrast material can interfere with later treatment of thyroid diseases.

Lymphoma

Both Hodgkin's and non-Hodgkin's lymphoma can cause mediastinal masses. Hodgkin's lymphoma, although less common overall, is more likely than non-Hodgkin's lymphoma to involve the mediastinum. Fifty percent to 80% of patients with Hodgkin's lymphoma present with mediastinal adenopathy.

The most typical presentation of Hodgkin's lymphoma is an anterior mediastinal mass without necrosis or calcification (most often the nodular sclerosing type of Hodgkin's) (Fig. 13-21). Hodgkin's disease may be confined to the anterior mediastinum but commonly presents with paratracheal and hilar adenopathy as well and on occasion spreads to the adjacent lung.

Compared with Hodgkin's disease, non-Hodgkin's lymphoma is more likely to involve

the lung and is more likely to show discontinuous involvement of nodes. For instance, the disease can skip the anterior mediastinum and instead cause isolated adenopathy in the middle and posterior mediastinum (Fig. 13-22). Non-Hodgkin's lymphoma also has a more variable appearance than Hodgkin's disease, depending on the grade of the lymphoma. Low-grade lymphomas, such as follicular non-Hodgkin's lymphoma, can involve intrathoracic lymph nodes but do not cause large masses. High-grade lymphomas may cause large mediastinal masses, sometimes mimicking the anterior mediastinal involvement of Hodgkin's (Fig. 13-23). These tumors are often more aggressive than Hodgkin's and are more likely to involve extranodal tissues, show signs of necrosis, and invade or compress adjacent structures such as the vena cava (causing superior vena cava syndrome). There are two types of non-Hodgkin's lymphoma that typically arise as large masses confined to the anterior mediastinum, mediastinal B-cell lymphoma (a type of diffuse large cell lymphoma) and lymphoblastic lymphoma. Mediastinal B-cell

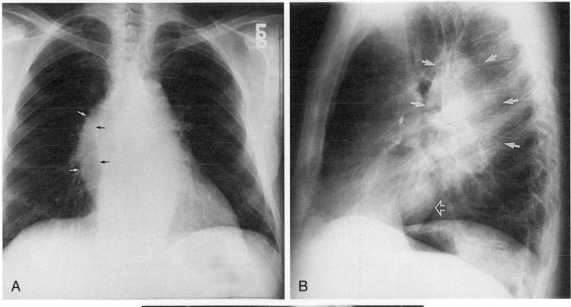

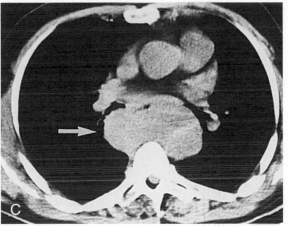

FIGURE 13-22 Posterior-anterior and lateral chest radiographs and contrast-enhanced computed tomography: non-Hodgkin's lymphoma involving the middle and posterior mediastinum.

A, Frontal chest radiograph demonstrates lobular mass *(white arrows)* that fills the azygoesophageal recess. It does not obliterate the right heart border *(black arrows)*, indicating that it does not extend to the anterior mediastinum.

B, Lateral chest radiograph reveals the mass to involve the middle and posterior mediastinum *(arrows)*. The *open arrow* indicates the posterior wall of the left ventricle.

C, Contrast-enhanced CT demonstrates the large lobular mass, centered in the middle mediastinum and extending into the posterior mediastinum. It causes convexity in the azygoesophageal space *(arrow)* and obliterates the soft tissue planes surrounding the esophagus and aorta. Unlike Hodgkin's lymphoma, the mass spares the anterior mediastinum.

lymphoma, like Hodgkin's disease, may be associated with a large amount of fibrosis and may be difficult to diagnosis from the limited tissue obtained by a needle biopsy. Lymphoblastic lymphomas occur in young adults and are more readily diagnosed on transthoracic needle biopsy (Fig. 13-24).

A mediastinal mass can persist after therapy for lymphoma. This is particularly likely in tumors that initially contained a large amount of fibrotic tissue, such as some types of Hodgkin's disease. In the past, gallium scanning and MRI were used to try to differentiate residual malignancy from residual benign fibrosis. More recently, fluorodeoxyglucose scanning with positron emission tomography has shown promise in this area. No imaging regimen is foolproof in making this determination. Often the clinician must obtain a biopsy to determine which lymph nodes are truly diseased.

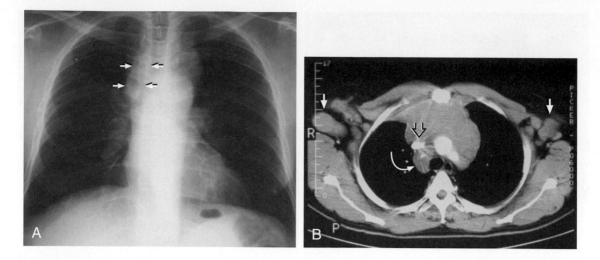

FIGURE 13-23 Posterior-anterior chest radiograph and contrast-enhanced computed tomography: mediastinal B-cell non-Hodgkin's lymphoma.

A, PA chest radiograph shows bilateral widening of the upper mediastinal contours. The outer border of the right tracheal wall is obscured by an adjacent mass *(arrows)*.

B, Contrast-enhanced CT shows a large anterior mediastinal mass as well as bilateral axillary adenopathy *(solid arrows)*. The mass extends into the middle mediastinum, where it is seen adjacent to the trachea *(curved arrow)*. Although the appearance of the mass is very similar to that of nodular sclerosing Hodgkin's disease, the presence of superior vena cava compression *(open arrow)* and possible chest wall invasion are more typical of an aggressive non-Hodgkin's lymphoma (such as a mediastinal B-cell lymphoma). Often an open biopsy is needed to differentiate the two diseases.

Special Sites in the Anterior Mediastinum

Two specific locations in the anterior mediastinum are worth additional attention, the internal mammary nodes and the cardiophrenic angles. Internal mammary nodes lie against the

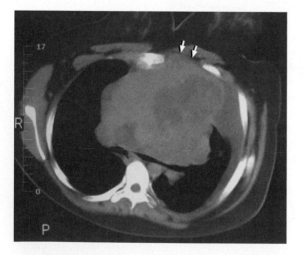

FIGURE 13-24 Contrast enhanced computed tomography: lymphoblastic lymphoma. CT shows a large, heterogeneous mass that obliterates fat planes as it involves the anterior and middle mediastinum. There is also definite invasion of the chest wall *(arrows)*. This is a more aggressive appearance than usually seen in nodular sclerosing Hodgkin's disease.

sternum, medial to the internal mammary artery and vein, and drain the medial portion of the breasts. Enlargement of these nodes without involvement of other lymph nodes in anterior mediastinum suggests metastatic breast cancer rather than lymphoma. Unfortunately, pathologically enlarged internal mammary nodes are difficult to detect on chest radiographs and can be seen only on the lateral view. This is an important area to examine on chest CT scans of patients with suspected metastatic breast carcinoma (Fig. 13-25).

Both cardiophrenic angles are common sites of a pericardial fat pad. Shadows in these areas are so common that physicians often overlook them on chest radiographs. Unfortunately, significant conditions can have a similar appearance. If the cardiophrenic contour changes over time, the mass appears more opaque than the usual fat pad, or the patient has a known malignancy, this area should be further evaluated with other imaging techniques such as CT scanning.

Enlargement of pericardial nodes can be mistaken for a pericardial fat pad on chest radiographs (Fig. 13-26). Pericardial nodes are found adjacent to the anterior aspect of the heart, just above the diaphragm. Nodal enlargement

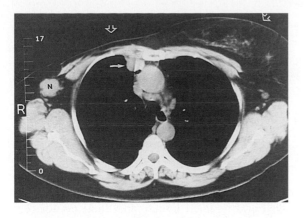

FIGURE 13-25 Contrast-enhanced computed tomography: breast carcinoma with enlarged right internal mammary nodes. Single axial view demonstrates enlarged right internal mammary lymph nodes *(arrow)*. Note asymmetry in breasts after mastectomy *(open arrows)* and right axillary lymph node metastasis (N).

is usually malignant in origin, typically caused by a lymphoma, rarely by a mesothelioma. Pericardial cysts and Morgagni's hernia can also mimic an epicardial fat pad. They are characteristically seen in the cardiophrenic angle, usually on the right.

A chest CT study can readily differentiate pericardial cysts and pericardial lymph nodes from a pericardial fat pad. A Morgagni hernia

and an epicardial fat pad may appear similar because they both contain fat. Clinically, the distinction is not crucial because both are benign processes (see Chapter 11).

Middle Mediastinum (Table 13-4)

Esophageal Disease

The most common radiographic abnormality of the middle mediastinum is a hiatal hernia (Fig. 13-27). It is commonly seen along the inferior margin of the middle mediastinum, posterior to the cardiac silhouette on lateral view. On frontal projection, hiatal hernias often widen the paraspinous lines. The presence of an air-fluid level is usually all that is necessary to make a definite diagnosis. If the hernia is fluid filled at the time of the radiograph and the diagnosis less certain, the presence of a hiatal hernia can be confirmed with a barium study of the esophagus and stomach. Although most hiatal hernias are asymptomatic, they are associated with gastroesophageal reflux, and this is important in some clinical settings. For instance, in a patient with recurrent basilar pneumonias the presence of a large hiatal hernia favors a diagnosis of recurrent aspiration.

Unlike hiatal hernias, most esophageal carcinomas cause serious symptoms before they produce a definite mediastinal abnormality on

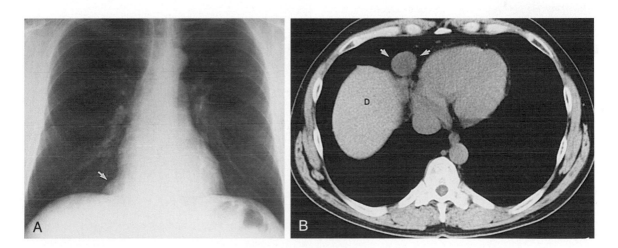

FIGURE 13-26 Posterior-anterior chest radiograph and non–contrast-enhanced computed tomography: pericardial lymph node in a patient with lymphoma.

A, Chest examination shows convex opacity at the right costophrenic angle *(arrow)* that mimics an epicardial fat pad.

B, Single non–contrast-enhanced CT section at the level of the dome of the right diaphragm (D) shows a smooth relatively low-attenuation mass adjacent to the right cardiac border *(arrows)*. Enhancement after administration of intravenous contrast material would help confirm that this mass is a pericardial lymph node rather than a pericardial cyst.

TABLE 13-4
Causes of Middle Mediastinal Masses

Metastatic adenopathy
Bronchogenic carcinoma
Metastases from nonthoracic malignancies
   (e.g., breast carcinoma)

Lymphoma
Hodgkin's
Non-Hodgkin's (includes AIDS-related lymphoma)

Inflammatory adenopathy
Tuberculosis
Histoplasmosis
Sarcoidosis
Anthrax

Vascular
Right aortic arch
Venous anomalies (e.g., azygous continuation of
   vena cava)

Esophageal pathology
Hiatal hernias
Achalasia
Carcinoma
Esophageal varices

Miscellaneous
Mediastinal lipomatosis
Bronchogenic cysts
Primary tracheal tumors

AIDS, acquired immunodeficiency syndrome.

chest radiographs. A distal esophageal carcinoma may cause widening of the paraspinous soft tissues, but in most patients the chest radiograph is normal. Benign obstructing lesions of the esophagus, such as achalasia, typically cause a greater degree of esophageal dilatation because of their indolent course (Fig. 13-28). On frontal projections a dilated esophagus appears as a long smooth contoured mass along the right side of the mediastinum that changes the azygoesophageal recess contour from concave to convex. On lateral view the thickened esophageal wall and retained intraluminal fluid lie adjacent to the trachea and cause apparent thickening of the posterior tracheal wall (>4 mm). The frequent presence of an air-fluid level makes the diagnosis much easier.

Neoplastic Adenopathy

Aside from hiatal hernias, most middle mediastinal masses are caused by mediastinal adenopathy, too often related to metastatic neoplasms. Bronchogenic carcinoma and breast carcinomas are the most common origins of these metastases, but genitourinary malignancies and melanoma can also metastasize to mediastinal nodes. Occasionally bronchogenic neoplasms cause extensive mediastinal adenopathy even

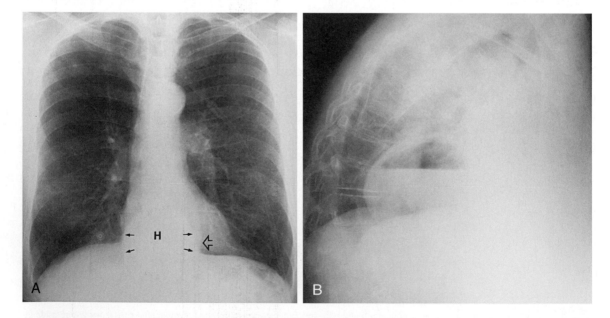

FIGURE 13-27 Posterior-anterior and lateral chest radiographs: hiatal hernia with and without air-fluid level.

    A, PA chest view demonstrates a retrocardiac mass (H) with well-defined convex lateral margins *(arrows).* No air-fluid level is identified in this radiograph. The *open arrow* indicates the margin of the descending aorta.

    B, Lateral radiograph (of same patient) shows a large hiatal hernia with a well-seen air-fluid level. The hernia is centered in the inferior aspect of the middle mediastinum.

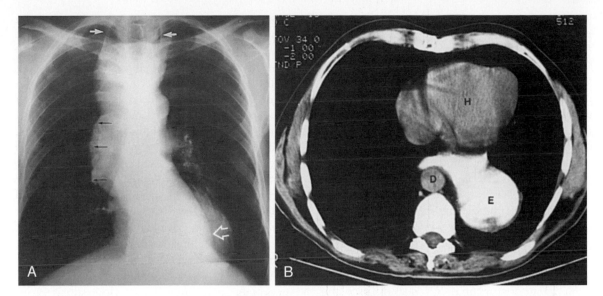

FIGURE 13-28 Posterior-anterior chest radiograph and contrast-enhanced computed tomography: achalasia.

A, The frontal chest radiograph demonstrates lobulated mediastinal opacity extending from the thoracic inlet to the diaphragm. Note the air outlining the outer margins of the esophageal walls in the supraclavicular regions *(white arrows)*; because the esophagus is posterior to the trachea, lung lies adjacent to it above the level of the clavicles. The azygoesophageal recess is convex, pushed laterally by the dilated midportion of the esophagus *(black arrows)*. There is also a retrocardiac opacity on the left caused by a dilated distal esophagus *(open arrow)*.

B, Noncontrast enhanced CT at the level of the cardiac ventricles (H) shows a dilated contrast material–containing esophagus (E) extending from the midline into the left paravertebral gutter. D, descending aorta.

though the primary tumor is not seen on the chest radiograph. This can mimic the appearance of a lymphoma. In these cases, the primary lung tumor may be endobronchial or may have originated near the mediastinum where it is difficult to distinguish from adjacent adenopathy. Small cell carcinomas typically produce extensive mediastinal adenopathy while the parenchymal origin of the neoplasm remains small and difficult to detect (see Fig. 9-19).

As discussed previously, both Hodgkin's and non-Hodgkin's lymphoma can invade the middle mediastinum. Although the bulkiest adenopathy of Hodgkin's lymphoma usually centers in the anterior mediastinum, contiguous nodal groups within the middle mediastinum or neck are often involved. High-grade non-Hodgkin's lymphoma may be confined to the mediastinum at the time of presentation, but low-grade lymphomas are likely to be at advanced stages, involving extrathoracic sites by the time they cause detectable mediastinal adenopathy. Similar to a low-grade lymphoma, chronic lymphocytic leukemia may also affect middle mediastinal nodes in its latter stages.

Inflammatory Adenopathy

Most of the inflammatory conditions that cause mediastinal adenopathy may also cause hilar adenopathy (and are discussed in the section on hilar masses). These include primary tuberculosis, histoplasmosis, silicosis, and sarcoidosis. Sarcoidosis seldom causes middle mediastinal adenopathy without causing concomitant bilateral hilar adenopathy. This observation is sometimes helpful in differentiating sarcoidosis from lymphoma (Table 13-5). Patients with adenopathy from sarcoidosis are also more likely than

TABLE 13-5
Adenopathy in Sarcoid and Lymphoma

	Unilateral Hilar	Paratracheal	Prevascular (anterior mediastinum)	Mediastinal >> Hilar
Sarcoid	Rare	Common	Uncommon	Almost Never
Lymphoma	Common	Common	Common	Common

lymphoma patients to remain asymptomatic despite having impressive radiographic findings.

Vascular Causes

Relatively common vascular causes of middle mediastinal masses include a right aortic arch, an abnormal azygous vein (from a variety of causes), and aortic dissections. These are discussed in Chapter 12. Aortic aneurysms may occur in the anterior, middle, or posterior compartments (and are discussed further in "Posterior Mediastinum" later). Hematomas are also a cause of middle mediastinal masses and occur after both blunt and penetrating injuries, including iatrogenic trauma such as complicated central line placement. Hematomas with convex borders suggest high-pressure bleeding from an arterial source. CT scanning of the hematoma shows multiple different densities within the hematoma if bleeding has remitted and recurred over time (Fig. 13-29). Primary vascular tumors, such as hemangiomas, are very rare. Occasionally, in the setting of severe portal hypertension, paraesophageal varices can become large enough to create an apparent mass on chest radiographs in the inferior portion of the middle mediastinum. The diagnosis is easily confirmed by CT with intravenous contrast.

Miscellaneous

As discussed in Chapters 9 and 10, congenital anomalies arise from varying combinations of abnormal bronchi and alveoli and abnormal pulmonary vasculature. Congenital cysts arise from the embryologic foregut, the precursor to bronchi, and therefore are at the opposite end of the spectrum from pulmonary arteriovenous malformations. These cysts are occasionally the cause of a mediastinal mass. Bronchogenic cysts are the most common congenital cyst within the middle mediastinum. They are usually located near the carina, are sharply marginated, and are filled with fluid that may be of various densities on CT (see Fig. 9-7). Complete absence of enhancement after administration of intravenous contrast material is an important diagnostic clue. Mediastinal bronchogenic cysts are less likely to become infected than bronchogenic cysts within the lung parenchyma. On rare occasions, a mediastinal cyst may cause symptoms by compressing adjacent structures.

A more common cause of an abnormal mediastinal contour, mediastinal lipomatosis, is not a true mass. The increase in mediastinal fat is usually diffuse, involving both the anterior and middle mediastinum, and can be associated

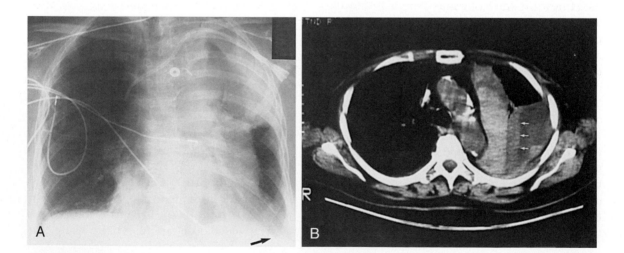

__FIGURE 13-29__ Posterior-anterior chest radiograph and contrast-enhanced computed tomography: mediastinal hematoma following central venous pressure line placement.

A, The chest radiograph shows opacification of the upper half of the left hemithorax caused by mediastinal widening and adjacent pleural fluid. There is also fluid blunting the left costophrenic angle *(arrow)*. Note the left subclavian catheter.

B, Contrast-enhanced CT at the level of the aortic arch shows multiple different densities in the left hemithorax, representing blood of different ages in the mediastinum and pleural spaces. *Arrows* point to an interface between hematomas of different ages. Hematomas from more recent hemorrhage are denser (whiter).

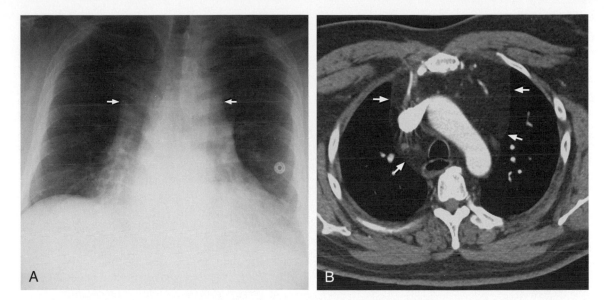

FIGURE 13-30 Posterior-anterior chest radiograph and contrast-enhanced computed tomography: mediastinal lipomatosis.

A, The mediastinal contours appear very wide on PA chest radiograph *(arrows)*. Note that the soft tissue opacities that widen the mediastinum are only slightly opaque.

B, Contrast-enhanced CT of the same patient at the level of the aortic arch. There is extensive mediastinal fat *(arrows)* that accounts for the widened contours seen on chest radiograph.

with obesity or increased levels of systemic corticosteroids (such as in Cushing's syndrome). The diagnosis may be suggested by the clinical history and the chest radiograph, but CT is needed for confirmation. CT shows the homogeneous fat density of the "mass" (Fig. 13-30). The malignant cause of a predominantly fat-containing mass, a liposarcoma, is extremely rare and contains some tissue with a higher density than fat on CT.

Posterior Mediastinum

According to Felson's method, the posterior mediastinum is divided from the middle mediastinum by a line connecting each thoracic vertebral body approximately 1 cm behind its anterior margin. Using this definition, the most common causes of posterior mediastinal masses are neural tumors (Table 13-6).

Neural Neoplasms

Tumors of neural origin occur in the posterior mediastinum because of the proximity of spinal nerve roots and sympathetic ganglia. Tumors of the sympathetic ganglia are rare in adults, although ganglioneuromas are occasionally seen. Neoplasms of the nerve sheath cells are

much more common and are usually benign. These include schwannomas and neurofibromas. Schwannomas (neurilemomas) are composed of nerve sheath cells (spindle cells), and neurofibromas contain nerve sheath cells, fibroblasts, and other tissue. Neurofibromas are associated with neurofibromatosis type 1.

TABLE 13-6
Causes of Posterior Mediastinal Masses

Neural neoplasms
Schwannoma
Neurofibroma
Ganglioneuroma

Non-neural neoplasms
Lymphoma
Metastasis (e.g., testicular)

Inflammation
Paraspinal abscess (e.g., tuberculous)

Vascular
Aortic aneurysm

Miscellaneous
Bochdalek's hernia
Extramedullary hematopoiesis
Meningoceles (rare)

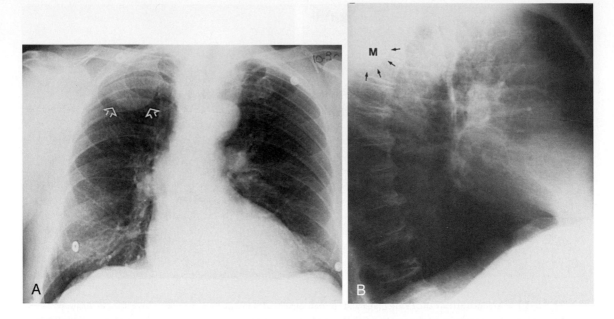

FIGURE 13-31 Posterior-anterior and lateral chest radiographs: neurofibroma.

A, A large mass projects in the right apex *(open arrows)*. It has a smooth distinct inferior margin and an imperceptible superior margin that makes broad contact with the chest wall, forming obtuse angles. These findings suggest that the mass did not arise in the lung parenchyma.

B, The lateral chest view demonstrates a barely perceptible mass projecting far posterior behind the anterior margin of the vertebra (M with *arrows*). The location suggests a neurogenic mass.

Other radiographic signs of this disease (e.g., scoliosis and multiple soft tissue nodules) can also be seen on chest radiographs. Most neurofibromas form rounded masses in the paravertebral gutters (Fig. 13-31). Classically, they cause widening of a neural foramen on lateral radiographs. They can extend into the spinal canal, creating dumbbell-shaped masses that can be seen with CT but are best evaluated with spinal MRI (Fig. 13-32).

Non-Neural Neoplasms

Lymphadenopathy from metastatic bronchogenic carcinoma, testicular carcinoma, or lymphoma may cause a posterior mediastinal mass (Fig. 13-33). Chest radiographs show widened paraspinal soft tissues. Although lymphoma affecting this portion of the chest may be contiguous with intra-abdominal disease, the silhouette of the lateral margins of the paraspinous soft tissues is obscured as it extends below the diaphragm (see Fig. 13-22). Felson termed this the thoracoabdominal sign, and it can occur with any mass that crosses the diaphragm (e.g., hiatal hernia, descending thoracic aortic aneurysm).

Aortic Aneurysms

Aortic aneurysms can involve any compartment of the mediastinum. Aneurysms related to syphilis (now very rare), cystic medial necrosis (e.g., Marfan's or annuloaortic ectasia), and vasculitis usually involve the ascending aorta in the

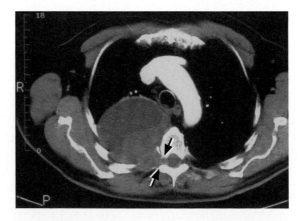

FIGURE 13-32 Contrast-enhanced chest computed tomography: neurofibroma. There is a large heterogeneous paraspinal mass in the right chest. A portion of the tumor extends into a right neuroforamina, widening it *(arrows)*.

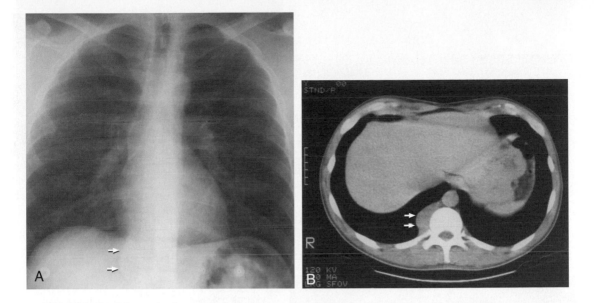

FIGURE 13-33 Posterior-anterior chest radiograph and non–contrast-enhanced computed tomography: testicular carcinoma metastases.
A, PA chest view shows widening of the paraspinal tissues *(arrows)* just above the level of the posterior aspect of the diaphragm.
B, Non–contrast-enhanced CT slice through the lowermost portion of the chest and the upper abdomen. There is a soft tissue mass in the right paraspinous area *(arrows)* caused by metastatic spread of testicular carcinoma along periaortic lymph nodes.

anterior compartment. Most aortic aneurysms are atherosclerotic in origin. Although they may occur in the ascending aorta, they more frequently occur in the arch and descending aorta, the latter coursing downward along the border between middle and posterior mediastinum. Diagnosis may be hampered by individual variation in the size of the descending aorta. It is helpful to remember that the descending aorta should never be larger in diameter than the ascending aorta. The usual ratio is 1:1.5.

The diameter of a normal descending aorta is 3 cm or less. A dilated thoracic aorta, however, is not labeled an aneurysm until its diameter is greater than 4 cm, and the risk of rupture probably does not increase significantly until the aortic diameter is greater than 5 cm. Some aneurysms are fusiform, involving the entire circumference of the aorta. Others are saccular, involving only a portion of the circumference. Saccular aneurysms are also shorter than fusiform aneurysms and are more easily mistaken for a solid mass on plain chest radiographs (Fig. 13-34).

Thoracic aneurysms are accurately diagnosed by CT or MRI, and both are useful for detecting a change in the size of the aneurysm over time. Either CT or MRI can also differentiate a fusiform aneurysm from a chronic type B aortic dissection with a dilated false lumen (see Chapter 12).

Miscellaneous

Both a tuberculous and a pyogenic paraspinal abscess may present as a posterior mediastinal mass. These are usually associated with spinal osteomyelitis and discitis. Plain radiographs characteristically show extensive destruction of the margins of the vertebral bodies adjacent to the infected disc space. Spinal MRI better shows the full extent of the disease (Fig. 13-35).

Bochdalek's hernias (see Chapter 11) and extramedullary hematopoiesis may also cause posterior mediastinal masses. The latter occurs in patients with several forms of hereditary anemias and in patients with myelofibrosis. Figure 13-36 is an algorithm for the evaluation of an abnormal mediastinum in adults.

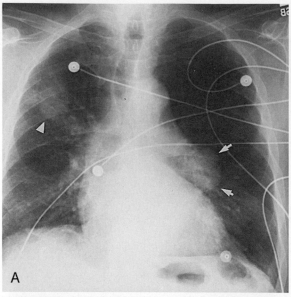

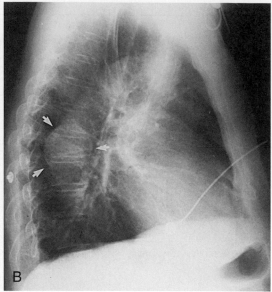

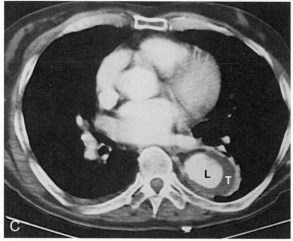

FIGURE 13-34 Posterior-anterior and lateral chest examinations and contrast-enhanced computed tomography: descending aortic aneurysm and bronchogenic carcinoma, right upper lobe.

A, Frontal radiograph demonstrates a left infrahilar "opacity" *(arrows)* that does not obscure the silhouette of the left heart border. Note also the right upper lobe mass *(arrowhead).*

B, Lateral radiograph demonstrates the left-sided opacity to be contiguous with the descending aorta *(arrows).* No calcification or effusion is seen.

C, Contrast-enhanced CT shows the left-sided mass to be a saccular aneurysm. There is contrast in the patent lumen (L) of the aorta and thrombus present in the periphery (T).

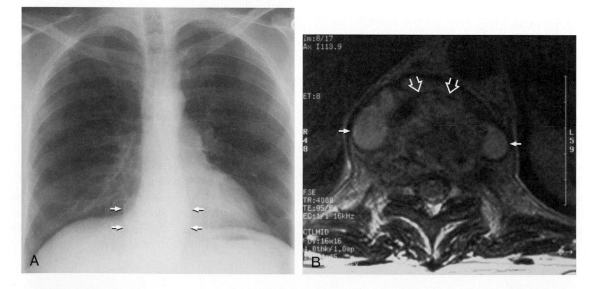

FIGURE 13-35 Posterior-anterior chest radiograph and axial magnetic resonance imaging of the spine: paraspinous abscess.

A, PA chest view shows lateral displacement of both the right and left paraspinous soft tissues *(arrows).*

B, Axial T2-weighted MRI of the lower thoracic spine shows the abscess fluid as high signal *(arrows)* adjacent to the vertebral body *(open arrows).*

ALGORITHM FOR MEDIASTINAL MASS SEEN ON CHEST RADIOGRAPH

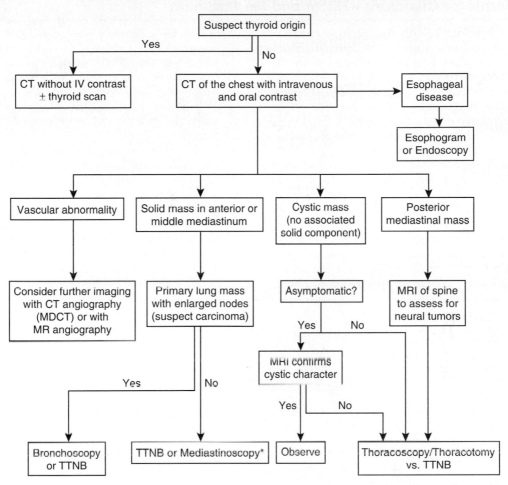

*Note: In the appropriate clinical setting anterior mediastinal masses that have CT findings consistent with a thymoma or teratoma may be excised without biopsy.

FIGURE 13-36 Algorithm: mediastinal mass. CT, computed tomography; IV, intravenous; MDCT, multidetector computed tomography; MRI, magnetic resonance imaging; TTNB, transthoracic needle biopsy.

Pearls for Clinicians—Hilum and Mediastinum

1. A chest radiograph that shows symmetric enlarged hila without an apparent mediastinal mass is most consistent with sarcoidosis or enlargement of pulmonary arteries (caused by pulmonary hypertension). If opacities encircle the hila on the lateral projection, they are probably caused by enlarged lymph nodes and sarcoidosis is therefore most likely.

2. Mediastinal masses several centimeters in size may present only subtle findings on chest radiographs. These masses can be detected with focused inspection of the right tracheal wall, aorticopulmonary window concavity, paraspinous soft tissues on the frontal view, and retrosternal space and Raider's angle on the lateral view.

3. Although there are many types of lymphoma, only three commonly arise as isolated anterior mediastinal masses in adults: nodular sclerosing Hodgkin's, mediastinal (diffuse, large) B-cell lymphoma, and lymphoblastic lymphoma. Lymphoblastic lymphoma occurs in younger patients and is more readily diagnosed with transthoracic needle biopsy than the other two.

4. Even if massive, nodal masses centered in the middle mediastinum are much more likely to be caused by lung carcinoma than lymphoma in patients with a history of extensive tobacco use.

5. MRI is useful for evaluation of suspected neural tumors and suspected congenital cysts and for the evaluation of vascular masses in the mediastinum if iodinated intravenous contrast material is contraindicated.

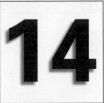

14

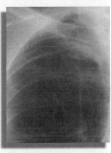

Chest Wall

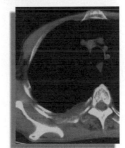

The major components of the chest wall are the ribs, spine, shoulder girdle, and extrapleural soft tissues. Many physicians neglect the chest wall when examining chest radiographs. This is unfortunate because routine observations aid in the diagnosis of many cardiopulmonary diseases. The chest wall is also important because it can be the source of many of the artifacts seen on chest radiographs. For example, a unilateral mastectomy is perhaps the most common cause for one hemithorax to appear diffusely more opaque than the other. Less common artifacts include heavily calcified fibroadenomas in the breast that may be mistaken for lung granulomas (Fig. 14-1) and soft tissue abscesses that are mistaken for intraparenchymal cavities (Fig. 14-2). Other examples or artifacts related to the chest wall are described in Chapter 2.

☐ ANATOMY

On posterior-anterior (PA) or anterior-posterior (AP) radiographs, it is easiest to examine the ribs by first following the course of the posterior segment of each rib as it travels laterally and downward from the spine. Along the inferior margin of the lower ribs there is a costal groove. This groove thins the inferior margins of the lower ribs, often making that margin less distinct and occasionally mimicking a destructive lesion.

Rib notching (see later discussion) and rib companion shadows are also seen along the posterior segments of the ribs. Rib companion shadows are linear opacities that parallel the inferior margin of the upper ribs and the axillary portions of lower ribs. Companion shadows are formed by the superimposition of intercostal soft tissue and are seen to some extent in most patients. These shadows may be confused with apical pneumothoraces. Pneumothoraces, however, rarely run exactly parallel to long segments of the rib margin (see Fig. 2-7).

The anterior aspect of the ribs is examined by following their course downward and medially. Between the anterior and posterior portions of the ribs, there is an "axial" segment that is foreshortened on PA chest radiographs. This segment (lateral rib arcs) is seen only end-on

261

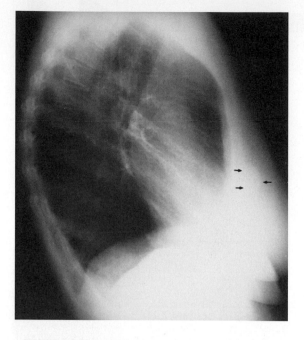

FIGURE 14-1 Lateral chest examination: calcification in fibroadenoma. An anterior chest wall mass with a large calcification *(arrows)* projects over the breast contour. The size, characteristics, and location suggest benign breast disease, either organizing hematoma or, as in this case, a fibroadenoma. The lesion projected over the lung parenchyma on the posterior-anterior view.

(in profile) in the frontal projection. Deformities in the axillary area are best seen by following the lateral-most chest wall from its superior to inferior aspect. Any deviation of this margin from a smooth arc suggests an abnormality. This is a good place to find subtle postoperative abnormalities and cough (tussive) fractures.

Sometimes it is useful to count the number of ribs (e.g., to help describe the location of a parenchymal lung lesion on the radiograph). On most chest radiographs, the inferior ribs are partially obscured, so it is easiest to count down from the top. The posterior aspect of the rib is seen more clearly than the anterior aspect. Unfortunately, shadows of the first three ribs overlap posteriorly. Mistakes in numbering can be avoided if the upper ribs are followed forward and their position is rechecked at the manubrium.

Special radiographs of the ribs can help to evaluate rib abnormalities. These radiographs are taken with a different radiographic technique than standard chest radiographs in order to improve the visualization of bone structures. The examination also includes oblique views of the chest on which the rib arcs (axial portion of the ribs) are better visualized because they are elongated.

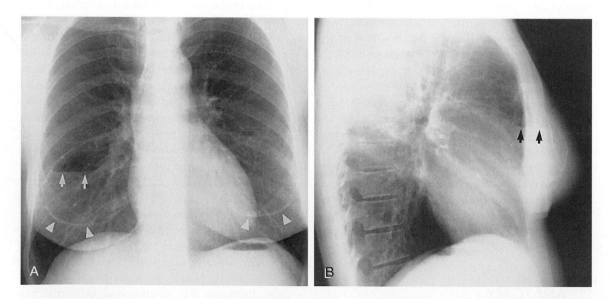

FIGURE 14-2 Posterior-anterior (**A**) and lateral (**B**) radiographs: breast abscess. The patient has had bilateral mammoplasties that are now surrounded by linear calcifications *(arrowheads)*. The air-fluid level seen *(arrows)* is from a superimposed breast abscess.

Routine PA chest radiographs do not show the thoracic spine as clearly as they do the ribs. Pedicles and other anatomic details may be difficult to see behind the heart and mediastinum. This is more problematic with portable radiography because it uses lower energy x-rays. It also can be difficult to assess vertebral body height (looking for compression fractures) on frontal views. Body height is better evaluated on the lateral projection. Anterior wedging, decreased height of the anterior aspect of the vertebral body, is commonly seen on the lateral projection. It may be caused by trauma but often is secondary to osteopenia, such as postmenopausal osteoporosis (see later discussion). Underlying osteopenia may not be evident because conventional radiographs (chest or dedicated spine studies) are not sensitive for detecting decreased bone density. Plain radiographs cannot reliably diagnose osteopenia until 35% to 50% of the cancellous bone has been lost. Conversely, overexposed images can sometimes give the impression of osteopenia when the bone density is in fact normal. Dual x-ray absorptiometry (DEXA) and CT densitometry are much more reliable than plain radiographs for diagnosing osteopenia.

The shoulder girdles are often, but not always, seen on chest radiographs. Sometimes they are obscured by labels or project off the side of the image on frontal projection. The distal clavicle and humeral head are more reliably seen on PA or AP projections, but the sternum is well evaluated only on the lateral projection. The sternoclavicular joints are difficult to see on both frontal and lateral views (see later discussion).

☐ CONGENITAL ABNORMALITIES

Congenital malformations of the ribs are common, occurring in about 3% of the population. One of the abnormalities, cervical ribs, occurs in 1 of 75 patients and is usually bilateral (Fig. 14-3). In a minority of patients, cervical ribs may be associated with a thoracic outlet syndrome. The syndrome manifests as upper extremity symptoms related to compression of the brachial plexus, subclavian vein, or artery.

Chest wall deformities affecting both the ribs and the sternum are also common. Pectus carinatum, or pigeon breast, is anterior protrusion of the sternum. Pectus excavatum is a

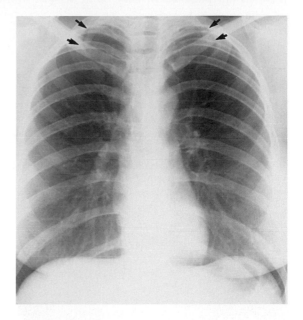

FIGURE 14-3 Posterior-anterior chest radiograph: cervical ribs. Asymmetric development of rudimentary ribs *(arrows)* at the C7 level bilaterally. These are usually an incidental asymptomatic finding, but 5% to 10% of cervical ribs can be associated with thoracic outlet syndrome.

depression of the sternum relative to the anterior ribs. Most patients with either deformity are asymptomatic, although a few individuals can have coexistent heart disease. For example, pectus carinatum is associated with atrial and ventricular septal defects and pectus excavatum is associated with mitral valve prolapse. Patients with Marfan's syndrome may also have pectus excavatum, but other skeletal abnormalities are often more striking (Fig. 14-4).

More commonly, chest wall deformities cause radiographic abnormalities that can be mistaken for pathology on PA or AP radiographs. In patients with pectus excavatum, the cardiac silhouette is shifted to the left, sometimes creating the illusion of cardiomegaly. The right heart border may be obscured by superimposition of soft tissues along the right margin of the sternum. This can be mistaken for right middle lobe disease. Both cardiomegaly and right middle lobe disease can usually be excluded by examination of the lateral chest radiograph. Lateral projections show that the heart is squeezed between the depressed sternum and the spine, accounting for its increased width. The lateral view also shows that the middle

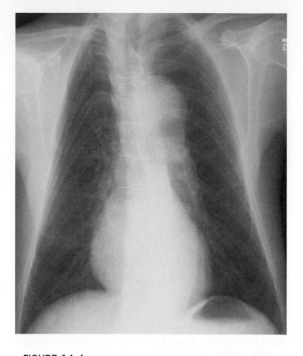

FIGURE 14-4 Posterior-anterior chest radiograph: Marfan's syndrome. The thoracic cage is markedly elongated and there is evidence of previous sternotomy for repair of ascending aortic aneurysm. The aortic arch is markedly dilated.

lobe is free of atelectasis or air space disease (Fig. 14-5).

Spinal deformity from scoliosis of the thoracic spine is occasionally seen on a chest radiograph. Most scoliosis is idiopathic and is most prevalent in young women. A minority of scoliosis is truly congenital, meaning that it is caused by a deformed vertebral body. Neuromuscular diseases (e.g., cerebral palsy, syringomyelia, or muscular dystrophy) also cause scoliosis. In patients with neuromuscular disease the spine often forms a gradual C-shaped curve instead of the S-shaped curve of idiopathic scoliosis.

Besides causing mobility and cosmetic problems, scoliosis can directly affect respiratory function. The volume of the thorax is reduced by lateral bending and by rotation of the ribs along the longitudinal axis of the spine. More important, these distortions in the architecture of the thorax disrupt normal function of the respiratory muscles, particularly the diaphragm. If the maximal angle of curvature (Cobb's angle) is less than 60 degrees, the resulting physiologic impairment is usually not significant. At angles greater than 60 degrees, the incidence

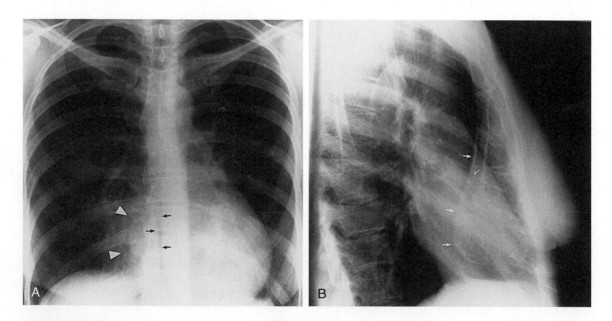

FIGURE 14-5 Posterior-anterior and lateral chest radiographs: pectus excavatum (funnel chest).

A, Frontal chest view demonstrates blurring of the right cardiac border *(arrowheads)* caused by the nearly sagittal orientation of the parasternal chest wall. The cardiac silhouette is displaced slightly to the left, and there is increased downward inclination of the anterior portion of the ribs. A small area of lucency is seen in the midline *(arrows)*, which is air outlined by the soft tissues of the breasts. This is a characteristic finding.

B, Lateral radiograph demonstrates marked posterior depression of the sternum *(arrows)*. Note that the cardiac margin is displaced somewhat posteriorly but is still anterior to the vertebral bodies.

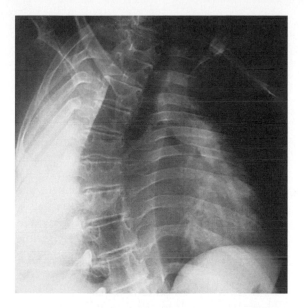

FIGURE 14-6 Posterior-anterior chest radiograph: scoliosis with atelectasis. There is marked dextroscoliosis with secondary atelectasis of almost the entire right lung. The broad C-shaped scoliosis is consistent with the patient's underlying muscular dystrophy.

ninth ribs at the anterior axillary line. (They have also been reported far posteriorly along the costovertebral junction.) The patient's pain can be pleuritic in nature and closely mimic the symptoms of pulmonary emboli. These fractures are minimally displaced and may not be evident on routine chest radiographs, leading to additional diagnostic procedures to exclude the diagnosis of pulmonary emboli (Fig. 14-7).

There are a few other instances in which identifying specific rib fractures may be important. Flail segments (ribs broken in two places) are signs of major blunt chest trauma and are often accompanied by pulmonary contusion. The presence of fractures of the lower ribs raises concern for concurrent injury of the liver or spleen. First or second rib fractures have been associated with great vessel injuries but are almost always accompanied by other radiographic signs of chest trauma. They are probably not a strong predictor of vascular injury if they are an isolated finding. Last, healed rib

of ventilatory abnormalities increases. When the deformity measures 120 degrees, respiratory failure and alveolar hypoventilation often occur. Secondary atelectasis is often present when the deformities are this extensive (Fig. 14-6).

☐ TRAUMA

Rib Trauma

Although rib fractures are a frequent injury, documenting the actual site of the break is usually not clinically important. The chest radiograph is the most useful study in assessing patients with suspected rib fractures because it can diagnose important injuries that may be associated with fracture, such as pneumothorax, hemothorax, and lung contusion. Special radiographs of the ribs taken in order to document the fracture are usually not necessary because the results rarely alter management of the patient.

Radiographs of the ribs are occasionally helpful in patients presenting with chest pain. Older patients may fracture ribs without major trauma, for example, by coughing. These post-tussive rib fractures most commonly occur in the fourth to

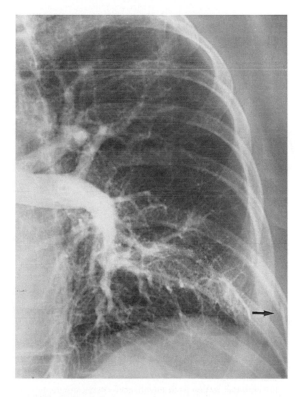

FIGURE 14-7 Pulmonary angiogram: rib fracture symptoms mistaken for symptoms of pulmonary embolus. The findings on this anterior-posterior pulmonary angiogram in the late arterial phase are normal. However, there is a post-tussive fracture of the lateral sixth rib *(arrow)* along the axillary line.

fractures can be mistaken for masses in the chest wall or in the lung parenchyma (see Chapter 2). Oblique views of the ribs can often determine whether the suspect opacity is caused by a healed rib fracture, and these plain radiographs can be much more cost effective than a chest CT scan. Healed fractures should have smooth well-defined cortical borders. Loss of the cortical margin suggests rib invasion by infection or tumor rather than a post-traumatic deformity (Fig. 14-8).

Sternum and Clavicle Trauma

Like rib fractures, clavicle fractures are also commonly caused by chest trauma and are usually evident on plain radiographs. The sternoclavicular joint, however, is difficult to visualize regardless of the projection used. If injury to this area is suspected, thin section CT of the sternoclavicular joints is the most useful study to obtain. The same study is useful in detecting nontraumatic sternoclavicular joint disease such as suspected septic arthritis of the sternoclavicular joint typically seen in intravenous drug abusers. Sternum fractures are not as common as clavicle or rib fractures. They are rarely visible on AP portable radiography, even when they can be diagnosed clinically by palpation. Other than CT, sternal fractures are best seen on lateral radiographs (Fig. 14-9). Sternal fractures imply significant blunt chest trauma with risk of other injuries including cardiac contusion. Fortunately, most of the resulting cardiac contusions remain asymptomatic.

Iatrogenic Trauma

Typically, patients who suffer iatrogenic chest wall trauma, such as a thoracotomy, are left with

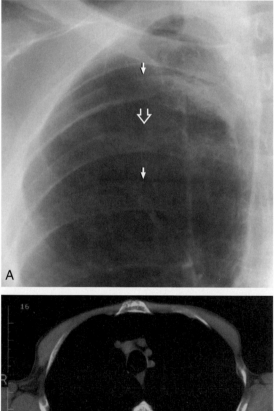

FIGURE 14-8 Detail from posterior-anterior chest radiograph and section from unenhanced chest computed tomography: adenocarcinoma of the lung.

A, Detail from a chest radiograph shows that the superior margins of the normal ribs are well defined *(arrows)*. The superior margin of the fifth rib is poorly defined *(open arrow)*.

B, Chest CT section shows that a pleural mass has invaded the fifth posterior rib.

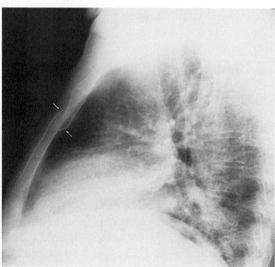

FIGURE 14-9 Lateral chest radiograph: sternal fracture. The lateral view best demonstrates the posteriorly displaced subacute fracture *(arrows)* through the body of the sternum, minimally depressed. Minimally displaced acute fractures can be difficult to identify even on lateral views; the only clue may be contiguous soft tissue swelling related to extrapleural hematoma.

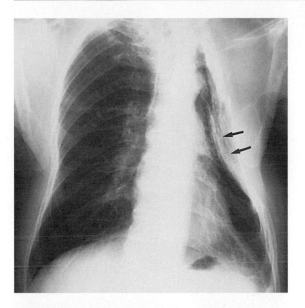

FIGURE 14-10 Posterior-anterior chest radiograph: thoracoplasty. Marked postsurgical deformity of the rib cage (resulting from treatment for tuberculosis prior to the antibiotic era) is present with associated pleural calcifications *(arrows)*. Note the significant volume loss associated with ipsilateral mediastinal shift.

only minor lasting deformity of the chest wall. Post-thoracoplasty deformity, however, is dramatic (Fig. 14-10). Several decades ago, surgeons routinely performed thoracoplasties as part of the treatment for tuberculosis. The operation involved the obliteration of a portion of the hemithorax by resection of multiple ribs. This procedure is only rarely necessary today. Chest wall resections are still occasionally performed in patients with bronchogenic carcinoma that has locally invaded the chest wall but has not spread to mediastinal nodes or distant sites. Localized rib resection may also be performed to allow drainage of a chronic empyema.

☐ TUMORS AND TUMOR-LIKE DISEASES

Diffuse osseous metastases can be detected on chest radiographs, appearing as a widespread increase in bone opacity, termed osteosclerosis. This pattern is most often caused by either breast or prostate carcinoma (Fig. 14-11). Some metabolic bone diseases, including secondary hyperparathyroidism and diseases associated with abnormal bone marrow, myelofibrosis, mastocytosis, and sickle cell anemia, can also cause diffuse osteosclerosis.

Neoplasms may also cause focal abnormalities of the chest wall. Benign osseous tumors such as enchondromas and tumor-like processes such as fibrous dysplasia can deform ribs (Fig. 14-12). These rib lesions are usually not associated with soft tissue masses. Destructive rib lesions that are accompanied by an extraosseous soft tissue mass are usually malignant.

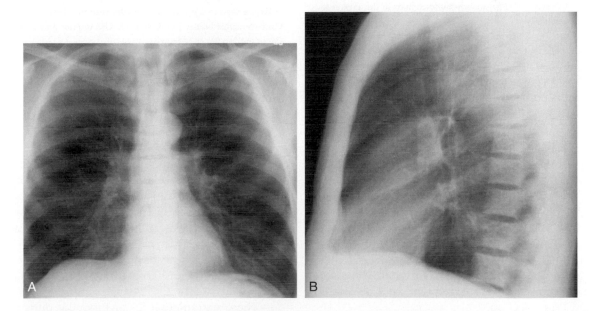

FIGURE 14-11 Posterior-anterior and lateral chest radiographs: prostate carcinoma. The bones of the thoracic cage are all more opaque than normal. The increased opacity of the bones is most evident in the appearance of the vertebral bodies on the lateral projection. Osteoblastic metastases have caused the increased opacity.

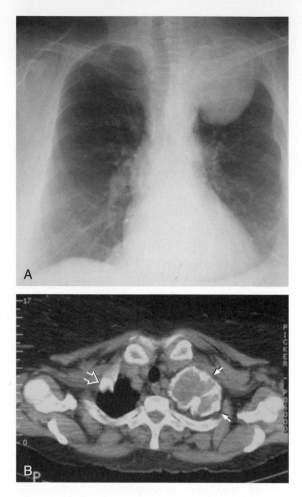

__FIGURE 14-12__ Posterior-anterior chest radiograph and computed tomography: fibrous dysplasia.

A, There is a large smooth-bordered mass in the apex of the left hemithorax.

B, CT section through the mass shows that this represents soft tissue that has expanded the left first rib *(arrows).* The normal right first rib is seen on the contralateral side *(arrowhead).* This mass is more expansile than seen in most cases of fibrous dysplasia occurring within a rib.

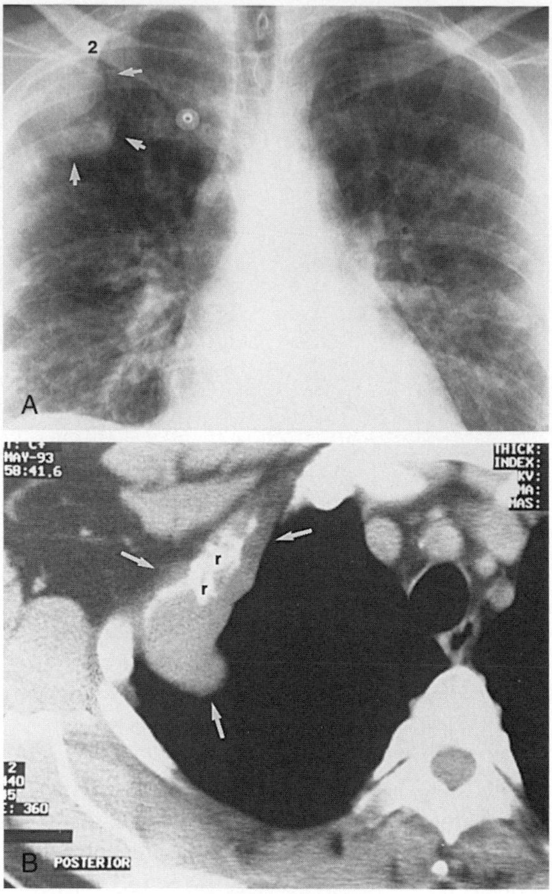

__FIGURE 14-13__ Posterior-anterior chest radiograph and contrast-enhanced computed tomography: myeloma involvement of ribs.

A, The frontal radiograph shows a large right apicolateral lesion *(arrows)* that forms obtuse angles with the chest wall. Only its medial border is well defined. The anterior portion of the second rib (2) is destroyed.

B, Contrast-enhanced CT. An axial scan reveals the marked destruction of the rib (r) and the associated soft tissue mass *(arrows).*

Myeloma or metastases (e.g., lung carcinoma, breast carcinoma) are most commonly responsible for this appearance in adults (Fig. 14-13). Masses in the sternum are usually malignant, either originating in the hematopoietic marrow within the sternum or spreading to the sternum through its rich blood supply The lateral chest radiograph must be carefully examined for sternal lesions, which are frequently not detectable on PA projection.

Some abnormalities begin in the soft tissues of the chest wall and affect the ribs secondarily.

Benign processes, such as neurofibroma, may cause erosion or sclerosis of a rib margin. Malignant diseases cause more destructive changes. Infectious diseases, such as actinomycosis, blastomycosis, tuberculosis, and, occasionally, nocardiosis, cause similar destructive lesions of the ribs or sternum. Their appearance may be indistinguishable from that of malignancy (Figs. 14-14 and 14-15).

These extrapleural lesions may be difficult to differentiate from pleural lesions on plain radiographs. Both types of lesions form broad

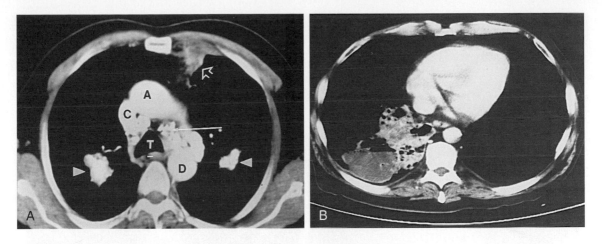

FIGURE 14-14 Contrast-enhanced computed tomography images: nocardial infection.

A, An irregular density *(open arrow)* is apparent in the left anterior chest wall extending from the lung periphery through the visceral and parietal pleura into the soft tissues adjacent to the sternum. Also demonstrated are focal areas of progressive massive fibrosis *(arrowheads)* and calcified anterior-posterior window nodes *(long arrow)*. A, ascending aorta; C, superior vena cava; D, descending aorta; T, trachea.

B, CT section from a different patient shows a more typical example of nocardial infection. Necrotizing infection of the lung parenchyma is manifest as a lung abscess and multiple air-filled cavities, but no chest wall invasion is evident.

and relatively flat masses (unlike spherical parenchymal nodules) adjacent to the pleural surface. When viewed in profile (narrow side of the mass facing the x-ray beam), the medial margin of the mass is well defined because it is tangential to the x-ray beam. The medial border of the mass may be seen to form obtuse angles with the chest wall. When viewed face on (broad side of the mass facing the x-ray beam), at least one border appears indistinct (Fig. 14-16). If the lesion is very flat, it may be nearly invisible when it is projected en face. Because pleural and extrapleural masses have similar radiographic appearances, it is useful to consider both entities when generating a differential diagnosis (Table 14-1).

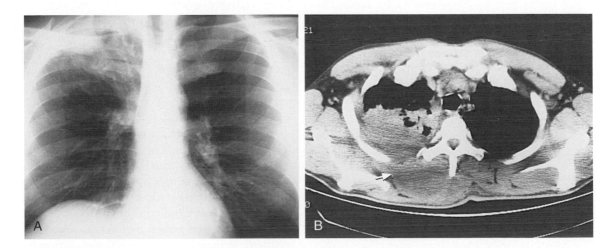

FIGURE 14-15 Posterior-anterior radiograph and computed tomography: actinomycosis.

A, Air space disease is present in the right upper lobe and there is adjacent pleural disease in the lung apex.

B, CT shows evidence of cavities within the lung and a pleural effusion. An area of fluid attenuation extends through the pleural surface into the chest wall *(arrow)*.

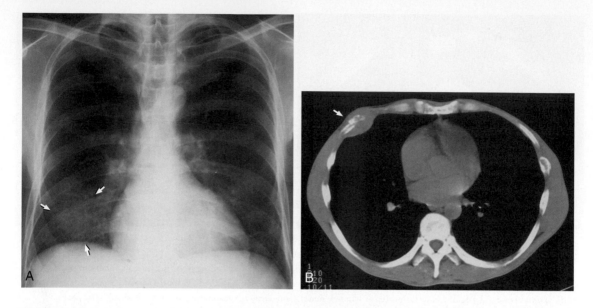

FIGURE 14-16 Posterior-anterior chest radiograph and computed tomography section: multiple myeloma.

A, PA radiograph shows an ill-defined opacity overlying the right lung base *(arrows)*. The borders of the mass are not well seen in this projection because the mass is seen face on (en face). The margins of the mass are not tangential to the x-ray beam.

B, CT shows a expanding mass of one of the right ribs that caused the opacity over the right lung.

☐ MISCELLANEOUS CONDITIONS AFFECTING THE SPINE

Vertebral body deformities are frequently seen with chest radiography. Some deformities are caused by acute major trauma. More commonly, vertebral body deformities result from minor

TABLE 14-1
Chest Wall and Pleural Masses

Masses originating from the pleura
Empyema or loculated effusion*
Metastases*
Plaques
Fibrous tumor of the pleura
Mesothelioma

Masses originating from the chest wall
Mesenchymal tumors
Lipoma*
Sarcoma
Desmoid
Myeloma/plasmacytoma*
Metastases*
Neural tumors

*Most common.

trauma to bone weakened by osteoporosis, osteomalacia, hyperparathyroidism, or malignancy. Hyperparathyroidism has a characteristic appearance, causing bands of increased radiopacity at the inferior and superior end plates of each vertebral body. This pattern is called the rugger-jersey spine (Fig. 14-17). In the past, these changes occurred more commonly in primary than secondary hyperparathyroidism. Now, however, primary hyperparathyroidism tends to be diagnosed at any earlier stage because of improvements in detecting hypercalcemia. Most rugger-jersey spines are now seen in patients with secondary hyperparathyroidism due to chronic renal failure.

Osteoporotic vertebral bodies often show delicate, linear, vertical opacities. These are the vertical trabeculae that have become more apparent than usual because the trabeculae in other orientations have been resorbed. Osteoporotic vertebral bodies may become biconcave (fish-mouthed vertebra), anteriorly wedged, or (less commonly) diffusely flattened (Fig. 14-18). Wedging and diffuse compression are caused by fractures of the weakened body, termed insufficiency fractures. Anterior wedging of one or more thoracic vertebral bodies is

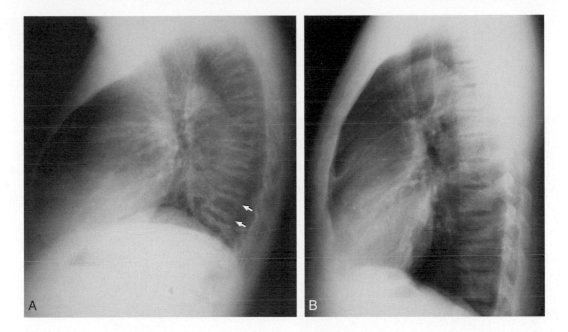

FIGURE 14-17 Two lateral chest radiographs: rugger-jersey spine in two patients.

   A, Lateral radiograph shows well-demarcated horizontal bands of dense osteosclerosis in the vertebral end plates, which gives this condition its name *(arrows).* This rugger-jersey appearance is most common with secondary hyperparathyroidism.

   B, Lateral radiograph of a second patient with renal osteodystrophy. The osteosclerosis in the vertebral bodies is more diffuse in this patient and the horizontal banding is not as evident.

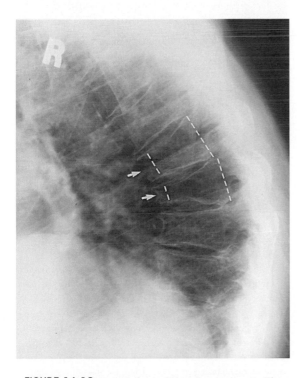

FIGURE 14-18 Lateral chest radiograph: osteoporosis. There is diffuse osteopenia and anterior wedging of two middle thoracic vertebral bodies *(arrows).* Severity of the wedging can be measured by comparing anterior and posterior body heights *(dashed lines).*

commonly seen on lateral radiographs of elderly patients, particularly women. Pain associated with vertebral insufficiency fractures can be mitigated by performance of a vertebroplasty, at which time acrylic cement (polymethylmethacrylate) is injected into the fractured vertebral body to stabilize its structure.

   Unfortunately, it can be difficult to distinguish fractures related to osteoporosis from those associated with malignant infiltration of the bone. Both of these conditions can lead to compression fractures of the vertebral body. Malignant infiltration may cause more loss in posterior height of the vertebral body than is typically seen in osteoporosis, but this is not a reliable finding. Loss of a pedicle outline on PA projection does strongly suggest malignant disease (Fig. 14-19).

   Osteomyelitis can also cause collapse of a vertebral body but is more commonly seen in the lumbar than the thoracic spine. Because the infection usually starts in the portion of the vertebral body adjacent to a intervertebral disc, the infection spreads through the disc space, destroying the inferior end plate of one vertebral body and the superior end plate of the vertebral body below it (Fig. 14-20).

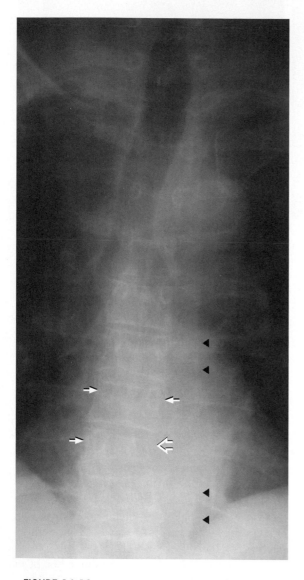

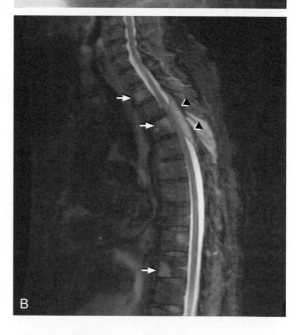

FIGURE 14-19 Anterior-posterior thoracic spine radiograph: metastatic carcinoma. The pedicles of the normal vertebra are seen on end, forming oval opacities *(arrows)*. The left pedicle of one of the lower thoracic vertebral bodies is absent *(open arrow)*. The interface between the paraspinous soft tissues and the adjacent lung *(arrowheads)* is also disrupted at this level, suggesting the presence of an adjacent soft tissue mass.

FIGURE 14-20 Lateral chest radiograph and magnetic resonance imaging: metastases to the thoracic spine.

A, In this patient, there is a pathologic compression fracture of a thoracic vertebral body *(arrow)*. The body is diffusely flattened, with marked loss of both anterior and posterior height.

B, Sagittal weighted magnetic resonance image of the spine in a different patient. The sequence is T2 weighted, showing the cerebrospinal fluid as a very high signal and the spinal cord as an intermediate signal (gray). There are areas of high signal *(arrows)* within multiple vertebral bodies, none of which have yet fractured. There is also an epidural tumor mass impinging on the spinal cord *(arrowheads)*.

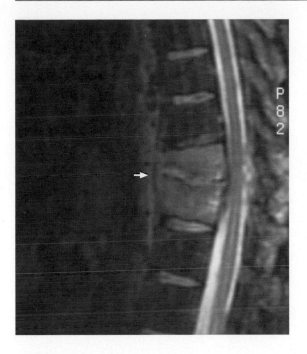

FIGURE 14-21 Sagittal magnetic resonance imaging: osteomyelitis. Sagittal T2-weighted MRI of the same patient imaged in Figure 13-35. Two adjacent vertebral bodies show high signal because of edema caused by osteomyelitis. The disc space between the two bodies is narrowed *(arrow)* and the adjacent vertebral end plates are destroyed.

Magnetic resonance imaging or a radionuclide bone scan can help diagnose underlying malignancy. Both studies can be useful in detecting malignancy by identifying other (noncollapsed) vertebrae as abnormal despite a normal appearance on plain radiographs. Magnetic resonance images may support the diagnosis of malignancy if they demonstrate abnormal marrow within portions of the collapsed vertebrae separate from the fracture (Fig. 14-21). The presence of a soft tissue mass also favors malignant disease rather than osteoporosis.

Myeloma is unlike other malignancies in several ways. It is more likely to involve the vertebral body and spare the pedicle, and it is frequently not detected on radionuclide bone scans. On plain radiographs, it can produce multiple well-circumscribed lytic lesions or diffuse osteopenia that are indistinguishable from osteoporosis.

Ankylosing spondylitis is another spinal disorder that is seen relatively frequently on chest radiographs. The disorder impairs pulmonary function by accentuating thoracic kyphosis and decreasing chest wall compliance. This results in a mixed pattern of restriction and hyperinflation on pulmonary function testing. A small number of patients with ankylosing spondylitis also develop apical fibrosis or aortic valve disease or both.

Typical osseous changes of ankylosing spondylitis occur at the thoracolumbar junction. Vertically oriented calcifications form along the margin of the intervertebral discs connecting adjacent vertebral bodies and causing the spine to appear similar to a bamboo pole (bamboo spine). These syndesmophytes may be seen on both lateral and AP views (Fig. 14-22). Syndesmophytes look different from the more triangular oblique bone outgrowths of spondylosis deformans (degenerative spinal disease). They are also thinner and hug the contour of the intervertebral discs more closely than the flowing ossifications of diffuse idiopathic skeletal hyperostosis (DISH). The latter disease occurs in older males and is often most pronounced along the right side of the thoracic spine (perhaps because the ossifications are not disturbed by pulsations of the descending aorta). Patients with DISH are usually asymptomatic (Fig. 14-23).

☐ OTHER

Extraspinal manifestations of arthropathies are only occasionally seen on chest radiographs. The distal ends of the clavicles can be eroded or "penciled" in patients with progressive systemic sclerosis, rheumatoid arthritis, and hyperparathyroidism (Fig. 14-24). The glenohumeral joints are often visualized on chest radiography. Degenerative arthritis is unusual in these joints because they are not weight bearing. Marked joint space narrowing suggests that trauma or some other agent (e.g., crystal deposition) has damaged the cartilage. If the humeral head is displaced upward so that it is only a few millimeters from the acromion, the patient probably has a chronic rotator cuff tear. This is a common finding in elderly patients.

These and similar subtle musculoskeletal findings are interesting, but they exceed the usual diagnostic realm of chest radiography. These also go beyond the scope of this text. Interested clinicians should consider consulting the bone radiology text in this series.

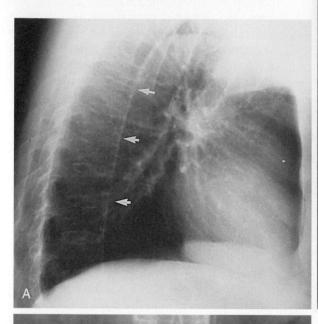

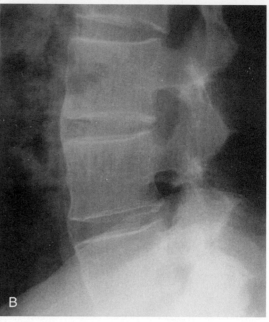

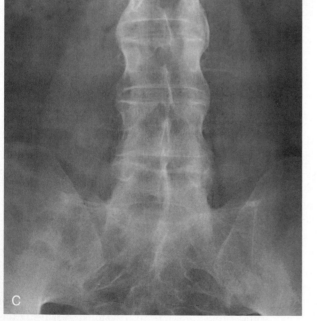

FIGURE 14-22 Lateral chest, anterior-posterior, and lateral lower lumbar spine radiographs: ankylosing spondylitis.

A, Lateral chest view: Thin paravertebral calcifications are seen anteriorly *(arrows).* The findings are pathognomonic of ankylosing spondylitis. These calcifications are called syndesmophytes and are oriented more vertically than the spinal calcifications seen in either osteoarthritis or diffuse idiopathic skeletal hyperostosis (see Fig. 14-18).

B and C, Typical ankylosing spondylitis of the lumbar spine.

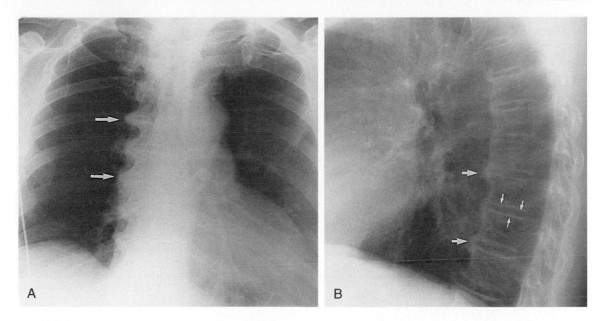

FIGURE 14-23 Posterior-anterior and lateral chest radiographs: diffuse idiopathic skeletal hyperostosis (DISH).

A, On frontal chest radiograph DISH is often more pronounced on the right side *(arrows)* (aortic pulsations may diminish ossification on the left).

B, Calcification of the anterior longitudinal ligament and flowing ossifications *(large arrows)* connecting multiple vertebral levels are the hallmarks of DISH in the spine. This condition is often unaccompanied by osteochondrosis (degenerative disc changes). Note the normal disc space *(small arrows)*.

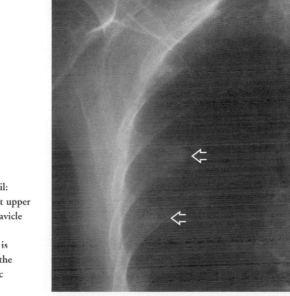

FIGURE 14-24 Posterior-anterior chest radiograph detail: penciling of clavicles in rheumatoid arthritis. Detail of right upper lobe and right shoulder girdle shows the penciling of the clavicle clearly *(arrows)*. The small nodules *(open arrows)* represent rheumatoid lung nodules. Note also that the humeral head is "high riding," obliterating the space normally taken up by the rotator cuff *(curved arrow)*. This finding indicates a chronic rotator cuff tear.

Pearls for Clinicians—Chest Wall

1. Masses originating from the chest wall often have at least one indistinct border on chest radiographs, appearing similar to masses arising from the pleura. Both masses of chest wall origin and masses of pleural origin can cause destruction of an adjacent rib.

2. Simple anterior wedging of thoracic vertebrae is most commonly due to underlying osteopenia in elderly patients. Focal loss of the outline of one or two vertebral pedicles (on frontal projection) is not caused by osteopenia and strongly suggests tumor invasion. Focal loss of opposing vertebral end plates usually indicates infection in the bone and intervening disc space.

3. Healed rib fractures may be mistaken for ill-defined lung masses on chest radiography. Oblique views of the ribs show these rib deformities to have smooth, well-defined cortical borders. If the affected ribs contain areas of bone lysis or if the cortical margin is disrupted, additional imaging is necessary.

4. Sternal abnormalities, such as trauma and pectus deformities, are easily seen on lateral radiographs but are often occult on frontal projections. Sternoclavicular joint trauma or infection is difficult to detect on either view and often requires evaluation with CT imaging.

Index

Page numbers followed by f indicate figures, t, tables.